HEALTH, DISEASE, AND ILLNESS

Health, Disease, ar

ARTHUR L. CAPLAN, JAMES J. McCARTN

lness CONCEPTS IN MEDICINE

OMINIC A. SISTI, EDITORS

With a Foreword by Edmund D. Pellegrino, M.D.

Georgetown University Press
Washington, D.C.

Georgetown University Press, Washington, D.C.

Printed in the United States of America

10 9 8 7 6 5 4 3 2 2009

This book is printed on acid-free, recycled paper meeting the requirements of the American National Standard for Permanence in Paper for Printed Library Materials.

Design by Jeff Clark and composition by Tag Savage at Wilsted & Taylor Publishing Services

Library of Congress Cataloging-in-Publication Data
Heath, disease, and illness : concepts in medicine / Arthur L. Caplan, James J. McCartney, and Dominic A. Sisti, editors ; with a foreword by Edmund D. Pellegrino.
p. cm.
Includes bibliographical references and index.
ISBN 1-58901-014-0 (pbk. : alk. paper)
1. Medicine—Philosophy. 2. Health—Philosophy. 3. Diseases—Philosophy. I. Caplan, Arthur L. II. McCartney, James J. III. Sisti, Dominic A.
R723.H398 2004
610'.1—dc22

2003019797

For Meg, who was both patient and understanding.

ARTHUR L. CAPLAN

Dedicated to my mother, Rita McCartney, who recently passed away and from whom I learned so much.

JAMES J. MCCARTNEY

To my family, friends, mentors, and colleagues who support and teach me.

DOMINIC A. SISTI

Contents

PART III: CLINICAL APPLICATIONS OF THE CONCEPTS OF HEALTH AND DISEASE: CONTROVERSIES/CONSENSUS

PART IV: NORMALCY, GENETIC DISEASE, AND ENHANCEMENT: THE FUTURE OF THE CONCEPTS OF HEALTH AND DISEASE

FOREWORD

Renewing Medicine's Basic Concepts

EDMUND D. PELLEGRINO

An ever-renewed analysis of basic concepts seems to me to be a central task of thought for it is the presupposition of an ever-renewed confrontation with reality. MARTIN BUBER

THE AIM OF THESE ESSAYS is to provide r medicine the kind of renewed analysis of basic concepts recommended ı the epigraph for thought in general. This was also the aim, two decades go, of a similar collection.[1] The dramatic changes in the realities of medine since then compel us today, once more, to reevaluate our underandings of the primal concepts of health and disease.

Concepts are the coin of philosophical discourse.[2] They structure our orldviews and define our perceptions of persons, things, and events. They ıstify our moral choices and reflect who, and what, we are. When conepts are seriously challenged, we are threatened with intellectual and ıoral disorientation.

Foreword

Medicine today is showing signs of this disorientation. There is no longer unanimity about its goals, meanings, or moral compass points. Its relationship to culture and society is in question.[3] Medicine is in the same conceptual state Heidegger detected in modern philosophy: "[T]he question about the nature of a thing awakens at those times when the thing whose nature is being questioned has become obscure and confused, when at the same time the relationship of men to what is being questioned has become uncertain or has been shattered."[4]

In light of its unquestioned power to affect human life, clarification of medicine's basic concepts is as much a moral as an intellectual obligation. Confusion about the nature of health and disease is ultimately confusion about the concept of medicine itself. Basic concepts shape what we think medicine *is*; and what we think medicine *is* in turn shapes those basic concepts.

For many centuries, the ideas of health and disease were the signature concepts that delimited the nature of medicine. The Hippocratic author of the treatise "On Art" used medicine's special preoccupation with disease to distinguish it from religion and philosophy: "First I will define what I conceive medicine to be. In general terms, it is to do away with the sufferings of the sick, to lessen the violence of their diseases, and to refuse to treat those who are overmastered by their diseases realizing that in such cases medicine is powerless."[5]

In a few words, we are told what medicine is, what its end should be, when it is futile, and when it ought not to be used. This is a concise philosophy of medicine based in the notion of disease as a cause of human suffering.

The Hippocratics defined diseases as specific entities exhibiting clusters of concrete signs, symptoms, and prognoses. Health was construed as the absence of discernible disease. These ancient notions persisted into the modern era.[6] As specific etiological causation was described, the old definitions were modified, but the centrality
of disease as an organizing concept persist
William Osler, the preeminent clinician of m
ern times, regarded disease as a concept shap
medicine pretty much as his ancient forbears d
"The whole life of the profession whether m
ing in its units or expressed in its great instituti
is controlled today as ever it was by what we thi
of the nature of disease."[7]

Osler and his contemporaries did not enga
the epistemological questions of whether dise
was an ontological, sociocultural, or histori
entity. These are the kinds of questions cons
ered in the earlier volume on the subject of co
cepts of health and disease.

Twenty years later, in the present volume, t
conceptual focus has shifted to a much more fu
damental level—not so much the epistemolo
cal theory of disease that should prevail, but wh
shall count as a disease in the first place, and h
much of human experience medicine should e
compass. This shift is the result of many compl
factors, three of which seem particularly pe
nent: (1) the enormous expansion and depth
our scientific understanding of the workings
life and the human organism, (2) enlarged e
pectations of medicine's powers to improve t
quality and duration of human life, and (3)
growing illusion of immortality through medi
progress.

Under this impetus, every disturbance of fun
tion, imperfection, or threat to life's "quality" b
comes a disease, a problem for resolution by t
technological prowess of medicine. Imperfe
tions, limitations of any kind, and gaps betwe
expectations and capabilities are no longer tol
able. Beyond this, there is the growing hope th
human finitude itself can be defeated, that agi
can be ameliorated so completely that perpetu
youth and full vigor are within the foreseeab
grasp of humanity.

Within this cultural climate, each new a
vance of medicine's scientific base raises ne
questions about health and disease and th
about the range of medicine. We are now unce

n about what constitutes normalcy, about the undaries where health ends and disease be-s. For example, when does being overweight, rying a deleterious gene, not living up to your ents' expectations, having less than an opti-l I.Q., being short of stature, or lacking ath-ic ability become a disease? Are menopause, ng, adolescence, hyperactivity in children, d infertility pathological entities? Is a disease fined by the availability of a treatment?

Has the definition of health really now be-me what the World Health Organization omised years ago—freedom from all physical, ental, and social aberrations? Is one unhealthy his imperfections could be cured by enhance-ent? Does wanting to be a superstar athlete en-le one to hormonal treatment? Should health surers reimburse only for "disease" defined as vious pathological manifestations, or should ey include quality-of-life enhancements as ell? How does cataract extraction to enhance ht differ from steroid use to enhance weight ting or memory pills to enhance academic ores? How much of human life should be med-alized?

Beyond these questions are the most profound estions of what it is to be human. When do we in or lose personhood? Is one still an individual ter a series of tissue transplants or when mi-ochips in the brain modify behavior? Our sci-tific and sociocultural metamorphoses now t the stage for the larger question "What is med-ine?" and, then, the even larger question of Vhat is it to be human?" How do these ques-ons get answered without some agreement on a ilosophical anthropology, a subject receiving tle attention in the United States?

Today, concepts of health and disease are early still important for medicine, but specify-g what they mean has become far more dif-cult in the past twenty years. They promise to ecome even more so during the next twenty, as edical science continues to stretch the bound-ies of health and disease.

What is apparent, as perhaps it was not in the earlier volume, is the need for a deeper interpen-etration of medicine and philosophy with each other, as Aristotle and Aquinas envisioned it: "For many natural philosophers complete their in-quiry with things that belong to medicine, and many physicians, who pursue the art of medicine philosophically, using not only experience but seeking causes, begin the medical inquiry where natural philosophers leave off. From which it is clear that the study of health and disease is com-mon to a philosopher and physician."[8]

This conjunction is today a reality. "Philoso-phers" are increasingly intrigued by the new knowledge of the genome or molecular biology generally. The implications for our conceptual understanding of human nature and human life are profound. On the other hand, thoughtful physicians and medical scientists are impelled by the nature of their discoveries and observations to ask what medicine is philosophically.[9]

In this respect, one needs only list such new re-alities as the mapping of the human genome, the potentialities of stem cell research and cloning, the permutations and combinations of reproduc-tive biology and the fundamental chemistry and physics of life. A deepening grasp of the mecha-nisms of health and disease will not eradicate the concepts, but it does demand their careful en-largement, refinement, and sophistication.

Future volumes will continue to reflect on the basic concepts of health and disease. They will need to probe ever more deeply into the concepts of body, psyche, mind, soul, and human nature. They will confront the more basic concept of hu-mans as a species of natural kind, and this will re-quire a reflection and analysis on the most basic concept underlying biology and medicine, the concept of man.

NOTES

1. Arthur L. Caplan, H. Tristram Engelhardt, Jr., and James J. McCartney, eds., *Concepts of Health and Dis-*

ease: Interdisciplinary Perspectives. Reading, Mass.: Addison-Wesley, 1981.

2. Gottlob Frege, "The Fundamental Laws of Arithmetic. II," in *Classics in Logic*, ed. Dagobert Runes. New York: Philosophical Library, 1962; Ludwig Wittgenstein, *Philosophical Investigations*, trans. G. E. M. Anscombe, with German and English indexes. New York: MacMillan, 1958; and Robert Brandom, "Reason, Expression, and the Philosophic Enterprise," in *What Is Philosophy?* eds. C. P. Ragland and Sarah Heidt. New Haven, Conn.: Yale University Press, 2001, 74–95.

3. Mark J. Hanson and Daniel Callahan, eds., *The Goals of Medicine: The Forgotten Issues in Health Care Reform*. Washington, D.C.: Georgetown University Press, 1999.

4. Martin Heidegger, *What Is Philosophy?* Trans. William Kloback and Jean T. Wilde. Albany, N.Y.: New College and University Press, 1956, cited in *What Is Philosophy?* eds. Ragland and Heidt.

5. Hippocrates, *The Art*, trans. W. H. S. Jones. Cambridge, Mass.: Harvard University Press, 1981, vol. 2: 193.

6. Knud Faber, *Nosography in Modern Internal Medicine*, with introduction by Rufus Cole. New York: P. B. Hoeber, 1923.

7. William Osler, *The Quotable Osler*, eds. Mark E. Silverman, T. Jock Murray, and Charles S. Bryan. Philadelphia: American College of Physicians, 2003, 109.

8. Thomas Aquinas, "Preface, Commentary on Sense and the Sensed Object," in *Thomas Aquinas: Selected Writings*, ed. and trans. Ralph McInerny. New York: Penguin, 1998, vol. 16: 453.

9. E. D. Pellegrino, "What the Philosophy of Medicine Is." *Theoretical Medicine and Bioethics* 1998, 19 (4): 315–36.

BIBLIOGRAPHY

Aquinas, Thomas. "Preface" to Commentary on *On Sense and the Sensed Object*. In *Thomas Aquinas: Selected Writings*. Edited and translated by Ralph Mc erny. New York: Penguin, 1998, 447–54.

Brandom, Robert. "Reason, Expression, and Philosophic Enterprise." In *What Is Philosophy?* ited by C. P. Ragland and Sarah Heidt. New Hav Conn.: Yale University Press, 2001, 74–95.

Caplan, Arthur L., H. Tristram Engelhardt, Jr., James J. McCartney, eds. *Concepts of Health and D ease: Interdisciplinary Perspectives*. Reading, Mass.: dison-Wesley, 1981.

Faber, Knud. *Nosography in Modern Internal M icine*. Introduction by Rufus Cole. New York: P. Hoeber, 1923.

Frege, Gottlob. "The Fundamental Laws of Ari metic. II." In *Classics in Logic*. Edited by Dagob Runes. New York: Philosophical Library, 1962, 329–

Hanson, Mark J., and Daniel Callahan, eds. *T Goals of Medicine: The Forgotten Issues in Health C Reform*. Washington, D.C.: Georgetown Univers Press, 1999.

Heidegger, Martin. *What Is Philosophy?* Transla by William Kloback and Jean T. Wilde. Albany, N. New College and University Press, 1956. Cited in *Wh Is Philosophy?* Edited by C. P. Ragland and Sar Heidt. New Haven, Conn.: Yale University Press, 20

Hippocrates. *The Art*. Translated by W. H. S. Jon Cambridge, Mass.: Harvard University Press, 1981.

Osler, William. *The Quotable Osler*. Edited Mark E. Silverman, T. Jock Murray, and Charles Bryan. Philadelphia: American College of Physicia 2003.

Pellegrino, E. D. "What the Philosophy of Me cine Is." *Theoretical Medicine and Bioethics* 1998, (4): 315–36.

Wittgenstein, Ludwig. *Philosophical Investigatio* Translated by G. E. M. Anscombe, with German a English indexes. New York: MacMillan, 1958.

PART I

Historical Discussions of Health, Disease, and Illness

PART I IS A SURVEY of various historical onstructions of health and disease. It begins with an excerpt from *On the latural Faculties* by GALEN OF PERGAMUM (ca. 150 CE). The Greek physi- an's framework had a profound impact on medicine, and his synthesis of ncient medical theories, such as Hippocrates' humors, and burgeoning natomical knowledge was accepted as dogma for centuries. In this brief election, Galen recounts descriptions of how the four humors—yellow nd black bile, blood, and phlegm—are formed and explains their presence relation to temperature. An imbalance of the humors results in disease.

In a similar way, an imbalance in what we might call "moral humors" nay lead to diseases of the soul. For MAIMONIDES (ca. 1150 CE), character traits that guide moderate and balanced deeds are the virtues of a healthy soul. The sick soul is directly analogous to the sick body: A person who is physically sick has a distorted palate and enjoys foods that are repugnant to healthy people. A person who is spiritually sick has a distorted vision of right conduct and acts immorally. Those who are physically ill and who do not seek treatment by a physician will die. And so, too, those who are spiritually ill and do not seek out healing of the Sages will die. The presentation by Maimonides highlights the conceptual interconnectedness of spiritual, moral, and physical health that is a latent feature of the nosological frameworks presented in other chapters of the book.

From classical humoral explanations to prototypes of the disease-as-entity framework, ROY PORTER AND G. S. ROUSSEAU present an historical survey of how gout was understood during the Renaissance. Among other Renaissance thinkers, the authors describe Swiss physician, alchemist, and philosopher Paracelsus' (ca. 1500) important move in rejecting the notion that gout and renal calculi were caused by an endogenous imbalance of the humors. Rather, they write, Paracelsus was the first to claim that a disease—gout—was of exogenous origin and was often later personified (and deified) as taking up residence with its victim. This development notwithstanding, therapeutic remedies tended to assume that gout was of a more humoral origin, and it was treated as such.

As another example of the moral dimension of disease, gout was construed as a biological manifestation of Maimonides' "diseases of the soul" brought on by excess and a lavish lifestyle. But although gout punished the extravagance of the rich, it also was the "disease of monarchs" and as such it was desirable to healthy plebeians. Indeed, Holy Roman Emperors, English lords, and even members of the Medici family were known to suffer from gout. The gouty sick role provided the well endowed with yet another excuse to avoid manual labor, assistance to others, or other social obligations. On the one hand, moral such as Petrarch welcomed an attack of gout as opportunity to lecture to victims on moral a spiritual growth by taming the excesses of the v tim. On the other hand, a gouty affliction wa sign of social status and upward mobility and v celebrated.

In what is now understood to be a paradigma example of a pseudoscientific just-so story that inforced a racist ideology, when taken in histo cal context SAMUEL CARTWRIGHT'S lecture is i portant on many levels. Cartwright's discussi illustrates the social-ladenness of the concept disease. Invoking the classic humoral theory disease, Cartwright claims that for "negroes" fully flourish, they ought to labor under the co trol of a white man. Cartwright argues that, blacks, "red, vital blood" is essential for tr human cogency and hard work infuses the bla man's blood with this vital force. Thus, ha working slaves are better off than free blac who are predisposed to malingering and "rasc ity" due to an excess of nonvital humors, "bla blood," and defective hemostasis. Cartwrig also develops his naturalistic vision of the desti of blacks as slaves on the basis of selective biblic and historical hermeneutics. In doing so, Ca wright medicalizes the unhealthy tendency some slaves to seek freedom, or run aw Drapetomania is the disease that causes slaves run away. Further developing the idea of that h moral excess or loss of hemostasis leading to m lingering and rascality, the disease, Dysaesthe Aethiopis, becomes part Cartwright's nosology a nosology that clearly illustrates how sociopoli cal power structures are at once legitimized a reinforced by the concept of disease. Cartwrigh lecture presents an early example of the medica ization of deviance, a phenomenon explored some detail in part III.

French historian, philosopher of science, a mentor of Michel Foucault, GEORGES CANGUI HEM reviews the various models of disease. T reader should approach this selection in the co

t of Canguilhem's influence on medical epis-
nology, especially that of Michel Foucault in
e *Birth of the Clinic*.

Two selections on the status of mental illness low. THOMAS SZASZ argues that there is no h thing as mental illness, or, at least, that ental illness" is a misnomer for a physiological ease of the brain. Further the phenomena typ-lly referred to as "mental illness" may be the allenges of one's life, a struggle that is alto-her normal. "Mental illness" has reached thic proportions in how it is applied and in-ked by patients and mental health profession-. Again the moral dimension of illness is em-asized, as Szasz vigorously argues that "mental ness" is often the result of shortfalls in the uggle to live the moral life and is a tool of self-ceit for those who avoid an authentic life.

GEORGE ENGEL questions the medical model toto, and, with particular regard to psychoso-l diseases, he introduces another set of funda-ental nosological problems. Should medicine al only with somato-organic diseases and not ychosocial distresses, or is such a clear dis-ction impossible to draw? How and why did e mind-body dualism, which is the foundation the medical model, develop and persist? Engel ces the thread of medical reductionism back the Cartesian tradition and the Catholic hurch's dogmatic influence on metaphysical atters. By espousing a biopsychosocial model, ngel seeks to integrate the social, historical, and ltural and in so doing account for the lived ex-rience of illness by some patients who show no apparent signs of disease. He seeks to move beyond the split of reductionists and exclusionists (Szasz being the latter) in hopes of fully recognizing the ills of those with anything from diabetes or schizophrenia to basic dysphoria. Engel presents the analogous case of the battle between molecular biologists (reductionists) and the psychosocialists as being resolved in part by the systems theorists who hold the holistic view that all levels of biological life are linked. He suggests applying this approach to medicine.

Finally, in a historical sketch of a practical problem, ROBERT A. ARONOWITZ discusses the criteria that are met when symptoms coalesce and are considered a disease. He recounts how various symptom clusters were construed as discrete diseases, which were discovered by physicians who sampled a very small number of patients. Indeed, the disciplinary matrix of institutional medicine of yesteryear created the potential for simpler disease recognition as (what might be seen today as) idiosyncratic signs and symptoms were accepted as diseases and reported out in medical journals and discussed among medical circles. Aronowitz presents asthma as an historical example of a symptom-based disease diagnosis. Despite individual variations in the symptoms of the disease, symptomatic asthma is a diagnosis that is well worth keeping for various institutional reasons. Aronowitz also asks us to consider how symptom clusters are transformed into legitimate diseases. He uses mental illness to craft his set of claims that legitimating factors are multidimensional.

CHAPTER 1

From *On the Natural Faculties, II, VIII*

GALEN *[Translated by Arthur John Brock, M.D.]*

NOW IN REFERENCE TO the *genesis of the umours,* I do not know that any one could add anything wiser than what as been said by Hippocrates, Aristotle, Praxagoras, Philotimus and many ther among the Ancients. These men demonstrated that when the nutri-ient becomes altered in the veins by the innate heat, blood is produced hen it is in moderation, and the other humours when it is not in proper roportion. And all the observed facts agree with this argument. Thus, iose articles of food, which are by nature warmer, are more productive of ile, while those which are colder produce more phlegm. Similarly of the eriods of life, those which are naturally warmer tend more to bile, and the older more to phlegm. Of occupations also, localities and seasons, and, above all, of natures themselves, the colder are more phlegmatic, and the warmer more bilious. Also cold diseases result from phlegm, and warmer ones from yellow bile. There is not a single thing to by found which does not bear witness to the truth of this account. How could it be otherwise? For, seeing that every part functions in its own special way because of the manner in which the four qualities are compounded, it is absolutely necessary that the function [activ should be either completely destroyed, or, at le hampered, by any damage to the qualities, a that thus the animal should fall ill, either a whole, or in certain of its parts.

Also the diseases which are primary and m generic are four in number, and differ from ea other in warmth, cold, dryness and moisture.

CHAPTER 2

Diseases of the Soul

MAIMONIDES *[From* The Essential Maimonides • *Translations of the Rambam* • *Translated by Avraham Yaakov Finkel]*

CHAPTER THREE

The Sick Soul

THE EARLY PHILOSOPHERS said that the ›ul, like the body, may be healthy or sick. The soul is healthy when its con-ıtion and that of its powers is such that it always does what is right and acts roperly. The soul is sick when its condition and that of its powers is such ıat it always does what is wrong and acts improperly. The science of med-ine studies the health of the body. People who are physically ill have dis-›rted tastes and, therefore, think that bitter things taste sweet and sweet ıings bitter. They imagine that wholesome things are unwholesome, and ıey have a rapacious appetite and a lust for things such as dust and coal, s well as for very sharp and sour foods, which healthy people loathe and eject because they do not enjoy them and may even find them harmful.

In the same way, people whose souls are sick—wicked and corrupt people—think that evil is good and that good is evil.[1] A wicked man constantly craves excess, which is harmful, but he believes it is beneficial because of the illness of his soul.

Healers of the Soul

When people who are unfamiliar with the science of medicine realize that they are sick, they consult a physician who tells them what they must do. He warns them not to eat certain things they mistakenly consider to be beneficial, and he prescribes things that they may find unpleasant and bitter. He does this so that their bodies may return to health and they will again choose the good and despise the bad.

Similarly, people whose souls become ill should consult the Sages, who are healers of the soul and will caution them not to indulge in evils that they mistakenly believe are good. In this manner, which I will discuss more fully in the following chapter, they may be cured by the art that heals man's moral qualities. However, if a person who is morally sick does not realize that he is sick but imagines that he is well, or if he is aware that he is sick but does not try to get healed, then his end will be the same as the person who suffers from a physical ailment and who continues to indulge himself and does not seek a cure. He will surely die.

Those who know that they are sick, but nevertheless indulge in their pleasures, are accurately described in the Torah. The pleasure seeker says, *"I will follow my heart's desires. Let me add some moisture to the dry"* (Devarim 29:18), meaning that he intends to satisfy his thirst [by satisfying his lusts], but thereby intensifies it.

A person who does not realize that he is sick is portrayed by King Solomon, *"The way of a fool is right in his own eyes, but the wise man accepts advice"* (Mishlei 12:15). Solomon is saying that the one who listens to the advice of the Sage is w for the Sage teaches the way that is truly right, the path that the person wrongly sees as ri Solomon also says, "*A road may seem right man, but in the end it is a road to death*" (Mis 14:12). Again, regarding those who are morall and do not know what is harmful or benefic Solomon says, *"The way of the wicked is all d ness; they do not know what will make them st ble"* (Mishlei 4:19).

I will deal with the art of healing the soul in next chapter.

CHAPTER FOUR

"Curing Diseases of the Soul": The Middle Road

Good deeds are balanced deeds, occupyin middle ground between two equally bad tremes: *too much*, excess[2] and *too little*, sufficiency.[3] Virtues are character traits, both born and acquired, that lie midway between two extremes of excess and insufficiency.[4] Go deeds are the direct result of these charac traits.

To illustrate: Self-control lies midway betwe intemperate passion and a total absence of fe ing for worldly enjoyment. Self-control is pro behavior, and the character trait that engend self-control is an ethical one. But immoder passion, which is at one extreme, and the total sence of feeling for worldly pleasure, at the ot extreme, are equally deplorable. The charac traits from which these two extremes result—temperate passion from immoderation and sence of feeling from insensibility—are mora imperfect qualities. Similarly, generosity is t middle road between stinginess and wastef ness; courage, between recklessness and co ardice; dignity, between haughtiness and bo ishness. Dignity is when one carries hims honorably and does not debase himself, haugh s is when one seeks honor more than is deved, boorishness is when one does things that unbecoming. Friendliness is the middle road ween aggressiveness and submissiveness.[5] mility is the middle course between conceit d self-abasement; contentedness, between ed and laziness; and goodheartedness, been meanness and extravagance. A goodrted man is one who is intent on doing good others, providing personal assistance, advice d money to the best of his ability, but without rming or disgracing himself. This is the middle d. The mean man, at one extreme does not nt to help others, even if he himself will not fer any loss, hardship, or damage through his nerosity. The extravagant man, on the other nd, goes to extremes of generosity, even to the ent of personal damage, disgrace, hardship, d loss.

Tolerance is the middle course between anger d indifference. Sensitivity is the middle course tween arrogance and timidness. According to r Sages, "A timid person cannot learn" (*Avos*); they did not say, "A sensitive person cannot rn." They also said, "The sensitive one goes to e Garden of Eden" (*Avos* 5:24) and did not say, he timid one goes to the Garden of Eden." erefore, I have made sensitivity the desirable ean and timidness the deplorable extreme. It is e same with the other qualities. We need to fine them in terms that everyone agrees on, so at these ideas are clearly understood....

The Cure for the Diseases of the Soul

ood as well as faulty character traits can only be quired or become embedded in the soul if one peatedly practices the acts that result from ese character traits over a long period of time. If ese acts are good, the person acquires a vire, but if they are bad, the person has a vice.[6] owever, no one is born with innate virtues or vices, as I shall explain in Chapter Eight, and everyone's conduct from childhood on is undoubtedly influenced by the behavior of relatives and countrymen.

This being so, a person may have a healthy soul from having followed the middle course in conduct. It is also possible that his actions may be leaning toward one extreme or the other, as we have discussed, in which case his soul is diseased. If that is so, he should seek a cure, just as he would if he were sick in his body. When the balance of one's physical health is disturbed, we must determine which way it is leaning in order to force it in the opposite direction until it returns to its proper condition. When it is straightened, we stop the treatment and feed the patient food that will maintain a physical balance. We must use exactly the same method to adjust an individual's moral equilibrium.

As an illustration, let us take the case of a man who has the trait of stinginess and uses it to deny himself every enjoyment in life. This is a defect of the soul that will result in immoral acts, as we explained. If we want to cure this sick man, it is not enough to order him to practice generosity; that would be as ineffective as a physician trying to cure a patient who is consumed by burning fever with mild medicines, which would not serve the purpose at all. Instead, we must encourage the miser to spend his money liberally, over and over again, until the tendency that brought on his avarice has totally disappeared. Then, when he reaches the point of almost becoming a spendthrift, we must put a stop to his wasteful spending and order him to continue with acts of generosity, watching him carefully all the while to make sure that he does not lapse either into extravagance or stinginess.

On the other hand, if a person is a spendthrift, we must order him to save money and repeat acts of miserliness. It is not necessary, however, for him to perform acts of avarice as many times as the stingy man should perform acts of wasteful spending. This novel idea, which is an established rule and secret of the science of healing the soul, tells us that it is easier for a spendthrift to become a generous donor than it is for a miser to adopt the habit of generosity. Likewise, it is easier for a person who is indifferent to pleasure to become pious and abstain from sin than it is for a man burning with passion to curb his desires. Therefore, the pleasure-seeker must be induced to practice restraint more than the indifferent man should be persuaded to indulge his passions. Similarly, the coward must be exposed to danger more frequently than the reckless man should be forced to practice restraint. The mean man needs to practice kindness to a greater degree than the overly generous person must practice meanness. This is a fundamental rule of the science of healing faulty character traits.

NOTES

1. Compare, "*Ah, those who call evil good and good evil; who present darkness as light and light as* darkness"(Isaiah 5:20).

2. An example of excess is a person who squanders his money.

3. An example of insufficiency is a miser.

4. The Rambam derived his doctrine of the mid
road (also called the Golden Mean) from the To
the Prophets, and the Sages of blessed memory, as
sented in this discourse. We read in Tanach, for ex
ple, "*Do not swerve to the right* or *the left; keep your*
from evil" (Mishlei 4:27); "*Do not overdo goodness*
don't act the wise man to excess, or you may be du
founded. Do not overdo wickedness..." (Koh
7:16,17); "*Give me neither poverty nor riches, but pro*
me with my daily bread" (Mishlei 30:8). The Sages
"The ways of the Torah may be compared to two ro
one of fire, the other of snow. If the traveler veers to
side, he will be burned to death; if he veers to the ot
he will perish in the snow. What is he to do? Let h
take the middle road" (*Yerushalmi Chagigah*, 1
Tosefta Chagigah, 2).

5. The Rambam here uses an old Spanish word t
means passivity. This trait stems from indifference
lethargy and is the opposite of aggressiveness, wh
stems from nervousness and hotheadedness.

6. "As the Sages put it, "Once a person has comn
ted a sin and repeated it, it becomes to him a permit
act" (*Yoma*, 86b).

CHAPTER 3

Prometheus's Vulture: The Renaissance Fashioning of Gout

ROY PORTER AND G. S. ROUSSEAU

[From Gout: The Patrician Malady*]*

...kills us with a lingering death, and like Prometheus's vulture, gnaws us into fresh torment. "A DISSERTATION ON THE GOUT," *LONDON MAGAZINE* (OCTOBER 1755), 612, LETTER FROM R. DRAKE TO EDITOR

THE INVENTION OF PRINTING and the spread of literacy, the growth of towns, affluence, courts, and universities created the conditions sustaining the vast sixteenth-century proliferation of medical learning and publishing. Elite physicians and surgeons promoted medical humanism, aiming to recover, perfect, and improve the authorities of Antiquity; meanwhile, books began to appear instructing the laity how to tend their health and treat their ailments.[1]

Among their ABCs of disease and head-to-foot anatomical charts, many such works included discussions of arthritic conditions and podagra, distilled and sometimes simplified from the masters of Antiquity and Islam, spelling out the nature and causes of those afflictions, and informing readers, professional and lay, about prevention and cure. Works even began to appear devoted exclusively or essentially to gout. The first of these was *Ob das Podagra Möglich zu Generen oder Nit. Nutzlich zu Wissen Allen dene die damit Behafft* (On whether it is possible to cure gout. Useful to know for all those who suffer from it). The work of a German physician, Dominicus Burgawer, it was printed in Strasburg by Mathias Apiarius in 1534.[2] Little is known about the author, except that his text shows him to have been an admirer of Rhazes and Avicenna and familiar with Paracelsus. It may serve as a window upon Renaissance views.

Asking "What is Podagra?" Burgawer responded that "it is a pain in the feet with or without swelling, which comes from dampness or draught." The generic term for the condition was "ARTHETICA" [*sic*], which, he said, may be rendered as "sickness of the limbs." In Latin its name was "GUTTA," which "means 'drop' because it is like the drops running down the roofs to the ground."[3] The correct word depended upon the terminus of the flow: "If the flux or matter goes into the hands it is called CIRAGIA, into the hip SCIATICA, into the knees GENUGRA, and into the feet PODAGRA."[4]

Burgawer then turned to aetiology, for "prevention is possible if one knows this." Podagra arose "from outward or inward sudden changes to extremes of cold or heat"—"cold" of course meant more within humoral theory than a temperature measurable by a thermometer. This dangerous cold, he explained, "can be caused by superfluous food, superfluous sleep and constant idleness." Rhazes had proved that pain did no tack "those who work, only those who do not h to work." There were also, he believed, ot causes of gout, intelligible in the light of Grae Roman teachings on the nonnaturals:

> The disease also comes from great sadness, a from excessive venery, especially after meals, Hippocrates and other philosophers say eunu and those who have nothing to do with wom do not get it. . . . Similarly harmful is inordin eating and drinking, mixing one's wines, wh stifles natural heat, whereby superfluous flu are collected in the body, and this happens to grand gentlemen who have all their heart sires.[5]

The point about gender was especially telli Burgawer concluded in good Renaissance ma ner by citing his source: "All this has been sa concisely by Rhazes."[6]

Burgawer's tract was representative of mu contemporary writing. It drew upon the author of Greek and Arab physicians; it offered a mu causal account of the disease, grounded in h moral philosophy and the individual consti tion; and it stressed temperamental (moral a emotional) as well as strictly physical factors.

Among the fullest discussions of podagra w that presented by the French surgeon Ambro Paré (1510–90), whose magisterial surgical wr ings contained a discussion "Of the Disease of t Joints Commonly Called the Gout." Paré wro eloquently, being himself like Sydenham a ce tury later, a sufferer. "The paines of the goute," explained, obviously describing his own cas "are rightly accounted amongst the most grevo and acute; so that through the vehemency of t agony many are almost mad, and wish them selves dead."[7] Paré held the natural duration an acute attack was forty days; it was either inhe ited or acquired; and, he pointed out in Galen mould, that what determined its severity was t venomousness of the peccant matter distill from the humours, as it "causeth intolerable to nting paine not by the abundance, because it ppens to many who have the gout, no signe of luxion appearing in the jointes."[8] Unlike Parasus, Paré was diffident about the chemistry of rbific matter: "It is not of a more knowne, or ily exprest nature than that which causeth the gue, Lues veneria or falling sicknesse."[9]

What triggered attacks? In most cases, Paré ggested, the affected joint must previously have en weakened, either by nature or by an accint. But the predisposing cause lay in overlulgence and luxury.[10] Discussing diet, he adcated chicken as easily digested—though with reservation, reflecting Renaissance theories out cosmic correspondences, that "some of the tients have disallowed of the eating of capons d the like birds, because they are subject to bee ubled by the goute in the feete." Folklore had that hawks also, mirroring their aristocratic sters, were subject to this complaint.[11]

Paré recommended a double defence. It was ential to follow a moderate regime—"such uty persons as remain intemperate and given gluttony and venerie (especially the old)," he sisted, "may hope for no health by the use of edicines."[12] But he also expressed some faith medical interventions, chiefly prophylactic: quent copious bloodletting, vomits, sweatg, purging and diuresis, including the use of rmodactyl (colchicum) pills. Gouty subjects ould not drink much, lest excess fluid chill the mach and so check digestion, thereby leaving rudities" which would collect in the blood and eate fresh poison. Though a surgeon, Paré was cumspect regarding external remedies, except utery and setons as counter-irritants. One of any practitioners who referred to it as the "opobrium medicorum," Paré took the view that, hile it might be prevented and treated, gout did ot admit radical cure.

With gout as with so much else, the great challnge to humanist orthodoxy came from the wiss iconoclast Paracelsus (1493–1541).[13] He was e first who radically rejected humoral ideas of gout and renal calculus, regarding the emphasis upon "catarrh" and "flux" as mere gammon, lacking anatomical plausibility. If black bile had its seat in the spleen, how could it descend to the legs, causing ulceration?[14] Each was a disease in its own right, though certain diseases, for example syphilis, would, however, develop only on top of others, by "transplantation."[15] Syphilis, for Paracelsus, was the pathological expression of the lewdness and luxury rife in those corrupt times, but it was also a "specific" poison.[16] Thus, there was the risk that gout would change into gouty syphilis.[17]

The image of "tartar" and "tartaric disease" occupies a prominent place among Paracelsus' nosological theories. It implied general pathological conceptions. Disease was a concrete entity which could be made visible and tangible, in contrast to disease in the Ancient sense, conceived as a mere humoral upset. It was seen as exogenous—due to indigestible matter introduced with food and drink—rather than endogenous, as with Hippocratic theory. The disease entity could be defined in chemical terms as the product of coagulation, connected with the action of "salt" on the deleterious substance entering from outside. It was a failure to separate "pure" from "impure," nourishment from waste. Furthermore, this process was "specific," a chemical operation in its own right, departing from the holistic model posited by Classical medicine. Overall disease was a local process.[18]

On the basis of such pathological convictions, Paracelsus advanced in *De Morbis Tartareis* (1531) a novel explanation of gout, via his concept of the diseases of tartar. Some local factor, such as water supply, probably influenced corporeal chemical depositions of this kind, he suggested, noting that in Switzerland, "the most healthy land, superior to Germany, Italy and France, nay all Western and Eastern Europe, there is no gout, no colic, no rheumatisms and no stone."[19] Gouty nodules consisted of calcined synovia or an excremental salt—tartar—coagulated in a joint.

The tartar found in wine casks was a result of fermentation. Such material could be compared to certain natural bodily deposits—encrustations on the teeth (still called, of course, "tartar"), gallstones and kidney stones.

Bodily tartar, Paracelsus believed, was derived from food and released through digestion. In some individuals it failed to be excreted, tending rather to be coagulated by "spirit of salt" and thereby transformed into stony substances. In the tartarous precipitation of the gout:

> The gluten, which was called synovia by the old wound surgeons, is sticky and gelatinous like egg-white. Now when salty matter comes into contact with and mixes itself with this, it coagulates at once into a solid.... The gout of the feet, hands, and knees has its origin in this coagulation.[20]

This theory of "tartarous disease"—a tendency to retain acrid substances—was one of the earliest attempts at a chemical aetiology for a malady. Paracelsus, however, made no practical advance in therapy. Moreover, the impact of his teachings upon later thinking is somewhat equivocal. Other learned doctors, including Théodore Turquet de Mayerne,[21] the French-trained physician to James I, adopted his views. In his *Treatise of the Gout*, translated by Thomas Sherley and published posthumously in 1676, Turquet Mayerne considered gout as one of the diseases of tartar, but his views did not prove influential.[22]

This is not to suggest that the Tudor and Stuart era did not bring discussions of gout among English physicians. These, however, chiefly summarized and popularized the commonplaces of learned medicine. Henry VIII's physician, Andrew Boorde (1490–1549), broached the question of podagra in two works, the *Dyetary of Health* (1542), and *The Breviary of Health* (1547).[23] Attempting to reconcile Greek and Latin sources and to find English equivalents for classical concepts, Boorde deplored the slovenly habit of giving the name arthritis to all aches in the joints, "whether the pain arise from a rheumatic flammation or a gouty humour": "all jointe nesses are not the goute."[24] He distinguished f types, namely chiagra (of hands, fingers a arms); podagra (of the feet, toes and legs); "Go arterycke, which involves jointes elsewhere"; a sciatica.

In matters therapeutic, Boorde endorsed H manist orthodoxies. Allopathic in his pre ences, he aimed at the removal of peccant h mours by prophylactic, spring and autu bleedings, as Galen had advocated, supported a moderate diet. During paroxysms, exter remedies should be used. He recommended wearing of dog-skin hose, perhaps taking a h from Soranus of Ephesus, who had sugges that gouty feet should be anointed with seal and then encased in seal-skin slippers. Boo also prescribed daily application to the pain joints of baked fermentations of ox-dung wrapp in cabbage leaves. Such external methods co be accompanied by strong scammony purg followed by generous quantities of treacle "weaken the virulency of the gouty mal nancy."[25] He was keen on an infusion of ash ba *(Fruxinus excelsior)*, a favourite recipe all o Europe for gout, scurvy and fevers until the troduction of the Peruvian bark (*cinchona*).[26] favoured assorted diuretics, including sor roots, parsley and other herbs stewed in broth Like many contemporaries, Boorde presented mixed bag of treatments, evidently responding the fact that gout itself was protean.

In 1560 there appeared a *Method of Phisicke* Phillip Barrough, a Fellow of the College Physicians, *Containing the Causes, Signs a Cures of Inward Diseases in Man's Body fro the Head to the Foot.*[28] By 1583 it had run to a se enth edition, dedicated to Lord Burghley, a cel brated martyr to the gout. In his chapter "Of t Goute in the Feet and the Jointes," Barrou gnawed at the taxonomic problem dogging co temporary physicians: that of distinguishing va joint afflictions, clarifying the terms used for m by Classical authors, and matching up old authorities against clinical reality. He ded to think of a diversity of words, a unity of ease:

odagra and arthritis in Latin be diseases of one ind, and therefore they differ not but in places iseased, for in both of them there is weakness of he joints and unnatural humour floweth to them, nd if that the fluxe of the humour do flow to the eet, that is called podagra in Latin, but if the humour flow to the joints, it is called in Greek arthriis, in Latin articularis morbis, the joint sickness.[29]

Precisely what should count as podagra troud him. Barrough also aired the causes of the ease and mentioned—with what, in the light he dedication, might be taken as a breathtak; want of tact—that "this disease is engendered continued crudities and drunkenness, and of moderate using of lechery." Alongside such ppocratic orthodoxies, he tabulated other preitants: an attack could come on by "vehement d swift deambulations and walkings, by supssions and stopping of accustomed excretions d fluxes and through intermission of familiar ercises. Perturbations of the mind do not only gender this evil, but also do breed hurtful and rrupt humours"—the well-worn mixture of disposing and exciting causes, physical and otional triggers.[30]

A popular work was Thomas Cogan's *The ven of Health* (1584), "for all those that have are for their health, amplified upon five words Hippocrates, Labour, Meat, Drink, Sleep d Venus."[31] Alongside attention to the nonturals, he counselled prudence and moderan: "Wherefore I say to the gentleman who have e gout, that although the forebearing of wine d women and other things noisome in that disse do not utterly take away the gout, yet it will ate quality and abridge the pain and make it ich more tolerable."[32] Cogan's book traded upon the intimate connections between kitchen and pharmacy, victuals and medicine. Discussing diet, he pointed out that *eating* old and hard cheese was taboo because it bred melancholy—but there was more to cheese than edibility: "an old hard cheese is good for some things, for Galen showeth that an old cheese cut in pieces and sodden with the broth of a gammon of bacone and made in the manner of a plaster and laid to the joint where the gout is, will break the skin and dissolve those hard knots which the gout causeth."[33] Without forbidding wine, Cogan urged abstinence at the onset of an attack. The link between gout and excess was clear: he would address "the Gentlemen that hath the gowt," and them alone, "for poore men seldome have it, because for the more part it groweth through excesse and ease."[34]

Much was proposed and used against gout. Drawing upon medieval authors such as Gilbertus Anglicus, who had recommended an ointment made of puppy boiled up with cucumber, rue and juniper, herbals offered remedies,[35] and there was always the wisdom of the Ancients to fall back upon. As Thomas Nash observed in *A Pleasant Comedie, Called Summers Last Will and Testament*:

> And well observe Hippocrates old rule
> The onely medicine for the foote is rest.[36]

The idea that luxurious living would bring nemesis in the form of vengeful maladies was a Humanist commonplace, particularly after the appearance of the new disease of syphilis.[37] "They foreshorten their lives considerably," commented Laurent Joubert, adopting the Hippocratic view that gout was the wages of sexual excess,

> just as do lascivious and wanton lechers, who do not live very long but fall quickly subject, prey, and victim to gout, colic, nephritis, apoplexy, paralysis, convulsions, and other disease of indigestion (the cause of phlegm, father of all these diseases).[38]

Pithily in The *Rape* of *Lucrece* Shakespeare anchored the malady to miserly, masculinist moorings that would hold up through to the era of the Georgians and Victorians:

> The aged man that coffers-up his gold,
> Is plagu'd with cramps, and gouts and painful fits.

This he achieved, as well, by highlighting its pains and perils,[39] implying, through the railings of Falstaff, that it was the old man's version of the pox: "A man can no more separate age and covetousness than 'a can part young limbs and lechery; but the gout galls the one, and the pox pinches the other."[40]

In Renaissance times it was a fantasy but also a visible fact that podagra haunted the pre-eminent. The muster of illustrious sufferers was imposing.[41] The Medici in Florence illustrated the links between gout and grandeur upon which many contemporaries remarked. Son of the gouty Giovanni, Cosimo de'Medici (1389–1464) was said to have grown "old very rapidly as he suffered very severely from the gout, and in his later years became very infirm, which caused him to leave the affairs of the state largely to others." Cosimo had two sons, one of whom, Piero il Gottoso (1416–69), succeeded him. Piero ("The Gouty") suffered from boyhood onwards with acute attacks; for long spells he was unable to address public business; he became very crippled; and late in life his incapacity was such that he could move only his tongue.[42]

The Holy Roman Emperor Charles V (1500–58) suffered his first gouty paroxysm at the age of twenty-eight. Severe attacks followed in 1536 and 1544–45, when he was immobilized for almost the whole winter. By 1550 he was almost completely physically disabled. Despite increasing incapacity, Charles failed to control the gluttony that fed his disease. Ignoring court physicians, he would follow the latest quack who would promise recovery without the need to curb his appetite. His recurrent bouts of gout influenced the fate of his Empire. Thus in French wars, plans to lay siege to Metz, the ke Lorraine, had to be postponed in 1552 becaus was sick. Physical incapacity was perhaps reason for his abdication in favour of his Philip: two years later he died miserably, "s and frustrated of the goute before the High A of his chapel in the Escorial."[43]

What treatments did Charles V try? A t porarily fashionable remedy for gout, as wel for other diseases like syphilis, was a decoctio guaiac wood, or *lignum vitae*, recently in duced from the New World via the Augsb banking family of Fugger. An alternative was "China root," the diuretic extract of the dried zome known later as *Smilax china*, brought b from the East by the Portuguese, for wh similar virtues were claimed.[44] With both, the tient was put to bed on a low diet in a hea room, and the decoction administered. The E peror was subjected to each of these "specifi he preferred China root, however, as fewer etary restrictions were thought necessary. N ther proved effective.[45]

In England, the pre-eminent gout sufferer w William Cecil, Lord Burghley.[46] Assorted lett to him survive in English, Latin, French and I ian, offering infallible cures. A note from a N Dyon dated 24 January 1553 recommended combination of diet and physic. Similar dir tions came from Lady Harington in a letter dat 4 February 1573, and an Italian letter dated 12 D cember 1575, concerned a secret gout powd Four years later Dr. Henry Landwer came with a Latin prescription for medicated slippe while Dr. Hector Nones, or Nuñez, a Fellow the College of Physicians and one of the lead of London's Spanish Jewish colony, showe him with cures culled from Averroes and othe In 1583 yet another letter from a certain Nicho Gybberd held out prospects of an infallible cu an alchemical tincture of gold. The Earl Shrewsbury also wrote begging His Lordship ıke trial of my OYLE OF STAGS BLUD, for I am ngly persuaded of the rare and great vertu reof. I know it to be a most safe thynge, yet ıe offence there is in the smell thereof."[47]

n a letter of 1592, Henry Bossevyle, an al-:mist living in Calais, offered in return for ferment and a fee of four or five hundred ınds to "furnish some infallible plaisters to e the gout":

Concernynge the applyinge thereof, one water solution] must bathe the place nere unto the ›ayne, leaving a joynte between the place of payne ınd the place bathed, if conveniently it maye be. Then must a peece of the sayd lether be cutte con-venient to make a plaister, which muste be well moystened in one of the sayde waters, and thereon several other powerful things spredde, which plaister muste be layde upon the place bathed, :here to remayne XII howers; and afterwards :here must be freshe bathinge and plaisters.[48]

cautious with regard to his own health as to the tion's, Burghley sent no answer.

To his son Robert, Earl of Salisbury, Burghley queathed not only several of his offices of state t also his affliction, from which Robert died on May 1612 on his return from a "cure" in Bath lered by Turquet de Mayerne, the royal physi-ın. Burghley's eldest son, Thomas (1542–1623), rl of Exeter, also suffered, leading to his un-ıely retirement from court and occasional nfinement in his house at Wimbledon.[49]

As gout took up residence with ministers and onarchs, it also became identified as the mon-:h among maladies—often being jocularly re-rred to, with echoes of Classical lore, as a quasi-ity born of the union of Bacchus and Venus.[50] e explanation as to why gout's abode lay within e palace, or at least the mansion and manor-use, was provided by the popular just-so story the travels of Monsieur Gout and the Spider.[51] "A Tale That is True Enough," Richard Hawes fered readers his *The Poore-Mans Plaster-Box. Furnished with Diverse Excellent Remedies for Sudden Mischances, and Usuall Infirmities, Which Happen to Men, Women, and Children in this Age* (1634), just one of many tellings.[52] The point of Hawes's tale was to explain why the gout "commonly keepes good company, as Bishops, Cardinals, Dukes, Earles, Lords, Knights, Judges, Gentlemen, and Merchants." It was all because of the wretched entertainment Monsieur Gout had once received at a peasant's cot. "A great while ago," Hawes began,

when Monsieur Gout was not so rich (as now he is), he was forced to travel, as other poor men are sometimes. In his travel he met with a spider, whose journey lay as Mr. Gout's did. They being both benighted, they sought lodging, and came to a poore man's house, which the Gout took up for his lodging, for he always being a lazy com-panion, would go no further; but the spider being more nimble, went to a rich man's house, and there took up his lodging for the night. The next day they met again, and asked each other of their entertainment the past night.

"Mine," said the Gout, "was the worst as ever I had, for I had no sooner touched the poor man's legs, thinking there to take my rest, but up he gets, and to thrashing he goes, so that I had no rest the whole night."

"And I," said the spider, "had no sooner begun to build my house in the rich man's chamber, but the maid came with a broom, and tore down all my work, and so fiercely did pursue me, that I had so much ado to save my life, as ever I had."

"Seeing it is so, then," said the Gout, "we will change lodging, I will go to the rich man's house, and thou shalt go to the poor man's." They both were well and content, and did so, and found such ease and rest in their lodging, that they resolved never to remove, for the spider built and was not troubled, the Gout he was enter-tained with a soft cushion, with down pillows, with dainty caudles, and delicate broths. In brief,

> he did like it so well, that ever since he takes up his lodging with rich men, where I desire that he should take his rest, rather than in my poor house.[53]

With a sting in the tail equally for *Dives* and *Lazarus,* the fable was often recycled, not least by La Fontaine.[54] Personification of diseases in this Aesopian manner, endowing them with moral messages, was a common rhetorical device.[55] Humanists liked to suck sermons out of sickness, and maladies formed a school of virtue.[56]

Petrarch (1304–74) had pioneered the genre two centuries earlier. In a letter written around 1338 from his retreat at Vaucluse he had offered his own rendition of the fable of the spider and the gout, drawing the uplifting conclusion that while the poor had to stomach certain nuisances—such as creepy-crawlies—their simple way of life protected them from the terrible retribution of the gout.[57] In a series of moral letters to a gouty friend, Colonna, he praised the disease for the opportunities it furnished for moral edification:[58]

> You will see that like the bridle for the untamed horse a gout was required for you. Perhaps it ought to be required for me too so that I might now learn to stay in one place and settle down. Without doubt, however, it was required for you more than anyone else I know. You would, if you could, have gone beyond the boundaries of the inhabited world; you would have crossed the ocean; you would have gone to the antipodes, and your reason would not have helped you seek a halt though it is powerful in other matters. What more need I say? You were able to stay still only with the help of the gout.[59]

In his *De remediis,* written 1357–60, Petrarch further moralized gout. In that series of dialogues, "Sorrow" complained of being "tortured by repulsive gout," made "unfit" and weakened: "I cannot stand on my feet."[60] "Reason" provided the moral corrective, explaining that it was to be expected that old age brought an "army of diseases"; but years also brought wisdom: gout encouraged to be ruled by one's head not one's feet. Not "this disease afflicts mostly the rich," provi the perfect inducement to "declare war not on the pleasures of Bacchus but of Venus."[6 short, "Reason" counseled that one's shield la temperance.[62] The best persuasive to contine gout was a fate against which the courage Christian philosopher should fortify himsel strengthening the mind: "even when you are ly down, your mind can stand up straight"; he of mind and soul paved the way for philosop meditation, which was of far greater value t the frivolities to which gout mercifully pu stop.[63]

The Petrarchan prescription for extract philosophy from podagra was pursued by prince of Humanist scholars, Erasmus. In 1511 *Encomium Moriae* (Praise of Folly) launc that brilliant genre of Humanist writing, mock encomium. Tracts in that mould too facetious praise for the subject being satiriz the principal "heroes" of encomia being wic men, loathsome creatures (lice, for examp various sins and vices, and disease. Among vices the most popular was drunkenness and the maladies, gout—subjects intimately in linked.[64]

Throughout his life, Erasmus suffered p health and hypochondriacal tendencies, frett about ruining his constitution by his dedicat to learning, while reading extensively in the m ical writings of Antiquity. "I can see also that own health is frail," he wailed as early as 1506, fore his first bout of renal colic, "and has be further weakened to a considerable degree by laborious studies."[65] Twenty years later he plained his kidney stones:

> I surmise that I know the cause of the illness. more than twenty years I have been in the ha of standing when I do my writing and hardly e sit down. . . . As it is inevitable that the stomach one who writes standing is somewhat bent, I s

nise that the stomach has begun to remove half-igested food because the gastric juices had been ed somewhere else and that is the cause that the tone does not keep enlarging.[66]

n 1522 his friend and fellow Humanist llibald Pirckheimer, after suffering gouty at-ks for about a decade, published his homage he *Encomium Moriae: Apologia seu Podagra us* (In Praise of Gout).[67] Pirckheimer iquely alluded to the *Praise of Folly* in the In-duction.[68] In her opening declamation, the iden Podagra asked: "For how can there pro-d any right judgment when Folly captivates sdom, Rashness rules Reason, Impotence of nd cashiers counsel?"[69]

Pirckheimer had earlier written that "The doc-s claim that my excessive studying is the cause my ailment. . . . However, for what does one when one may not study?"[70] The pair of Hu-nists thus both experienced wry satisfaction in ving acquired the gout, considering it a testa-nt to unstinted scholarly labours. Erasmus ced their joint feelings to his comrade. "In ny which usually is unbearable," he wrote:

> because this tyrant with its cruel retinue moves from the loins through the haunches to the region of the spleen, from there it goes with the intention of breaking through into the bladder, tearing, twisting and throwing everything along the way into disorder; how used to violence are princes who delight more in being feared than in being loved.[71]

Shortly afterwards, in May 1525, Erasmus pub-hed an edition of St. John Chrysostom's *De cerdotio*. Its preface included a brief "En-mium to the Gout and the Stone,"[72] involving expansion of the letter written to Pirckheimer o months earlier. It expounded a philosophy licing Stoicism with Christianity, and praising e "glory" of disease.[73]

Launched by Petrarch and refined by Erasmus d Pirckheimer, the Renaissance gout eulogy continued with Geronimo Cardano's *Podagrae Encomium*. "What a man gout makes! devout, morally pure, temperate, circumspect, wakeful," he commented: "No one is so mindful of God as the man who is in the clutches of the pains of gout. He who suffers gout cannot forget that he is mortal, because it affects him in every part of his being."[74] The genre reached its elaborate apogee in *Ritterorden des podagrischen Fluss* (Order of the Gouty Humour), an allegorical poem composed by Georg Fleissner in 1594.[75] Further editions in 1596, 1600 and 1611 attest its popularity. Nothing is known about its author, except the information on the title page which indicates he was a captain from Schönberg living in Schlackenwerth, both towns near Carlsbad.

Prefaced by an epigram stating that "the strong must pay for their frivolity with hardship and must suffer great pain and be martyred for many years," Fleissner's encomium involved elaborate parodies operating upon several assumptions. Podagra was herself noble; those upon whom she bestowed her favours were thereby ennobled; by rendering her devotees sick, Podagra did them a huge favour, by preventing folly and crime and affording leisure for reflection.

Purportedly written by the Order Of Knights of the Gouty Humour, the encomium claimed to tell of the "delicate maiden and goddess PODAGRA's origin, birth, name, appearance, manner, upbringing, education, position, her playmates and servants, companions, amusement and principal pleasure." Many aspired to social distinction—but typically they failed![76] "No one thinks much of such nobility," the reader is told, hence effort was wasted in pursuit of gold and glory. But not so with gout:

> because the gouty are noble not in pretense but in deed. They do not chase after nobility, nor purchase it for money, but are soon raised to the nobility and gentry by their feet and hands. They then do not presume that there may be a respite from Podagra but realize that she is a noble, deli-

> cate maiden, born of the gods, who will not be so forgetful as to have relations with a coarse peasant man.[77]

Who, in any case, would want to be healthy? Good health was hopelessly plebeian, and a sure recipe for disaster: "Someone who lives in health is not master of his body even though he be of good means, but is unceasingly plagued with others' business. He is almost a serf."[78]

By contrast, what brought true dignity and distinction was disease and, among diseases, the princess was Podagra. Gout conferred the ultimate aristocratic luxury, ease:

> When friends presently appeal to him for aid, he can counter with the excuse that he really cannot move, because Podagra with a cramp has already challenged him to another fight, or has already attacked him, so that he cannot stand on his feet. . . . Now please tell me whether such a person is not without doubt in control of his body—is he not a mighty lord over it? Oh, Podagra, you are justly praised for all time![79]

Podagra did not merely confer ease. She also inspired religious faith and other nobler virtues:

> Podagra also encourages piety at all times: no one is more devout, moderate, or chaste than the gouty because they are always wide awake in bed and are not likely to sleep without prayer. They think much more about the hour of death than healthy people do.[80]

These were not the only pronouncements. Later encomia followed in the footsteps of these familiar twists of didactic irony, typically praising gout on two grounds. It afforded proof of social superiority, while compelling a life of ease preserving the victim from vices and temptation. Cutting the persiflage, the moral message was that gout was a consequence of venery, gluttony and drunkenness, and folks were victims of their own folly. Fools, folly, vice, pleasure: the very stuff of the Menippean tradition of Lucian, as we shall see over and again in the evolution of g
and its representations.

A late instance of this "Fools' Literature
Podagra by Gottfried Rogg (1669–1742) of A
burg, Bavaria, a publisher and engraver. An e
orate copperplate engraving, it has some of
features of the modern comic strip.[81] Presen
an apology for the ravages caused by gout, Po
gra is praised for her twenty virtues in a text
so uncommonly found that we cite the virtue
their entirety:

1. *The Podagra is a fashionable ailment.* Because he who is burdened by it does not run around all over town with other ambitious persons, but remains elegantly at home.
2. *It takes care of itself all alone.* Since it doe
not especially care about foreign things, having enough to do by itself.
3. *It is humble.* Because it attaches itself to th
patient's feet.
4. *Wakeful.* Because it permits little rest or sleep.
5. *Moderate.* Because the patient is repelled by almost all foods.
6. *Temperate.* Because such a patient often drinks water rather than wine.
7. *Obedient.* In that one in this condition let
himself be greased, have incense burned, and have the feet bandaged.
8. *Taciturn.* One sighs more than one reads, while all conversation becomes annoying.
9. *It is patient.* Because whether such a patie
may sit, lie, or stand, it is a constant effort for him.
10. *Prudent.* As long as one avoids or discards a
that from which it originates.
11. *Pious.* It teaches the person to pray and to direct his thoughts toward heaven.
12. *Shaming.* When it develops in a patient, h
attempts, as much as possible, to conceal h

illness and to masquerade under the name of another misfortune.

It helps the person to the greatest virtue. Because it stimulates him to abide by the commandments of heaven as much as possible, and finally brings him so far that he can derive a steady comfort from their possession.

Chaste. Since it does not even like to be touched.

It enriches the person in temporal and eternal values. In that it restrains him from many sins, it deters him from all feasts, toasts, dances, immoderate lovemaking, and so forth, whereby the structure of the human body becomes virtually shattered and decrepit, wherefore the healthy days of life are then frequently shortened by a great many disorders.

It is devout. Since it creates devout people, teaches them to live piously, and also brings about certain cessation of sin.

It is faithful. Because it seldom leaves its patient entirely.

It is wise. Since, in tormenting the person, it teaches him to know himself and to move others to sympathy.

It is loving. Because it attracts the evil vapors unto itself, consumes the humours, cleanses the body including the head, and thus brings about quite a different disposition in the person, and so proves its faithful services.

It finally is also majestic. One lies in bed like a king on his throne, one goes to meet no one, one arises for no one, one accompanies no one, and one finally visits no one, even when one has been visited.[82]

Taking all score of such benefits into consider-
on, only one conclusion was possible: celebra-
n of the blessed malady.[83]

NOTES

1. See Siraisi (1990) [N. G. Siraisi. 1990. *Medieval and Early Renaissance Medicine.* Chicago, Ill.: Chicago University Press]; Katherine Park (1985) [Katherine Park. 1985. *Doctors and Medicine in Early Renaissance Florence.* Princeton, N.J.: Princeton University Press]; Slack (1979) [Paul Slack. 1979. "Mirrors of Health and Treasures of Poor Men: Uses of the Vernacular Medical Literature of Tudor England." In C. Webster, ed. *Health, Medicine and Mortality in the Sixteenth Century.* Cambridge: Cambridge University Press, 237–74]; Roy Porter, ed. (1992) [Roy Porter, ed. 1992. *The Popularization of Medicine, 1650–1850.* London: Routledge]. For printing, see Eisenstein (1979) [Elizabeth L. Eisenstein. 1979. *The Printing Press as an Agent of Change,* 2 vols. Cambridge: Cambridge University Press].

2. Copeman and Winder (1969) [W. S. C. Copeman and Marianne Winder. 1969. "The First Medical Monograph on the Gout." *Medical History.* xiii, 288–93]. Copeman and Winder reproduce the text in translation, and we have drawn our account from theirs. Burgawer states that "The majority of people believe that gout [podagra] cannot be cured" adding, "Daily experience has convinced them of that" (A2r). This implies that "podagra" was a familiar condition.

3. In architectural English, "gutta" is the word for the little drops underneath triglyphs on Doric entablatures.

4. Burgawer, A2; Copeman and Winder (1969), 289.

5. Copeman and Winder (1969), 289 (all these somewhat eccentric spellings are as in the translation); Benedek (1987) [Thomas G. Benedek. 1987. "Popular Literature on Gout in the 16th and 17th Centuries". *Journal of Rheumatology.* xiv, 186], 186. On the non-naturals see Neibyl (1971) [P. Niebyl. 1971. "The Non-Naturals." *Bulletin of the History of Medicine.* xlv, 486–92]; Rather (1968) [L. J. Rather. 1968. "The 'Six Things Non-Natural': A Note on the Origins and Fate of a Doctrine and a Phrase." *Clio Medica.* iii, 337–47].

6. Rhazes (al-Razi, c. 850–932) was born in Persia. His twenty-volume masterpiece *Al-Hawi* or *El Hawi* contains medical knowledge from Greece, the Roman

Empire, India, Syria and Persia, supplemented by his personal experiences.

7. Paré's works will be cited in the translation by Thomas Johnson (1634), Book xviii [Ambroise Paré. 1634. *The Workes of that Famous Chirurgeon Ambrose Parey.* Trans. Thomas Johnson. London: Thomas Cotes and R. Young]. See Malgaigne (1965) [J. F. Malgaigne. 1965. *Surgery and Ambroise Paré.* Trans. W. B. Hamby. Norman, Okla.: University of Oklahoma Press]. Following apprenticeship to a barber-surgeon, Ambroise Paré (1510–90) completed his training in Paris. He is best known for his treatment of battle wounds.

8. Paré (1634), 698. See the discussion in Copeman (1964), 53ff [W. S. C. Copeman. 1964. *A Short History of the Gout and the Rheumatic Diseases.* Berkeley, Calif.: University of California Press].

9. Paré (1634), 697.

10. Ibid.

11. Ibid., 707.

12. Ibid., 710.

13. Swiss-born, Paracelsus (Philippus Aureolus Theophrastus Bombastus von Hohenheim, 1493–1541) trained in medicine with his father. He traveled widely, but later went to Basel as city physician. He advocated simplicity in his recipes and his experiences in chemistry prompted him to use heavy metals. He left Basel as his teachings were considered too unorthodox. For his writings on gout, see "Das Buch von den Tartarischen Krankheitten," in Paracelsus (1589–90) [Theophrastus von Hohenheim Paracelsus. 1589–90. *Die Bucher und Schriften . . . , an tag Geben Durch J. H. Brisgoium.* Basel: C. Waldkirch]. His works may be found in Sudhoff, ed. (1922–33) [Karl Sudhoff, ed. 1922–33. *Paracelsus: Sämtliche Werke,* 14 vols. Munich: R. Oldebourg] and Bernard Aschner, ed. (1975–77) [Bernard Aschner, ed. 1975–77. *Paracelsus: Sämtliche Werke,* 4 vols. Leipzig: Zentralantiquariat der Deutschen Demokratischen Republik]. For scholarship, see Pagel (1958a) [Walter Pagel. 1958a. *Paracelsus: An Introduction to Philosophical Medicine in the Era of the Renaissance.* Basel: Karger]; Debus (1977) [Allen G. Debus. 1977. *The Chemical Philosophy; Paracelsian Science and Medicine in the Sixteenth and Seventeenth Centuries.* New York: Science History Publicatic idem (1991) [Allen G. Debus. 1991. *The French Par sians: The Chemical Challenge to Medical and entific Tradition in Early Modern France.* Cambri Cambridge University Press]; idem (1965) [Aller Debus. 1965. *The English Paracelsians.* London: (bourne].

14. See Pagel (1958a), 135.

15. Ibid., 139.

16. Ibid., 140.

17. Ibid.

18. Ibid., 157.

19. The formation of stones within the human b was widely viewed as an expression of living nature. Rudwick (1976), ch. i [Martin J. S. Rudwick. 1976. *Meaning of Fossils: Episodes in the History of Pala tology.* New York: Scientific History Publicatio Pagel (1984), 33 [Walter Pagel. 1984. *The Smi Spleen: Paracelsianism in Storm and Stress.* Basel New York: Karger].

20. Cited and translated in Rodnan (1965) [Geral Rodnan. 1965. "Early Theories Concerning Etiol and Pathogenesis of the Gout." *Arthritis and Rheu tism.* viii, 599–610], 601, and in Pagel (1984), 33–34. Paracelsus (1574), 28–37, which may be found Aschner, ed. (1975–77), ii, 6–27. Paracelsus' ideas re being translated into modern chemical equivale Contextualization of Paracelsus' writings within naissance natural philosophy is offered in Goodri Clarke (1990) [Nicholas Goodrick-Clarke. 19 *Paracelsus: Artsen, Staat & Volksgezondheid in Ne land, 1840–1890.* London: Crucible]; idem tra (1990b) [Nicholas Goodrick-Clarke. 1990. *Paracels Essential Readings.* London: Crucible]; Paracel (1941) [Theophrastus von Hohenheim Paracels 1941. *Four Treatises of Theophrastus von Hohenhe Called Paracelsus.* Ed. Henry E. Sigerist. Baltimc Md.: Johns Hopkins University Press]; idem (19 [Theophrastus von Hohenheim Paracelsus. 19 *Paracelus: Selected Writings.* Trans. N. Guterm New York: Pantheon Books].

21. Theodore Turquet de Mayerne (1573–1655) v born in Geneva and studied at the University of H delberg, later at Montpellier, where he gradua

). in 1597. Moving to Paris he lectured on anatomy pharmacy and was appointed King's physician. He le use of chemical remedies, drawing condemna- from the Paris College of Physicians. Visiting Eng- l in 1606 he was appointed physician to Queen e of Denmark and returning in 1611 became physi- to four successive monarchs. In 1618 he wrote the ication to the King of the *Pharmacopoea Londi- sis* (1618). He was knighted in 1624.

2. Turquet de Mayerne (1676), 14–15 [Theodore quet de Mayerne. 1676. *A Treatise of the Gout*. Lon- : D. Newman]. See Debus (1965), 150–56, though unfortunately does not mention gout; for the acelsian tradition, idem (1977); idem (1991); Web- (1975) [Charles Webster. 1975, *The Great Instaura- : Science, Medicine, and Reform, 1626–1660*. Lon- : Duckworth].

3. Boorde (1562a) [Andrew Boorde. 1562a. *Dyetary Health*. London: T. Colwel]; idem (1587) [Andrew orde. 1587. *Breviary of Helthe for All Manner of Syck- sses and Diseases*. London: W. Middleton]. See peman (1964), 50–51. For surveys of early-modern glish medicine, see idem (1960) [W. S. C. Cope- n. 1960. *Doctors and Disease in Tudor Times*. Lon- : William Dawson & Sons]; Nagy (1988) [Doreen enden Nagy. 1988. *Popular Medicine in Seventeenth- ntury England*. Bowling Green, Ohio: Bowling een State University Popular Press]; Beier (1987) M. Beier. 1987. *Sufferers and Healers: The Experi- ce of Illness in Seventeenth-Century England*. Lon- n: Routledge & Kegan Paul].

24. Boorde (1587). Andrew Boorde (1490–1549) en- ed the Carthusian order. He left this in 1528 and died medicine on the Continent. He returned to gland in 1542 and set up a medical practice in Win- ester. His main works were: *Dyetery of Health* (1562), *eviary of Helthe for all Manner of Syckenesses and seases* (1587) and a travel guide, *The First Boke of the troduction of Knowledge* (1562).

25. Boorde (1587). Treacle is theriac, a complex ium preparation, with a multitude of ingredients: see atson (1966) [Gilbert Watson. 1966. *Theriac and ithidatium: A Study in Therapeutics*. London: The ellcome Historical Medical Library]. Scammony is the Syrian bindweed (*Convulvulus scammonia*). It is a strong cathartic, somewhat similar to jalap.

26. On cinchona (Jesuit's bark, Peruvian bark, the basis of quinine) see Jarcho (1993) [Saul Jarcho. 1993. *Quinine's Predecessor: Francesco Torti and the Early History of Cinchona*. Baltimore, Md.: Johns Hopkins University Press]. *Fraxinus excelsior*, the bark and seeds of ash, is an astringent, its seeds an aperient.

27. Boorde's contemporary, Sir Thomas Elyot, issued warnings on that score, however, to the effect that "Radysh rootes . . . causes to breake wynde and to pysse . . . they be unwholesome for theym, that have continually the goute or peynes in the joyntes": Elyot (1937) [Sir T. Elyot. 1541, 1937. *The Castel of Helath*. London: T. Berthelet; Reprint Ed. S. A. Tennenbaum, New York: Scholars Facsimiles and Reprints], 28. Elyot wrote of "reumes" as a synonym of catarrh.

28. Graham and Graham (1955) [Wallace Graham and K. M. Graham. 1955. "Men and Books. Our Gouty Past." *Canadian Medical Association Journal*. lxxiii, 485–93].

29. Barrough (1590), 210. The 1st edn appeared in 1583; the 3rd in 1596; the 4th in 1610; the 5th in 1617; the 6th in 1624; the 7th in 1634; the 8th in 1639 [Philip Barrough. *The Method of Phisick, Conteining the Causes, Signes, and Cures of Inward Diseases in Mans Bodie from the Head to the Foote*. London: Thomas Vautroullier].

30. Ibid.

31. Cogan (1584), title page (in Latin) [Thomas Cogan. 1584. *The Haven of Health Made for the Comfort of Students*. London:Henrie Midleton for William Norton]. The reference to Hippocrates shows Cogan was stressing the non-naturals. See Niebyl (1971); Rather (1968). Thomas Cogan (1545?–1607) studied in Oxford and became a fellow of Oriel in 1563. His works include *The Well of Wisedome . . .* (1577), and *The Haven of Health Made for the Comfort of Students* (1584).

32. Cogan (1584), Epistle Dedicatorie (at beginning).

33. Ibid., 161. The cheese-and-bacon poultice long continued popular.

34. Ibid., facing p. 4 of the Epistle Dedicatorie.

35. For an overview on treatment, see Ackerknecht (1973) [E. H. Ackerknecht. 1973. *Therapeutics from the Primitives to the 20th Century. With an Appendix: The History of Dietetic.* New York: Hafner] and Urdang (1944) [G. Urdang. 1944. *Pharmacopoeia Londinensis of 1618.* Madison, Wisc.: State Historical Society of Wisconsin]. For herbal cures, see Arber (1938) [Agnes Arber. 1938. *Herbals.* Cambridge: Cambridge University Press]; Foust (1992) [Clifford Foust. 1992. *Rhubarb: The Wonder Drug.* Princeton, N.J.: Princeton University Press]; B. Griggs (1981) [B. Griggs. 1981. *Green Pharmacy: A History of Herbal Medicine.* London: Jill Norman & Hobhouse]. For folk remedies, see W. G. Black (1883) [W. G. Black. 1883. *Folk Medicine: A Chapter in the History of Culture.* London: Folklore Society]; Chamberlain (1981) [Mary Chamberlain. 1981. *Old Wives' Tales: Their History, Remedies and Spells.* London: Virago]; Loux (1978) [Françoise Loux. 1978. *Sagesse du Corps: Santé et maladie dans les proverbs réginaux franyaises.* Paris: Maisonneuve et Larose]; idem (1979) [Françoise Loux. 1979. *Practiques et saviors populaires: le corps dans la société traditionelle.* Paris: Berger-Levrault]; idem (1988) [Françoise Loux. 1988. "Popular Culture and Knowledge of the Body: Infancy and the Medical Anthropologists." In R. Porter and A. Wear, eds. *Problems and Methods in the History of Medicine.* London: Croom Helm, 81–97]; idem (1993) [Françoise Loux. 1993. "Folk Medicine." In W. F. Bynum and R. Porter, eds. *Companion Encyclopedia of the History of Medicine.* London: Routledge, 661–75]. In twentieth-century America, folk cures for gout have included angelica, birch leaves (as a blood purifier), holly, strawberry, primose root and various other bitters: see Crellin and Philpott (1991) [John K. Crellin and Jane Philpott. 1991. *Herbal Medicine Past and Present,* 2 vols. Durham, N.C.: Duke University Press]; Barton and Castle (1877), 108f [Benjamin H. Barton and Thomas Castle. 1877. *The British Flora Medica.* London: Chatto & Windus].

36. Nash (1600), p. E [Thomas Nash. 1600. *A Pleasant Comedie, Called Summers Last Will and Testament.* London: Simon Stafford].

37. Gilman (1989) [Sander Gilman. 1989. *Sexuality: An Illustrated History.* New York: Wiley]; Andreski (1990) [Stanislav Andreski. 1990. *Syphilis, Puritanism and Witchcraft: A Historical Explanation in Lig[illegible] Medicine and Psychoanalysis.* New York: St. Ma[illegible] Press]; Quétel (1990) [Claude Quétel. 1990. *The [illegible]tory of Syphilis.* Trans. Judith Braddock and Brian [illegible] Oxford: Basil Blackwell.].

38. Joubert (1989), 260 [Laurent Joubert. 1989. [illegible] *ular Errors.* Trans. and Ed. Gregory David de Roc[illegible] Tuscaloosa, Ala., and London: University of Alab[illegible] Press].

39. "Yet I am better Than one that's sick o' th' g[illegible] since he had rather Groan so in perpetuity tha[illegible] cur'd By th' sure physician, Death," proclaims the [illegible]prisoned Posthumus in *Cymbeline* (V.iv.4). In *H[illegible] IV, Part 2* (I.ii.273) Falstaff declares: "A pox of this g[illegible] Or, a gout of this pox! For the one or the other p[illegible] the rogue with my great toe." Kail (1986), 232; see [illegible] Hoeniger (1992).

40. *Henry IV,* Part 2, I.ii.256.

41. This and the following come from Cope[illegible] (1964), 54–55; see also Appelboom and Bennett (19[illegible] [T. Appelboom and J. C. Bennett. 1986. "Gout of [illegible] Rich and Famous." *Journal of Rheumatology.* [illegible] 618–22].

42. Dying at fifty-three, he was succeeded by [illegible] young son, Lorenzo the Magnificent (1449–92), w[illegible] although inheriting the family gout, was less hars[illegible] afflicted than his father and grandfather, becoming [illegible] Italian Maecenas. On gout and the Medici, see Sch[illegible] (1950), chap. vii [Ferdinand Schevil. 1950. *The Me[illegible]* London: V. Gollancz].

43. On Charles V see Alvarez (1975) [Manuel [illegible]nandez Alvarez. 1975. *Charles V: Elected Emperor [illegible] Hereditary Ruler.* London: Thames and Hudson].

44. See Estes (1990), 46, 92 [J. Worth Estes. 19[illegible] *Dictionary of Protopharmacology: Therapeutic P[illegible]tices, 1700–1850.* Canton, Mass.: Science History P[illegible]lications and Watson Publishing International]. [illegible] guaiacum, see Hutten (1536) [Ulrich von Hutten. 15[illegible] 2nd ed. *Of the Wood Called Guaiacum, that Heal[illegible] the Frenche Pocks, and also Helpeth the Goute in [illegible] Feet, the Stoone, the Palsey and Other Dyseases.* L[illegible]doni: Berthelet.].

45. Weatherall, "Drug Therapies," in Bynum a[illegible] Porter, eds. (1993).

46. The following paragraphs distil Copeman (19[illegible]

S.C. Copeman. 1957. "The Gout of William il—The First Lord Burghley (1520–98)." *Medical tory*. i, 262–64].

7. Ibid. In ancient medicine, weird, wonderful and n repugnant treatments were standard, especially ng adepts of the esoteric arts. For the arcane back- ınd, see Eamon (1994) [William Eamon. 1994. *Sci- e and the Secrets of Nature: Books of Secrets in Me- al and Early Modern Culture*. Princeton, N.J.: ıceton University Press]. There is little information Nones (Nunez); he was admitted a Fellow of the lege of Physicians in 1554 and was a censor in 1562 1563.

8. Ibid. Copeman is citing Lansdowne Manu- pts (British Library), no. 69, art 60.

49. See also Alan G. R. Smith, ed. (1990) [Alan G. R. ith, ed. 1990. *The Anonymous Life of William Cecil, d Burghley*. Lewistown Me.: E. Mellen Press]; ynes (1989) [Alan Haynes. 1989. *Robert Cecil, Earl alisbury, 1563–1612: Servant of Two Sovereigns*. Lon- ı: Peter Owen]. For Mayerne's views, see Turquet de yerne (1676)

50. For this divine pedigree, see Benedek and Rod- ı (1963b) [Thomas G. Benedek and Gerald P. Rod- ı. 1963b. "'Podagra' by Gottfried Rogg: An Illus- ed Encomium on the Gout." *Journal of the History Medicine*. xviii, 349–52].

51. Idem (1970).

52. Hawes (1634), 31 [Richard Hawes. 1634. *The Poor- ıns Plaster-Box. Furnished with Diverse Excellent medies for Sudden Mischances, and Usuall Infirmi- , Which Happen to Men, Women, and Children in s Age*. London: Thomas Cotes for Franceis Grove]. e Eamon (1981). The same class point was made by preacher Henry Smith. Waving aside objections ong upper-class ladies that they were not physically apable of breast-feeding their babies, he demanded: ıt whose breasts have this perpetual drought? For- th it is like the goute, no beggars may have it, but cit- ns or Gentlewomen": Henry Smith (1598) [Henry ıith. 1598. *Four Sermons*. London: P. Short], quoted Fildes (1985), 101 [Valerie Fildes. 1985. *Breasts, Bot- s and Babies: A History of Infant Feeding*. Edin- rgh: Edinburgh University Press].

53. Hawes (1634), 31.

54. LaFontaine (1966) [Jean de La Fontaine. 1966. *Fables*. Ed. Antoine Adam. Paris: Flammarion]. Rodnan and Benedek have traced the "gout and the spider" tale back to the ninth century. In La Fontaine's telling of 1668, "when given a choice of earthly resting place, the spider first selected a palace, and the gout, to avoid physicians, chose a mean hut. They then traded places. The spider took to the peasant's shack where she could live undisturbed, while the gout, craving nourishment and attention, went straight, as lodger, To the palace of a bishop, who was bedbound Thereafter, her helpless prisoner." (Rodnan and Benedek [1970]) [Gerald P. Rodnan and Thomas G. Benedek. 1970. "Gout and the Spider." *Journal of the American Medical Association*. ccxi, 2157].

55. Also personified was venereal disease, thanks to Fracastoro's poem, *Syphilis, sive morbus gallicus* (1530) [Girolamo Fracastoro. 1530. *Syphilis, Sive Morbus Gallicus*. Verona: S. Nicolini da Sabbio]. In that pastoral myth, syphilis was a shepherd.

56. For such beliefs, see Ficino (1989) [Marsilio Ficino. 1989. *Three Books on Life*. Trans. Carol V. Kaske and John R. Clark. Binghamton, N.Y.: Renaissance Society of America]; Kristeller (1979) [Paul Kristellar. 1979. *Renaissance Thought and its Sources*. New York: Columbia University Press]; Barkan (1975) [L. Barkean. 1975. *Nature's Work of Art: The Human Body as Image of the World*. New Haven, Conn.: Yale University Press]. On Death teaching lessons, see Ariès (1981) [Philippe Ariès. 1981. *The Hour of Our Death*. Trans. H. Weaver. London: Allen Lane]; Geddes (1981) [Gordon E. Geddes. 1981. *Welcome Joy: Death in Puritan New England*. Ann Arbor, Mich: UMI Research Press]. For piety and sickness, see Wear (1985b) [Andrew Wear. 1985b. "Puritan Perceptions of Illness in Seventeenth-Century England." In Roy Porter, ed. *Patients and Practitioners*. Cambridge: Cambridge University Press, 55–99]; idem (1987) [Andrew Wear. 1987. "Interfaces: Perceptions of Health and Illness in Early Modern England." In Roy Porter and Andrew Wear, eds. *Problems and Methods in the History of Medicine*. London: Croom Helm, 230–55].

57. Benedek and Rodnan (1963a) [Thomas G. Benedek and Gerald P. Rodnan. 1963a. "Petrarch on Medicine and the Gout." *Bulletin of the History of*

Medicine, xxxvii, 397–416]. Francesco di Petrarch (1304–74) was the key figure in the early Italian Renaissance. He studied the humanities between 1315 and 1319 while in Montpellier. He moved to Vaucluse in 1337 where he wrote much of his most important work. In 1347 he set up home in Parma were he pursued the vocations of a poet and idealistic politician.

58. Petrarch (1975–85), bk vi, letter 3, p. 309 [Petrarch. 1975–1980. *Letters on Familiar Matters.* 3 vols. Trans. Aldo S. Bernardo. Baltimore Md.: Johns Hopkins University Press], cited in and discussed by Benedek and Rodnan (1963a).

59. Petrarch (1975–85), bk vi, letter 3, p. 309.

60. Petrarch (1991), 198–200, p. 198 [Petrarch. 1991. *Petrarch's Remedies for Fortune Fair and Foul,* 3 vols. Trans. and commentary Conrad H. Rawski. Bloomington, Ind.: Indiana University Press].

61. Ibid., chap. 84, p. 199.

62. Ibid., p. 200.

63. Ibid.

64. For the encomium, see Kaiser (1963) [W. Kaiser. 1963. *Praisers of Folly.* Cambridge, Mass.: Harvard University Press.]; Benedek (1962) [T. G. Benedek. 1962. "Doctors and Patients in 'The Ship of Fools'." *Journal of the American Medical Association.* clxxxi, 236–42], 236–42. Desiderius Erasmus (1466–1536) was educated at Gouda and Deventer. He was ordained in 1492 but left his order in 1494. The remainder of his life he traveled in Europe, writing, studying and teaching. As a Humanist, he encouraged interest in learning, self-knowledge and simple devotion. His writings include *In Praise of Folly* (1519); *Encomium artis medicae* (1518); *In Novam Testamentum ab eodem denuo recognitum* (1519). See Mynors and Thomson, eds (1974–79), ii, 110–11, no. 189 [R. A. Mynors and D. F. Thomson, trans. 1974–1994. *The Correspondence of Erasmus,* 11 vols. Toronto: University of Toronto Press].

65. Erasmus to Servatus Rogerus, 1 April 1506; and Benedek (1983) [Thomas G. Benedek. 1983. "The Gout of Desiderius Erasmus and Willibald Pirckheimer: Medical Autobiography and its Literary Reflections." *Bulletin of the History of Medicine.* lvii, 526–44].

66. Allen and Allen, eds (1906–47), vi, 422–44, no. 1759: Erasmus to John Francis, October 1526 [Percy S. Allen and H. M. Allen, eds. 1906–47. *Opus epistola[rum] Des. Erasmi Roterodami,* 11 vols. Oxford: Claren[don] Press]. Erasmus' letters are here presented as transl[ated] by Krivasy in an excellent article: "Erasmus's Me[dical] Milieu" (1973) [Peter Krivasy. 1973. "Erasmus's M[edical] Milieu." *Bulletin of the History of Medicine.* x[lvii], 113–54].

67. Eckert and Imhoff (1971); Krivasy (1973), The Humanist Willibald Pirckheimer (1470–1[530]) spent his youth in Munich then studied Gree[k in] Padua and law in Pavia. He returned to Nurem[berg] without graduating and remained there all his life[. He] suffered from acute gout.

68. Eckert and Imhoff (1971) [Willebad P. Ec[kert] and Christoph von Imhoff. 1971. *Willibald Pi[rck]heimer: Dürer Freund im Spiegel seines Lebens, se[iner] Werke und seiner Umwelt.* Cologne: Wiena[nd];] Benedek (1983).

69. Pirckheimer (1617) [Willibald Pirckhei[mer.] 1617. *The Praise of the Gout, Or, The Gouts Apologi[e. A] Paradox, Both Pleasant and Profitable, Written Firs[t in] the Latine Tongue, by that Famous and Noble Ger[-] man Bilibaldus Pirckheimerus Councellor unto [the] Emperours, Maximillian the first and Charles the Fi[ft.] And now Englished by William Est, Master of Arts.* L[on-] don: printed by G. P. for John Budge].

70. Reicke (1930), 56: Pirckheimer to Konrad A[del]mann [Enuk Reucje, 1930. *Willibald Pirckheir[mer.] Leben, Familie und Persönlichkeit.* Jena: Diederichs].

71. Allen and Allen, eds (1906–47), vi, 47–48, 1558.

72. Erasmus, Preface to St. John Chrysostom, tra[ns]lated in Benedek (1983), 537.

73. Ibid.

74. Cardano (1653) [Girolamo Cardano. 1653. *[In] aphorismos Hippocratis commentaria.* Ed. Pau[lus] Frambottus. Padua: Apud Paulum Frambottu[m].] Jerome Cardan (1501–76) studied medicine at Pa[dua] and held the chairs of medicine in Pavia in 1543 a[nd] Bologna in 1562. He is remembered for his contri[bu]tions to chemical thought and his work in algebra. [It is] believed that he gave an accurate early picture of rh[eu]matic fever and differentiated it clearly from gout.

75. Benedek (1969): the following quotations [a]

n from Benedek's translation. See also idem 7), 186 [Thomas G. Benedek. 1969. "The Gout Enium of Georg Fleissner, 1594." *Bulletin of the History of Medicine*. xliii, 116–37].

6. Benedek (1969), 126.

7. Ibid., 126–27.

8. Ibid., 129.

9. Ibid., 129–30.

o. Ibid., 130.

1. Benedek and Rodnan (1963b). Gottfried Rogg of Augsburg (1669–1742) was a draftsman, publisher and engraver, working between 1704 and 1732. Most of his illustrations are views of towns; *Podagra* seems to be his only work pertaining to a disease. See also Googe (1990) [Barnaby Googe. 1990. *The Overthrow of the Gout, and A Dialogue Betwixt the Gout and Christopher Ballista.* Ed. and introduced by Simon McKeown. London: Indelible Inc].

82. Benedek and Rodnan 1963b), 350–52.

83. Ibid., 352.

CHAPTER 4

Report on the Diseases and Physic Peculiarities of the Negro Race

SAMUEL A. CARTWRIGHT

GENTLEMEN: ON THE PART of the Co mittee, consisting of Doctors Copes, Williamson, Browning and myself, investigate the diseases and physical peculiarities of our negro populatio we beg leave TO REPORT—

That, although the African race constitutes nearly a moiety of our sout ern population, it has not been made the subject of much scientific inv tigation, and is almost entirely unnoticed in medical books and schoo It is only very lately, that it has, in large masses, dwelt in juxtapositi with science and mental progress. On the Niger and in the wilds of Afric it has existed for thousands of years, excluded from the observation of th ntific world. It is only since the revival of ning, that the people of that race have been oduced on this continent. They are located in se parts of it not prolific in books and medical hors. No medical school was ever established r them until a few years ago; hence, their dis- es and physical peculiarities are almost un- wn to the learned. The little knowledge that thern physicians have acquired concerning m, has not been derived from books or med- l lectures, but from facts learned from their n observation in the field of experience, or ked up here and there from others.

Before going into the peculiarities of their dis- es, it is necessary to glance at the anatomical l physiological differences between the negro l the white man; otherwise their diseases can- t be understood. It is commonly taken for nted, that the color of the skin constitutes the in and essential difference between the black l the white race; but there are other differ- ces more deep, durable and indelible, in their atomy and physiology, than that of mere color. the albino the skin is white, yet the organiza- n is that of the negro. Besides, it is not only in skin, that a difference of color exists between negro and white man, but in the membranes, muscles, and tendons and in all the fluids and retions. Even the negro's brain and nerves, the yle and all the humors, are tinctured with a ide of the pervading darkness. His bile is of a eper color and his blood is blacker than the ite man's. There is the same difference in the sh of the white and black man, in regard to lor, that exists between the flesh of the rabbit d the hare. His bones are whiter and harder an those of the white race, owing to their con- ning more phosphate of lime and less gelatine. s head is hung on the atlas differently from the ite man; the face is thrown more upwards and e neck is shorter and less oblique; the spine ore inwards, and the pelvis more obliquely out- rds; the thigh-bones larger and flattened from fore backwards; the bones more bent; the legs curved outwards or bowed; the feet flat; the gas- trocnemii muscles smaller; the heel so long, as to make the ankle appear as if planted in the middle of the foot; the gait, hopper-hipped, or what the French call *l'allure déhanchée*, not unlike that of a person carrying a burden. The projecting mouth, the retreating forehead, the broad, flat nose, thick lips and wooly hair, are peculiarities that strike every beholder. According to Soem- merring and other anatomists, who have dis- sected the negro, his brain is a ninth or tenth less than in other races of men, his facial angle smaller, and all the nerves going from the brain, as also the ganglionic system of nerves, are larger in proportion than in the white man. The nerves distributed to the muscles are an exception, being smaller than in the white race. Soemmerring re- marks, that the negro's brain has in a great mea- sure run into nerves. One of the most striking dif- ferences is found in the much greater size of the *foramen magnum* in the negro than the white man. The foramen, or orifice between the brain and the spinal marrow, is not only larger, but the medulla oblongata, and particularly the nerves supplying the abdominal and pelvic viscera. Al- though the nose is flat, the turbinated bones are more developed, and the pituitary membrane, lining the internal cavities of the nose, more ex- tensive than in the white man, and causing the sense of smell to be more acute. The negro's hearing is better, his sight is stronger, and he sel- dom needs spectacles.

The field of vision is not so large in the negro's eye as in the white man's. He bears the rays of the sun better, because he is provided with an anatomical peculiarity in the inner canthus, con- tracting the field of vision, and excluding the sun's rays, —something like the membrana nicti- tans, formed by a preternatural development of the plica lunaris, like that which is observed in apes. His imitative powers are very great, and he can agitate every part of the body at the same time, or what he calls *dancing all over.* From the diffusion of the brain, as it were, into the various

organs of the body, in the shape of nerves to minister to the senses, everything, from the necessity of such a conformation, partakes of sensuality at the expense of intellectuality. Thus, music is a mere sensual pleasure with the negro. There is nothing in his music addressing the understanding; it has melody, but no harmony; his songs are mere sounds, without sense or meaning—pleasing the ear, without conveying a single idea to the mind; his ear is gratified by sound, as his stomach is by food. The great development of the nervous system, and the profuse distribution of nervous matter to the stomach, liver and genital organs, would make the Ethiopian race entirely unmanageable, if it were not that this excessive nervous development is associated with a deficiency of red blood in the pulmonary and arterial systems, from a defective atmospherization or arterialization of the blood in the lungs—constituting the best type of what is called the lymphatic temperament, in which lymph, phlegm, mucus, and other humors, predominate over the red blood. It is this defective hematosis, or atmospherization of the blood, conjoined with a deficiency of cerebral matter in the cranium, and an excessive nervous matter distributed to the organs of sensation and assimilation, that is the true cause of that debasement of mind, which has rendered the people of Africa unable to take care of themselves. It is the true cause of their indolence and apathy, and why they have chosen, through countless ages, idleness, misery and barbarism, to industry and frugality, —why social industry, or associated labor, so essential to all progress in civilisation and improvement, has never made any progress among them, or the arts and sciences taken root on any portion of African soil inhabited by them; as is proved by the fact that no letters, or even hieroglyphics—no buildings, roads or improvements, or monuments of any kind, are any where found, to indicate that they have ever been awakened from their apathy and sleepy indolence, to physical or mental exertion. To the same physiological causes, deeply rooted
in the organization, we must look for an expl
tion of the strange facts, why none of the
guages of the native tribes of Africa, as pro
by ethnographical researches, have risen ab
common names, standing for things and actio
to abstract terms or generalizations; —why
form of government on abstract principles, w
divisions of power into separate departments,
ever been instituted by them; —why they have
ways preferred, as more congenial to their natu
a government combining the legislative, judi
and executive powers in the same individual
the person of a petty king, a chieftain or mas
—why, in America, if let alone, they always p
fer the same kind of government of their fo
thers, as it gives them more tranquility and s
sual enjoyment, expands the mind and impro
the morals, by arousing from the natural in
lence so fatal to mental and moral progress. Ev
if they did not prefer slavery, tranquility, a
sensual enjoyment, to liberty, yet their organi
tion of mind is such, that if they had their libe
they have not the industry, the moral virtue,
courage and vigilance to maintain it, but wo
relapse into barbarism, or into slavery, as th
have done in Hayti. The reason of this is found
in unalterable physiological laws. Under the co
pulsive power of the white man, they are made
labor or exercise, which makes the lungs perfo
the duty of vitalizing the blood more perfec
than is done when they are left free to indu
in idleness. It is the red, vital blood, sent to
brain, that liberates their mind when un
the white man's control; and it is the want o
sufficiency of red vital blood, that chains th
mind to ignorance and barbarism, when in fr
dom.

The excess of organic nervous matter, and
deficiency of cerebral—the predominance of
humors over the red blood, from defective
mospherization of the blood in the lungs, imp
to the negro a nature not unlike that of a ne
born infant of the white race. In children,
nervous system predominates, and the tempe

nt is lymphatic. The liver, and the rest of the ndular system, is out of proportion to the san-neous and respiratory systems, the white ds predominating over the red; the lungs con-ne less oxygen, and the liver separates more bon, than in the adult age. This constitution, well marked in infancy, is the type of the iopian constitution, of all ages and sexes. It is l known, that in infancy, full and free respira-n of pure fresh air in repose, so far from being uired, is hurtful and prejudicial. Half smoth-d by its mother's bosom, or the cold external carefully excluded by a warm room or external ering over the face, the infant reposes—re-athing its own breath, warmed to the same nperature as that of its body, and loaded with bonic acid and aqueous vapor. The natural ef-t of this kind of respiration is, imperfect at-spherization of the blood in the lungs, and a betude of intellect, from the defective vitaliza-n of the blood distributed to the brain. But it s heretofore escaped the attention of the sci-tific world, that the defective atmospheriza-n of the blood, known to occur during sleep in ancy, and to be the most congenial to their nstitutions, is the identical kind of respiration ost congenial to the negro constitution, of all es and sexes, when in repose. This is proved by e fact of the universal practice among them of vering their head and faces, during sleep, with blanket, or any kind of covering that they can t hold of. If they have only a part of a blanket, ey will cover their faces when about to go to ep. If they have no covering, they will throw eir hands or arms across the mouth and nose, d turn on their faces, as if with an instinctive sign to obstruct the entrance of the free exter-l air into the lungs during sleep. As in the case th infants, the air that negroes breathe, with eir faces thus smothered with blankets or other vering, is not so much the external air as their vn breath, warmed to the same temperature as at of their bodies, by confinement and reinspi-tion. This instinctive and universal method of breathing, during sleep, proves the similarity of organization and physiological laws existing between negroes and infants, as far as the important function of respiration is concerned. Both are alike in re-breathing their own breath, and in requiring it to be warmed to their own temperature, by confinement which would be insupportable to the white race after passing the age of infancy. The inevitable effect of breathing a heated air, loaded with carbonic acid and aqueous vapor, is defective hematosis and hebetude of intellect.

Negroes, moreover, resemble children in the activity of the liver and in their strong assimilating powers, and in the predominance of the other systems over the sanguineous; hence they are difficult to bleed, owing to the smallness of their veins. On cording the arm of the stoutest negro, the veins will be scarcely as large as a white boy's of ten years of age. They are liable to all the convulsive diseases, cramps, spasms, colics, etc., that children are so subject to.

Although their skin is very thick, it is as sensitive, when they are in perfect health, as that of children, and like them they fear the rod. They resemble children in another very important particular; they are very easily governed by love combined with fear, and are ungovernable, vicious and rude under any form of government whatever, not resting on love and fear as a basis. Like children, it is not necessary that they be kept under the fear of the lash; it is sufficient that they be kept under the fear of offending those who have authority over them. Like children, they are constrained by unalterable physiological laws, to love those in authority over them, who minister to their wants and immediate necessities, and are not cruel or unmerciful. The defective hematosis, in both cases, and the want of courage and energy of mind as a consequence thereof, produces in both an instinctive feeling of dependence on others, to direct them and to take care of them. Hence, from a law of his nature, the negro can no more help loving a kind master, than the child can help loving her who gives it suck.

Like children, they require government in every thing; food, clothing, exercise, sleep—all require to be prescribed by rule, or they will run into excesses. Like children, they are apt to over-eat themselves or to confine their diet too much to one favorite article, unless restrained from doing so. They often gorge themselves with fat meat, as children do with sugar.

One of the greatest mysteries to those unacquainted with the negro character, is the facility with which an hundred, even two or three hundred, able-bodied and vigorous negroes are kept in subjection by one white man, who sleeps in perfect security among them, generally, in warm weather, with doors and windows open, with all his people, called slaves, at large around him. But a still greater mystery is the undoubted fact of the love they bear to their masters, similar in all respects to the love that children bear to their parents, which nothing but severity or cruelty in either case can alienate. The physiological laws on which this instinctive and most mysterious love is founded in the one case, are applicable to the other. Like children, when well behaved and disposed to do their duty, it is not the arbitrary authority over them that they dread, but the petty tyranny and imposition of one another. The overseer among them, like the school-master among children, has only to be impartial, and to preserve order by strict justice to all, to gain their good will and affections, and to be viewed, not as an object of terror, but as a friend and protector to quiet their fears of one another.

There is a difference between infant negroes and infant white children; the former are born with heads like gourds, the fontinelles being nearly closed and the sutures between the various bones of the head united, —not open and permitting of overlapping, as in white children. There is no necessity for the overlapping of the bones of the head in infant negroes, as they are smaller, and the pelvis of their mothers larger than in the white race. All negroes are not equally black—the blacker, the healthier and stronger; any deviation from the black color, in the p race, is a mark of feebleness or ill health. W heated from exercise, the negro's skin is cove with an oily exudation that gives a dark colo white linen, and has a very strong odor. The o is strongest in the most robust; children and aged have very little of it.

I have thus hastily and imperfectly noti some of the more striking anatomical and ph ological peculiarities of the negro race. The q tion may be asked, Does he belong to the sa race as the white man? Is he a son of Adam? D his peculiar physical conformation stand in position to the Bible, or does it prove its tru These are important questions, both in a m ical, historical and theological point of view. T can better be answered by a comparison of facts derived from anatomy, physiology, hist and theology, to see if they sustain one anoth We learn from the Book of Genesis, that N had three sons, Shem, Ham and Japheth, a that Canaan, the son of Ham, was doomed to servant of servants unto his brethren. From h tory, we learn, that the descendants of Cana settled in Africa, and are the present Ethiopia or black race of men; that Shem occupied As and Japheth the north of Europe. In the 9th ch ter and 27th verse of Genesis, one of the most a thentic books of the Bible, is this remarka prophecy: "God shall enlarge Japheth, and shall dwell in the tents of Shem; and Cana *shall be* his servant." Japheth has been greatly e larged by the discovery of a new world, the co tinent of America. He found in it the India whom natural history declares to be of Asia origin, in other words, the descendants of She he drove out Shem, and occupied his tents: a now the remaining part of the prophecy is in t process of fulfilment, from the facts every wh before us, of Canaan having become his serva The question arises, Is the Canaanite, or Eth pian, qualified for the trying duties of servitu and unfitted for the enjoyment of freedom? If be, there is both wisdom, mercy and justice in t ree dooming him to be servant of servants, as decree is in conformity to his nature. atomy and physiology have been interrogated, the response is, that the Ethiopian, or naanite, is unfitted, from his organization and physiological laws predicated on that organi- on, for the responsible duties of a free man, , like the child, is only fitted for a state of pendence and subordination. When history is errogated, the response is that the only gov- ment under which the negro has made any provement in mind, morals, religion, and only government under which he has led appy, quiet and contented life, is that under ich he is subjected to the arbitrary power of heth, in obedience to the Divine decree. hen the original Hebrew of the Bible is inter- gated, we find, in the significant meaning of original name of the negro, the identical fact forth, which the knife of the anatomist at the secting table has made appear; as if the revela- ns of anatomy, physiology and history, were a re re-writing of what Moses wrote. In the He- w word "Canaan," the original name of the hiopian, the word *slave by nature,* or language the same effect, is written by the inspired pen- n. Hence there is no conflict between the rev- tions of the science of medicine, history, and inductions drawn from the Baconian philos- hy, and the authority of the Bible; one supports other.

As an illustration, it is known that all the He- w names are derived from verbs, and are nificant. The Hebrew verb *Canah,* from ich the original name of the negro is derived, erally means *to submit himself—to bend the ee.* Gesenius, the best Hebrew scholar of mod- n times, renders both the Kal, Hiphil and phal form of the verb from which Canaan, the iginal name of the negro is derived, in the fol- wing Latin: *Genu flexit*—he bends the knee; *genua procidet*—he falls on his knees; *depres- s est animus*—his mind is depressed; *submisse gessit*—he deports himself submissively; *fractus est*—he is crouched or broken; or in other words, *slave by nature,* the same thing which anatomy, physiology, history, and the inductions drawn from philosophical observations, prove him to be.

A knowledge of the great primary truth, that the negro is a slave by nature, and can never be happy, industrious, moral or religious, in any other condition than the one he was intended to fill, is of great importance to the theologian, the statesman, and to all those who are at heart seeking to promote his temporal and future welfare. This great truth, if better known and understood, would go far to prevent the East Indian Company and British government from indulging in any expectation of seeing their immense possessions in Asia enhanced in value, by the overthrow of slave labor in America, through the instrumentality of northern fanaticism; or of seeing the Union divided into two or more fragments, hostile to each other; or of gaining any advantages, that civil commotion on this side of the Atlantic would give to the tottering monarchies of Europe. With the subject under this aspect, the science of Medicine has nothing to do, further than to uncover its light, to show truth from error.

Without a knowledge of the physical differences between the Ethiopian and the Caucasian, the Queen of England's medical advisers would not be much better qualified to prescribe for a negro, than her parliament to legislate for him; or her subjects to dictate to us what position he should occupy in our republican Union of Sovereign States....

DRAPETOMANIA, OR THE DISEASE CAUSING SLAVES TO RUN AWAY

Drapetomania is from δραπετης, a runaway slave, and μανια, *mad or crazy.* It is unknown to our medical authorities, although its diagnostic symptom, the absconding from service, is well known to our planters and overseers, as it was to the ancient Greeks, who expressed by the single word δραπετης the fact of the absconding, and the relation that the fugitive held to the person he fled from. I have added to the word meaning runaway slave, another Greek term, to express the disease of the mind causing him to abscond. In noticing a disease not heretofore classed among the long list of maladies that man is subject to, it was necessary to have a new term to express it. The cause, in the most of cases, that induces the negro to run away from service, is as much a disease of the mind as any other species of mental alienation, and much more curable, as a general rule. With the advantages of proper medical advice, strictly followed, this troublesome practice that many negroes have of running away, can be almost entirely prevented, although the slaves be located on the borders of a free State, within a stone's throw of the abolitionists. I was born in Virginia, east of the Blue Ridge, where negroes are numerous, and studied medicine some years in Maryland, a slave State, separated from Pennsylvania, a free State, by Mason & Dixon's line—a mere air line, without wall or guard. I long ago observed that some persons, considered as very good, and others as very bad masters, often lost their negroes by their absconding from service; while the slaves of another class of persons, remarkable for order and good discipline, but not praised or blamed as either good or bad masters, never ran away, although no guard or forcible means were used to prevent them. The same management which prevented them from walking over a mere nominal, unguarded line, will prevent them from running away anywhere.

To ascertain the true method of governing negroes, so as to cure and prevent the disease under consideration, we must go back to the Pentateuch, and learn the true meaning of the untranslated term that represents the negro race. In the name there given to that race, is locked up the true art of governing negroes in such a manner that they cannot run away. The correct translation of that term declares the Creator's will in regard to the negro; it declares him to be the s missive knee-bender. In the anatomical con mation of his knees, we see *"genu flexit"* wri in the physical structure of his knees, being m flexed or bent, than any other kind of man. If white man attempts to oppose the Deity's will trying to make the negro anything else than ' *submissive knee-bender,"* (which the Almighty clared he should be,) by trying to raise him level with himself, or by putting himself on equality with the negro; or if he abuses the po which God has given him over his fellowman being cruel to him or punishing him in anger by neglecting to protect him from the wan abuses of his fellow-servants and all others, or denying him the usual comforts and necessa of life, the negro will run away: but if he ke him in the position that we learn from the Sc tures he was intended to occupy, that is, the p tion of submission, and if his master or overs be kind and gracious in his bearing towards h without condescension, and at the same ti ministers to his physical wants and protects h from abuses, the negro is spell-bound, and c not run away. *"He shall serve Japheth"*; he sh be his servant of servants; —on the conditi above mentioned—conditions that are clea implied, though not directly expressed. Acco ing to my experience, the "genu flexit"— awe and reverence, must be exacted from the or they will despise their masters, become ru and ungovernable and run away. On Mason a Dixon's line, two classes of persons were apt lose their negroes; those who made themsel too familiar with them, treating them as equa and making little or no distinction in regard color; and, on the other hand, those who trea them cruelly, denied them the common nec saries of life, neglected to protect them agai the abuses of others, or frightened them by a bl tering manner of approach, when about to pu ish them for misdemeanors. Before negroes r away, unless they are frightened or panic-stru they become sulky and dissatisfied. The cause

sulkiness and dissatisfaction should be in-
red into and removed, or they are apt to run
y or fall into the negro consumption. When
y and dissatisfied without cause, the experi-
e of those on the line and elsewhere was de-
edly in favor of whipping them out of it, as a
ventive measure against absconding or other
conduct. It was called whipping the devil out
hem.

f treated kindly, well fed and clothed, with
l enough to keep a small fire burning all night,
arated into families, each family having its
n house—not permitted to run about at night,
o visit their neighbors, or to receive visits, or to
intoxicating liquors, and not overworked or
osed too much to the weather, they are very
ily governed—more so than any other people
he world. When all this is done, if any one or
re of them, at any time, are inclined to raise
ir heads to a level with their master or over-
r, humanity and their own good require that
y should be punished until they fall into that
missive state which it was intended for them
ccupy in all after time, when their progenitor
eived the name of Canaan, or "submissive
eebender." They have only to be kept in that
te, and treated like children, with care, kind-
ss, attention and humanity, to prevent and
re them from running away.

DYSAESTHESIA AETHIOPIS, OR HEBETUDE OF MIND AND OBTUSE SENSIBILITY OF BODY—A DISEASE PECULIAR TO NEGROES—CALLED BY OVERSEERS, "RASCALITY"

ysaesthesia Aethiopis is a disease peculiar to ne-
oes, affecting both mind and body, in a manner
well expressed by dysaesthesia, the name I
ve given it, as could be by a single term. There
both mind and sensibility, but both seem to be
fficult to reach by impressions from without. There is partial insensibility of the skin, and so great a hebetude of the intellectual faculties as to be like a person half asleep, that is with difficulty aroused and kept awake. It differs from every other species of mental disease, as it is accompanied with physical signs or lesions of the body, discoverable to the medical observer, which are always present and sufficient to account for the symptoms. It is much more prevalent among free negroes living in clusters by themselves, than among slaves on our plantations, and attacks only such slaves as live like free negroes in regard to diet, drinks, exercise, etc. It is not my purpose to treat of the complaint as it prevails among free negroes, nearly all of whom are more or less afflicted with it, that have not got some white person to direct and to take care of them. To narrate its symptoms and effects among them would be to write a history of the ruins and dilapidation of Hayti and every spot of earth they have ever had uncontrolled possession over for any length of time. I propose only to describe its symptoms among slaves.

From the careless movements of the individuals affected with the complaint, they are apt to do much mischief, which appears as if intentional, but is mostly owing to the stupidness of mind and insensibility of the nerves induced by the disease. Thus, they break, waste and destroy everything they handle, —abuse horses and cattle, —tear, burn or rend their own clothing, and paying no attention to the rights of property, they steal other's to replace what they have destroyed. They wander about at night, and keep in a half-nodding sleep during the day. They slight their work, —cut up corn, cane, cotton or tobacco when hoeing it, as if for pure mischief. They raise disturbances with their overseers and fellow servants without cause or motive, and seem to be insensible to pain when subjected to punishment. The fact of the existence of such a complaint, making man like an automaton or senseless machine, having the above or similar symptoms, can be clearly established by the most direct and positive testimony. That it should have escaped the attention of the medical profession, can only be accounted for because its attention has not been sufficiently directed to the maladies of the negro race. Otherwise, a complaint of so common occurrence on badly-governed plantations, and so universal among free negroes, or those who are not governed at all, —a disease radicated in physical lesions and having its peculiar and well-marked symptoms, and its curative indications, would not have escaped the notice of the profession. The northern physicians and people have noticed the symptoms, but not the disease from which they spring. They ignorantly attribute the symptoms to the debasing influence of slavery on the mind, without considering that those who have never been in slavery, or their fathers before them, are the most afflicted, and the latest from the slave-holding South the least. The disease is the natural offspring of negro liberty—the liberty to be idle, to wallow in filth, and to indulge in improper food and drinks.

In treating of the anatomy and the physiology of the negro, I showed that his respiratory system was under the same physiological laws as that of an infant child of the white race; that a warm atmosphere, loaded with carbonic acid and aqueous vapor, was the most congenial to his lungs during sleep, as it is to the infant; that, to insure the respiration of such an atmosphere, he invariably, as if moved by instinct, shrouds his head and face in a blanket or some other covering, when disposing himself to sleep; that if sleeping by the fire in cold weather, he turns his head to it, instead of his feet, evidently to inhale warm air; that when not in active exercise, he always hovers over a fire in comparatively warm weather, as if he took a positive pleasure in inhaling hot air and smoke when his body is quiescent. The natural effect of this practice, it was shown, caused imperfect atmospherization or vitalization of the blood in the lungs, as occurs in infancy, and a hebetude or torpor of intellect—from blood not sufficiently vitalized being distributed to the

brain; also, a slothfulness, torpor and disinc
tion to exercise, from the same cause—the
of blood sufficiently treated or vitalized in th
culating system. When left to himself, the n
indulges in his natural disposition to idleness
sloth, and does not take exercise enough t
pand his lungs and to vitalize his blood, but d
out a miserable existence in the midst of filth
uncleanliness, being too indolent and havin
little energy of mind to provide for himself pr
food and comfortable lodging and clothing.
consequence is, that the blood becomes so hi
carbonized and deprived of oxygen, that i
only becomes unfit to stimulate the brain t
ergy, but unfit to stimulate the nerves of sens
distributed to the body. A torpor and insensi
pervades the system; the sentient nerves di
uted to the skin lose their feeling to so great
gree, that he often burns his skin by the fir
hovers over, without knowing it, and frequ
has large holes in his clothes, and the shoes o
feet burnt to a crisp, without having been
scious of when it was done. This is the di
called dysaesthesia—a Greek term expre
the dull or obtuse sensation that always att
the complaint. When aroused from his slot
the stimulus of hunger, he takes anything h
lay his hands on, and tramples on the righ
well as on the property of others, with perfe
difference as to consequences. When driv
labor by the compulsive power of the white
he performs the task assigned him in a head
careless manner, treading down with his fe
cutting with his hoe the plants he is put to
vate—breaking the tools he works with, and s
ing everything he touches that can be injur
careless handling. Hence the overseers c
"rascality," supposing that the mischief is i
tionally done. But there is no premeditated
chief in the case, —the mind is too torpid to
itate mischief, or even to be aroused by the a
passions to deeds of daring. Dysaesthesia, o
betude of sensation of both mind and body,
vails to so great an extent, that when the unf

ɛ individual is subjected to punishment, he :her feels pain of any consequence, or shows unusual resentment, more than by a stupid :iness. In some cases, anaesthesiae would be a re suitable name for it, as there appears to be almost total loss of feeling. The term "rascal-" given to this disease by overseers, is founded an erroneous hypothesis and leads to an in-rect empirical treatment, which seldom or r cures it.

The complaint is easily curable, if treated on nd physiological principles. The skin is dry, :k and harsh to the touch, and the liver inac-:. The liver, skin and kidneys should be stimu-:d to activity, and be made to assist in decar-nising the blood. The best means to stimulate skin is, first, to have the patient well washed h warm water and soap; then, to anoint it all :r with oil, and to slap the oil in with a broad ther strap; then to put the patient to some hard d of work in the open air and sunshine, that l compel him to expand his lungs, as chopping od, splitting rails or sawing with the crosscut or ip saw. Any kind of labor will do that will cause l and free respiration in its performance, as lift-; or carrying heavy weights, or brisk walking; object being to expand the lungs by full and ep inspirations and expirations, thereby to vi-ize the impure circulating blood by introduc-; oxygen and expelling carbon. This treatment ould not be continued too long at a time, be-use where the circulating fluids are so impure in this complaint, patients cannot stand pro-cted exercise without resting frequently and inking freely of cold water or some cooling bev-age, as lemonade, or alternated with pepper tea eetened with molasses. In bad cases, the blood s always the appearance of blood in scurvy, and mmonly there is a scorbutic affection to be en on the gums. After resting until the palpita-n of the heart caused by the exercise is allayed, e patient should eat some good wholesome od, well seasoned with spices and mixed with getables, as turnip or mustard salad, with vine-gar. After a moderate meal, he should resume his work again, resting at intervals, and taking re-freshments and supporting the perspiration by partaking freely of liquids. At night he should be lodged in a warm room with a small fire in it, and should have a clean bed, with sufficient blanket covering, and be washed clean before going to bed; in the morning, oiled, slapped and put to work as before. Such treatment will, in a short time, effect a cure in all cases which are not complicated with chronic visceral derange-ments. The effect of this or a like course of treat-ment is often like enchantment. No sooner does the blood feel the vivifying influences derived from its full and perfect atmospherization by ex-ercise in the open air and in the sun, than the negro seems to be awakened to a new existence, and to look grateful and thankful to the white man whose compulsory power, by making him inhale vital air, has restored his sensation and dis-pelled the mist that clouded his intellect. His in-telligence restored and, his sensations awakened, he is no longer the *bipedum nequissimus*, nor ar-rant rascal, he was supposed to be, but a good negro that can hoe or plow, and handle things with as much care as his other fellow-servants.

Contrary to the received opinion, a northern climate is the most favorable to the intellectual development of negroes, those of Missouri, Ken-tucky, and the colder parts of Virginia and Mary-land, having much more mental energy, more bold and ungovernable than in the Southern lowlands; a dense atmosphere causing a better vi-talization of their blood.

Although idleness is the most prolific cause of dysaesthesia, yet there are other ways that the blood gets deteriorated. I said before that negroes are like children, requiring government in every-thing. If not governed in their diet, they are apt to eat too much salt meat and not enough bread and vegetables, which practice generates a scorbutic state of the fluids and leads to the affection under consideration. This form of the complaint always shows itself in the gums, which become spongy and dark, and leave the teeth. Uncleanliness of skin and torpid liver also tend to produce it. A scurvy set of negroes means the same thing, in the South, as a disorderly, worthless set. That the blood, when rendered impure and carbonaceous from any cause, as from idleness, filthy habits, unwholesome food or alcoholic drinks, affects the mind, is not only known to physicians, but was known to the Bard of Avon when he penned the lines—"We are not ourselves when Nature, being oppressed, commands the mind to suffer with the body."

According to unalterable physiological laws, negroes, as a general rule, to which there are but few exceptions, can only have their intellectual faculties awakened in a sufficient degree to receive moral culture, and to profit by religious or other instruction, when under the compulsatory authority of the white man; because, as a general rule, to which there are but few exceptions, they will not take sufficient exercise, when removed from the white man's authority, to vitalize and decarbonize their blood by the process of full and free respiration, that active exercise of some kind alone can effect. A northern climate remedies, in a considerable degree, their naturally indolent disposition; but the dense atmosphere of Boston or Canada can scarcely produce sufficient hematosis and vigor of mind to induce them to labor. From their natural indolence, unless under the stimulus of compulsion, they doze away their lives with the capacity of their lungs for atmospheric air only half expanded, from the want of exercise to superinduce full and deep respiration. The inevitable effect is, to prevent a sufficient atmospherization or vitalization of the blood, so essential to the expansion and the freedom of action of the intellectual faculties. The black blood distributed to the brain chains the mind to ignorance, superstition and barbarism, and bolts the door against civilization, moral culture and religious truth. The compulsory power of the white man, by making the slothful negro take active exercise, puts into active play the lungs, through whose agency the vitalized b is sent to the brain, to give liberty to the mind, to open the door to intellectual improven The very exercise, so beneficial to the negro, i pended in cultivating those burning fields in ton, sugar, rice and tobacco, which, but fo labor, would, from the heat of the climate, go cultivated, and their products lost to the w Both parties are benefited—the negro as we his master—even more. But there is a third benefitted—the world at large. The three lions of bales of cotton, made by negro labo ford a cheap clothing for the civilized world. laboring classes of all mankind, having less to for clothing, have more money to spend in cating their children, and in intellectual, m and religious progress.

The wisdom, mercy and justice of the de that Canaan shall serve Japheth, is proved b disease we have been considering, becau proves that his physical organization, and laws of his nature, are in perfect unison with ery, and in entire discordance with liberty— cordance so great as to produce the loaths disease that we have been considering, as o its inevitable effects, —a disease that locks u understanding, blunts the sensations and ch the mind to superstition, ignorance and barism. Slaves are not subject to this dis unless they are permitted to live like free neg in idleness and filth—to eat improper food, indulge in spirituous liquors. It is not their ters' interest that they should do so; as they w not only be unprofitable, but as great a nuis to the South, as the free negroes were four be in London, whom the British governm more than half a century ago, colonized in S Leone to get them out of the way. The ma naticism that British writers, lecturers and e saries, and the East India Company, plante our Northern States, after it was found by tried experiments, that free negroes in Engl in Canada, in Sierra Leone and elsewhere, a perfect nuisance, and would not work as fre ers, but would retrograde to barbarism, was planted there in opposition to British policy. atever was the motive of Great Britain in sow- the whirlwind in our Northern States, it is v threatening the disruption of a mighty em- e of the happiest, most progressive and Chris- people, that ever inhabited the earth—and only empire on the wide earth that England ads as a rival, either in arts or in arms.

Our Declaration of Independence, which was wn up at a time when negroes were scarcely isidered as human beings, *"That all men are nature free and equal,"* and only intended to ly to white men, is often quoted in support the false dogma that all mankind possess same mental, physiological and anatomical anization, and that the liberty, free institu- ns, and whatever else would be a blessing to e portion, would, under the same external cumstances, be to all, without regard to any ginal or internal differences, inherent in the anization. Although England preaches this ctrine, she practises in opposition to it everywhere. Instance, her treatment of the Gypsies in England, the Hindoos in India, the Hottentots at her Cape Colony, and the aboriginal inhabitants of New Holland. The dysaesthesia aethiopis adds another to the many ten thousand evidencies of the fallacy of the dogma that abolitionism is built on; for here, in a country where two races of men dwell together, both born on the same soil, breathing the same air, and surrounded by the same external agents—liberty, which is elevating the one race of people above all other nations, sinks the other into beastly sloth and torpidity; and the slavery, which the one would prefer death rather than endure, improves the other in body, mind and morals; thus proving the dogma false, and establishing the truth that there is a radical, internal, or physical difference between the two races, so great in kind, as to make what is wholesome and beneficial for the white man, as liberty, republican or free institutions, etc., not only unsuitable to the negro race, but actually poisonous to its happiness.

CHAPTER 5

The Normal and the Pathological—Introduction to the Problem

GEORGES CANGUILHEM *[From* A Vital Rationalist: Selected Writings from Georges Canguilhem, *edited by F. Delaporte, translated by A. Goldhammer]*

INTRODUCTION TO THE PROBLEM

TO ACT, IT IS NECESSARY at least to localize. For example, how do we take action against an earthquake or hurricane? The impetus behind every ontological theory of disease undoubtedly derives from therapeutic need. When we see in every sick man someone whose being has been augmented or diminished, we are somewhat reassured, for what a man has lost can be restored to him, and what has entered him can also leave. We can hope to conquer disease even if doing so is the result of a spell, or magic, or possession; we have only to ember that disease happens to man in order to lose all hope. Magic brings to drugs and in-tation rites innumerable resources stemming n a profoundly intense desire for cure. Henry st Sigerist has noted that Egyptian medicine bably universalized the Eastern experience of asitic diseases by combining it with the idea of ase-possession: throwing up worms means ng restored to health.[1] Disease enters and ves man as through a door.

A vulgar hierarchy of diseases still exists today, ed on the extent to which symptoms can—or not—be readily localized, hence Parkinson's ease is more of a disease than thoracic shin-s, which is, in turn, more so than boils. With-wishing to detract from the grandeur of Louis teur's tenets, we can say without hesitation t the germ theory of contagious disease has tainly owed much of its success to the fact that mbodies an ontological representation of sick-s. After all, a germ can be seen, even if this re-ires the complicated mediation of a micro-pe, stains and cultures, while we would never able to see a miasma or an influence. To see an tity is already to foresee an action. No one will ject to the optimistic character of the theories infection insofar as their therapeutic applica-n is concerned. But the discovery of toxins and recognition of the specific and individual thogenic role of *terrains* have destroyed the autiful simplicity of a doctrine whose scientific neer for a long time hid the persistence of a re-tion to disease as old as man himself.

If we feel the need to reassure ourselves, it is cause one anguish constantly haunts our oughts; if we delegate the task of restoring the eased organism to the desired norm by techni-l means, either magical or matter of fact [posi-e], it is because we expect nothing good from ture itself.

By contrast, Greek medicine, in the Hippo-atic writings and practices, offers a conception disease which is no longer ontological, but dy-mic, no longer localizationist, but totalizing. Nature (*physis*), within man as well as without, is harmony and equilibrium. The disturbance of this harmony, of this equilibrium, is called "dis-ease." In this case, disease is not somewhere in man, it is everywhere in him; it is the whole man. External circumstances are the occasion but not the causes. Man's equilibrium consists of four humors, whose fluidity is perfectly suited to sus-tain variations and oscillations and whose quali-ties are paired by opposites (hot/cold, wet/dry); the disturbance of these humors causes disease. But disease is not simply disequilibrium or dis-cordance; it is, perhaps most important, an effort on the part of nature to effect a new equilibrium in man. Disease is a generalized reaction de-signed to bring about a cure; the organism devel-ops a disease in order to get well. Therapy must first tolerate and, if necessary, reinforce these he-donic and spontaneously therapeutic reactions. Medical technique imitates natural medicinal action (*vis medicatrix naturae*). To imitate is not merely to copy an appearance but, also, to mimic a tendency and to extend an intimate movement. Of course, such a conception is also optimistic, but here the optimism concerns the way of na-ture and not the effect of human technique.

Medical thought has never stopped alternating between these two representations of disease, between these two kinds of optimism, always finding some good reason for one or the other attitude in a newly explained pathogenesis. Deficiency diseases and all infectious or parasitic diseases favor the ontological theory, while en-docrine disturbances and all diseases beginning with *dys-* support the dynamic or functional the-ory. However, these two conceptions do have one point in common: in disease, or better, in the ex-perience of being sick, both envision a polemical situation—either a battle between the organism and a foreign substance, or an internal struggle between opposing forces. Disease differs from a state of health, the pathological from the normal, as one quality differs from another, either by the presence or absence of a definite principle, or by an alteration of the total organism. This heterogeneity of normal and pathological states persists today in the naturalist conception, which expects little from human efforts to restore the norm, and in which nature will find the ways toward cure. But it proved difficult to maintain the qualitative modification separating the normal from the pathological in a conception that allows, indeed expects, man to be able to compel nature and bend it to his normative desires. Wasn't it said repeatedly after Bacon's time that one governs nature only by obeying it? To govern disease means to become acquainted with its relations with the normal state, which the living man—loving life—wants to regain. Hence, the theoretical need, delayed by an absence of technology, to establish a scientific pathology by linking it to physiology. Thomas Sydenham (1624–1689) thought that in order to help a sick man, his sickness had to be delimited and determined. There are disease species just as there are animal or plant species. According to Sydenham, there is an order among diseases similar to the regularity Isidore Geoffroy Saint-Hilaire found among anomalies. Philippe Pinel justified all these attempts at classification of disease (nosology) by perfecting the genre in his *Nosographie philosophique* (1797), which Charles Victor Daremberg described as more the work of a naturalist than a clinician.

Meanwhile, Giovanni Battista Morgagni's (1682–1771) creation of a system of pathological anatomy made it possible to link the lesions of certain organs to groups of stable symptoms, such that nosographical classification found a substratum in anatomical analysis. But just as the followers of William Harvey and Albrecht von Haller "breathed life" into anatomy by turni into physiology, so pathology became a nat extension of physiology. The end result of evolutionary process is the formation of a th of the relations between the normal and pathological, according to which the pathol cal phenomena found in living organisms nothing more than quantitative variati greater or lesser according to corresponding p iological phenomena. Semantically, the pat logical is designated as departing from the mal not so much by *a-* or *dys-* as by *hyper* *hypo-*. While retaining the ontological theo soothing confidence in the possibility of tec cal conquest of disease, this approach is far fr considering health and sickness as qualitati opposed, or as forces joined in battle. The n to reestablish continuity in order to gain m knowledge for more effective action is such t the concept of disease would finally vanish. T conviction that one can scientifically restore norm is such that, in the end, it annuls the pat logical. Disease is no longer the object of angu for the healthy man; it has become instead object of study for the theorist of health. It is pathology, writ large, that we can unravel teachings of health, rather as Plato sought in institution of the State the larger and more ea readable equivalent of the virtues and vices of individual soul. [*The Normal and the Pathol cal (NP)*, pp. 11–13]

NOTE

1. Henry E. Sigerist, *Man and Medicine: An In duction to Moral Knowledge*, trans. Margaret C Boise (New York: Norton, 1932), p. 102.

CHAPTER 6

The Myth of Mental Illness

THOMAS S. SZASZ

MY AIM IN THIS ESSAY is to raise the ques-
)n "Is there such a thing as mental illness?" and to argue that there is not. nce the notion of mental illness is extremely widely used nowadays, in-
iiry into the ways in which this term is employed would seem to be espe-
ally indicated. Mental illness, of course, is not literally a "thing"—or
iysical object—and hence it can "exist" only in the same sort of way in
hich other theoretical concepts exist. Yet, familiar theories are in the
ıbit of posing, sooner or later—at least to those who come to believe in
iem—as "objective truths" (or "facts"). During certain historical periods,
:planatory conceptions such as deities, witches, and microorganisms ap-
eared not only as theories but as self-evident *causes* of a vast number

of events. I submit that today mental illness is widely regarded in a somewhat similar fashion, that is, as the cause of innumerable diverse happenings. As an antidote to the complacent use of the notion of mental illness—whether as a self-evident phenomenon, theory, or cause—let us ask this question: What is meant when it is asserted that someone is mentally ill?

In what follows I shall describe briefly the main uses to which the concept of mental illness has been put. I shall argue that this notion has outlived whatever usefulness it might have had and that it now functions merely as a convenient myth.

MENTAL ILLNESS AS A SIGN OF BRAIN DISEASE

The notion of mental illness derives its main support from such phenomena as syphilis of the brain or delirious conditions—intoxications, for instance—in which persons are known to manifest various peculiarities or disorders of thinking and behavior. Correctly speaking, however, these are diseases of the brain, not of the mind. According to one school of thought, *all* so-called mental illness is of this type. The assumption is made that some neurological defect, perhaps a very subtle one, will ultimately be found for all the disorders of thinking and behavior. Many contemporary psychiatrists, physicians, and other scientists hold this view. This position implies that people *cannot* have troubles—expressed in what are *now called* "mental illnesses"—because of differences in personal needs, opinions, social aspirations, values, and so on. *All problems in living* are attributed to physicochemical processes which in due time will be discovered by medical research.

"Mental illnesses" are thus regarded as basically no different than all other diseases (that is, of the body). The only difference, in this view, between mental and bodily diseases is that the former, affecting the brain, manifest themselves by means of mental symptoms; whereas the la affecting other organ systems (for example, skin, liver, etc.), manifest themselves by mear symptoms referable to those parts of the b This view rests on and expresses what are, in opinion, two fundamental errors.

In the first place, what central nervous sys symptoms would correspond to a skin eruptio a fracture? It would *not* be some emotion or c plex bit of behavior. Rather, it would be blind or a paralysis of some part of the body. The c of the matter is that a disease of the brain, an gous to a disease of the skin or bone, is a ne logical defect, and not a problem in living. example, a *defect* in a person's visual field ma satisfactorily explained by correlating it with tain definite lesions in the *nervous* system. On other hand, a person's *belief*—whether this b belief in Christianity, in Communism, or in *idea* that his internal organs are "rotting" and his body is, in fact, already "dead"—cannot be plained by a defect or disease of the nervous tem. Explanations of this sort of occurrence— suming that one is interested in the belief it and does not regard it simply as a "symptom" expression of something else that is *more inter ing*—must be sought along different lines.

The second error in regarding complex p chosocial behavior, consisting of communi tions about ourselves and the world about us mere symptoms of neurological functioning *epistemological*. In other words, it is an error p taining not to any mistakes in observation or r soning, as such, but rather to the way in which organize and express our knowledge. In the pr ent case, the error lies in making a symmetri dualism between mental and physical (or bodi symptoms, a dualism which is merely a habit speech and to which no known observations c be found to correspond. Let us see if this is so. medical practice, when we speak of physical c turbances, we mean either signs (for example fever) or symptoms (for example, pain). We sp of mental symptoms, on the other hand, when r to a patient's *communications about himself, ers, and the world about him.* He might state he is Napoleon or that he is being persecuted he Communists. These would be considered ntal symptoms *only* if the observer believed t the patient was *not* Napoleon or that he was being persecuted by the Communists. This kes it apparent that the statement that "X is nental symptom" involves rendering a judgnt. The judgment entails, moreover, a covert nparison or matching of the patient's ideas, ncepts, or beliefs with those of the observer l the society in which they live. The notion of ntal symptom is therefore inextricably tied to *social* (including *ethical*) *context* in which it nade in much the same way as the notion of lily symptom is tied to an *anatomical* and *geic context* (Szasz, 1957a, 1957b).

To sum up what has been said thus far: I have ed to show that for those who regard mental nptoms as signs of brain disease, the concept of ntal illness is unnecessary and misleading. For at they mean is that people so labeled suffer m diseases of the brain; and, if that is what they an, it would seem better for the sake of clarity say that and not something else.

MENTAL ILLNESS AS A NAME FOR PROBLEMS IN LIVING

e term "mental illness" is widely used to deribe something which is very different than a ease of the brain. Many people today take it for nted that living is an arduous process. Its hardip for modern man, moreover, derives not so uch from a struggle for biological survival as m the stresses and strains inherent in the social tercourse of complex human personalities. In is context, the notion of mental illness is used identify or describe some feature of an individl's so-called personality. Mental illness—as a formity of the personality, so to speak—is then garded as the *cause* of the human disharmony. It is implicit in this view that social intercourse between people is regarded as something *inherently harmonious,* its disturbance being due solely to the presence of "mental illness" in many people. This is obviously fallacious reasoning, for it makes the abstraction "mental illness" into a *cause,* even though this abstraction was created in the first place to serve only as a shorthand expression for certain types of human behavior. It now becomes necessary to ask: "What kinds of behavior are regarded as indicative of mental illness, and by whom?"

The concept of illness, whether bodily or mental, implies *deviation from some* clearly *defined norm.* In the case of physical illness, the norm is the structural and functional integrity of the human body. Thus, although the desirability of physical health, as such, is an ethical value, what health *is* can be stated in anatomical and physiological terms. What is the norm deviation from which is regarded as mental illness? This question cannot be easily answered. But whatever this norm might be, we can be certain of only one thing: namely, that it is a norm that must be stated in terms of *psychosocial, ethical,* and *legal* concepts. For example, notions such as "excessive repression" or "acting out an unconscious impulse" illustrate the use of psychological concepts for judging (so-called) mental health and illness. The idea that chronic hostility, vengefulness, or divorce are indicative of mental illness would be illustrations of the use of ethical norms (that is, the desirability of love, kindness, and a stable marriage relationship). Finally, the widespread psychiatric opinion that only a mentally ill person would commit homicide illustrates the use of a legal concept as a norm of mental health. The norm from which deviation is measured whenever one speaks of a mental illness is a *psychosocial and ethical one.* Yet, the remedy is sought in terms of *medical* measures which—it is hoped and assumed—are free from wide differences of ethical value. The definition of the disorder and the terms in which its remedy are sought are therefore at serious odds with one another. The practical significance of this covert conflict between the alleged nature of the defect and the remedy can hardly be exaggerated.

Having identified the norms used to measure deviations in cases of mental illness, we will now turn to the question: "Who defines the norms and hence the deviation?" Two basic answers may be offered: *(a)* It may be the person himself (that is, the patient) who decides that he deviates from a norm. For example, an artist may believe that he suffers from a work inhibition; and he may implement this conclusion by seeking help *for* himself from a psychotherapist. *(b)* It may be someone other than the patient who decides that the latter is deviant (for example, relatives, physicians, legal authorities, society generally, etc.). In such a case a psychiatrist may be hired by others to do something *to* the patient in order to correct the deviation.

These considerations underscore the importance of asking the question "Whose agent is the psychiatrist?" and of giving a candid answer to it (Szasz, 1956, 1958). The psychiatrist (psychologist or nonmedical psychotherapist), it now develops, may be the agent of the patient, of the relatives, of the school, of the military services, of a business organization, of a court of law, and so forth. In speaking of the psychiatrist as the agent of these persons or organizations, it is not implied that his values concerning norms, or his ideas and aims concerning the proper nature of remedial action, need to coincide exactly with those of his employer. For example, a patient in individual psychotherapy may believe that his salvation lies in a new marriage; his psychotherapist need not share this hypothesis. As the patient's agent, however, he must abstain from bringing social or legal force to bear on the patient which would prevent him from putting his beliefs into action. If his *contract* is with the patient, the psychiatrist (psychotherapist) may disagree with him or stop his treatment; but he cannot engage others to obstruct the patient's aspirations. Similarly, if a chiatrist is engaged by a court to determine sanity of a criminal, he need not fully share legal authorities' values and intentions in reg to the criminal and the means available for d ing with him. But the psychiatrist is expre barred from stating, for example, that it is not criminal who is "insane" but the men who w the law on the basis of which the very actions are being judged are regarded as "crimin Such an opinion could be voiced, of course, not in a courtroom, and not by a psychiatrist makes it his practice to assist the court in forming its daily work.

To recapitulate: In actual contemporary so usage, the finding of a mental illness is made establishing a deviance in behavior from cert psychosocial, ethical, or legal norms. The ju ment may be made, as in medicine, by the tient, the physician (psychiatrist), or others. medial action, finally, tends to be sought i therapeutic—or covertly medical—framew thus creating a situation in which *psychosoc ethical,* and/or *legal deviations* are claimed to correctible by (so-called) *medical action.* Si medical action is designed to correct only m ical deviations, it seems logically absurd expect that it will help solve problems whose v existence had been defined and established nonmedical grounds. I think that these consid ations may be fruitfully applied to the pres use of tranquilizers and, more generally, to w might be expected of drugs of whatever type in gard to the amelioration or solution of proble in human living.

THE ROLE OF ETHICS IN PSYCHIATRY

Anything that people *do*—in contrast to thir that *happen* to them (Peters, 1958)—takes pla in a context of value. In this broad sense, human activity is devoid of ethical implicatio en the values underlying certain activities are ely shared, those who participate in their pur- may lose sight of them altogether. The disci- e of medicine, both as a pure science (for mple, research) and as a technology (for ex- ple, therapy), contains many ethical consider- ns and judgments. Unfortunately, these are n denied, minimized, or merely kept out of us; for the ideal of the medical profession as l as of the people whom it serves seems to be ing a system of medicine (allegedly) free of ical value. This sentimental notion is ex- ssed by such things as the doctor's willingness reat and help patients irrespective of their re- ous or political beliefs, whether they are rich poor, etc. While there may be some grounds this belief—albeit it is a view that is not im- ssively true even in these regards—the fact re- ins that ethical considerations encompass a t range of human affairs. By making the prac- of medicine neutral in regard to some spe- c issues of value need not, and cannot, mean t it can be kept free from all such values. The ctice of medicine is intimately tied to ethics; d the first thing that we must do, it seems to me, o try to make this clear and explicit. I shall let s matter rest here, for it does not concern us cifically in this essay. Lest there be any vague- ss, however, about how or where ethics and dicine meet, let me remind the reader of such ues as birth control, abortion, suicide, and eu- nasia as only a few of the major areas of cur- nt ethicomedical controversy.

Psychiatry, I submit, is very much more inti- tely tied to problems of ethics than is medi- e. I use the word "psychiatry" here to refer to at contemporary discipline which is concerned th *problems in living* (and not with diseases of e brain, which are problems for neurology). oblems in human relations can be analyzed, terpreted, and given meaning only within en social and ethical contexts. Accordingly, it *es* make a difference—arguments to the contrary notwithstanding—what the psychiatrist's socioethical orientations happen to be; for these will influence his ideas on what is wrong with the patient, what deserves comment or interpretation, in what possible directions change might be desirable, and so forth. Even in medicine proper, these factors play a role, as for instance, in the divergent orientations which physicians, depending on their religious affiliations, have toward such things as birth control and therapeutic abortion. Can anyone really believe that a psychotherapist's ideas concerning religious belief, slavery, or other similar issues play no role in his practical work? If they do make a difference, what are we to infer from it? Does it not seem reasonable that we ought to have different psychiatric therapies—each, expressly recognized for the ethical positions which they embody—for, say, Catholics and Jews, religious persons and agnostics, democrats and Communists, white supremacists and Negroes, and so on? Indeed, if we look at how psychiatry is actually practiced today (especially in the United States), we find that people do seek psychiatric help in accordance with their social status and ethical beliefs (Hollingshead & Redlich, 1958). This should really not surprise us more than being told that practicing Catholics rarely frequent birth control clinics.

The foregoing position which holds that contemporary psychotherapists deal with problems in living, rather than with mental illnesses and their cures, stands in opposition to a currently prevalent claim, according to which mental illness is just as "real" and "objective" as bodily illness. This is a confusing claim since it is never known exactly what is meant by such words as "real" and "objective." I suspect, however, that what is intended by the proponents of this view is to create the idea in the popular mind that mental illness is some sort of disease entity, like an infection or a malignancy. If this were true, one could *catch* or get a "mental illness," one might *have* or *harbor* it, one might *transmit* it to others, and finally one could get *rid* of it. In my opinion, there is not a shred of evidence to support this idea. To the contrary, all the evidence is the other way and supports the view that what people now call mental illnesses are for the most part *communications* expressing unacceptable ideas, often framed, moreover, in an unusual idiom. The scope of this essay allows me to do no more than mention this alternative theoretical approach to this problem (Szasz, 1957c).

This is not the place to consider in detail the similarities and differences between bodily and mental illnesses. It shall suffice for us here to emphasize only one important difference between them: namely, that whereas bodily disease refers to public, physicochemical occurrences, the notion of mental illness is used to codify relatively more private, sociopsychological happenings of which the observer (diagnostician) forms a part. In other words, the psychiatrist does not stand *apart* from what he observes, but is, in Harry Stack Sullivan's apt words, a "participant observer." This means that he is *committed* to some picture of what he considers reality—and to what he thinks society considers reality—and he observes and judges the patient's behavior in the light of these considerations. This touches on our earlier observation that the notion of mental symptom itself implies a comparison between observer and observed, psychiatrist and patient. This is so obvious that I may be charged with belaboring trivialities. Let me therefore say once more that my aim in presenting this argument was expressly to criticize and counter a prevailing contemporary tendency to deny the moral aspects of psychiatry (and psychotherapy) and to substitute for them allegedly value-free medical considerations. Psychotherapy, for example, is being widely practiced as though it entailed nothing other than restoring the patient from a state of mental sickness to one of mental health. While it is generally accepted that mental illness has something to do with man's social (or interpersonal) relations, it is paradoxically m tained that problems of values (that is, of eth do not arise in this process.[1] Yet, in one se much of psychotherapy may revolve aro nothing other than the elucidation and weigh of goals and values—many of which may be tually contradictory—and the means wher they might best be harmonized, realized, or linquished.

The diversity of human values and the m ods by means of which they may be realized i vast, and many of them remain so unackno edged, that they cannot fail but lead to confl in human relations. Indeed, to say that hum relations at all levels—from mother to ch through husband and wife, to nation and tion—are fraught with stress, strain, and dis mony is, once again, making the obvious expli Yet, what may be obvious may be also poorly derstood. This I think is the case here. Fo seems to me that—at least in our scientific th ries of behavior—we have failed to *accept* simple fact that human relations are inheren fraught with difficulties and that to make th even relatively harmonious requires much tience and hard work. I submit that the idea mental illness is now being put to work to obsc certain difficulties which at present may be herent—not that they need be unmodifiable— the social intercourse of persons. If this is tr the concept functions as a disguise; for instead calling attention to conflicting human needs, pirations, and values, the notion of mental illn provides an amoral and impersonal "thing" ("illness") as an explanation for *problems in liv* (Szasz, 1960). We may recall in this connecti that not so long ago it was devils and witches w were held responsible for men's problems in cial living. The belief in mental illness, as som thing other than man's trouble in getting alo with his fellow man, is the proper heir to the lief in demonology and witchcraft. Mental ness exists or is "real" in exactly the same sense which witches existed or were "real."

:HOICE, RESPONSIBILITY, ,ND PSYCHIATRY

ile I have argued that mental illnesses do not t, I obviously did not imply that the social and :hological occurrences to which this label is rently being attached also do not exist. Like personal and social troubles which people l in the Middle Ages, they are real enough. It ne labels we give them that concerns us and, ing labeled them, what we do about them. ile I cannot go into the ramified implications his problem here, it is worth noting that a de-nological conception of problems in living e rise to therapy along theological lines. lay, a belief in mental illness implies—nay, re-res—therapy along medical or psychothera-tic lines.

What is implied in the line of thought set forth e is something quite different. I do not intend offer a new conception of "psychiatric illness" r a new form of "therapy." My aim is more odest and yet also more ambitious. It is to sug-t that the phenomena now called mental ill-sses be looked at afresh and more simple, that y be removed from the category of illness, and t they be regarded as the expressions of man's uggle with the problem of *how* he should live. e last mentioned problem is obviously a vast e, its enormity reflecting not only man's in-ility to cope with his environment, but even ore his increasing self-reflectiveness.

By problems in living, then, I refer to that truly plosive chain reaction which began with man's l from divine grace by partaking of the fruit of e tree of knowledge. Man's awareness of him-f and of the world about him seems to be a adily expanding one, bringing in its wake an er larger *burden of understanding* (an expres-n borrowed from Susanne Langer, 1953). *This rden,* then, *is to be expected and must not be isinterpreted.* Our only *rational* means for light-ing it is *more understanding,* and appropriate *tion* based on such understanding. The main alternative lies in acting as though the burden were not what in fact we perceive it to be and taking refuge in an outmoded theological view of man. In the latter view, man does not fashion his life and much of his world about him, but merely lives out his fate in a world created by superior beings. This may logically lead to pleading nonresponsibility in the face of seemingly unfathomable problems and difficulties. Yet, if man fails to take increasing responsibility for his actions, individually as well as collectively, it seems unlikely that some higher power or being would assume this task and carry this burden for him. Moreover, this seems hardly the proper time in human history for obscuring the issue of man's responsibility for his actions by hiding it behind the skirt of an all-explaining conception of mental illness.

CONCLUSIONS

I have tried to show that the notion of mental illness has outlived whatever usefulness it might have had and that it now functions merely as a convenient myth. As such, it is a true heir to religious myths in general, and to the belief in witchcraft in particular; the role of all these belief-systems was to act as *social tranquilizers,* thus encouraging the hope that mastery of certain specific problems may be achieved by means of substitutive (symbolic-magical) operations. The notion of mental illness thus serves mainly to obscure the everyday fact that life for most people is a continuous struggle, not for biological survival, but for a "place in the sun," "peace of mind," or some other human value. For man aware of himself and of the world about him, once the needs for preserving the body (and perhaps the race) are more or less satisfied, the problem arises as to what he should do with himself. Sustained adherence to the myth of mental illness allows people to avoid facing this problem, believing that mental health, conceived as the absence of mental illness, automatically insures the making of right and safe choices in one's conduct of life. But the facts are all the other way. It is the making of good choices in life that others regard, retrospectively, as good mental health!

The myth of mental illness encourages us, moreover, to believe in its logical corollary: that social intercourse would be harmonious, satisfying, and the secure basis of a "good life" were it not for the disrupting influences of mental illness or "psychopathology." The potentiality for universal human happiness, in this form at least, seems to me but another example of the I-wish-it-were-true type of fantasy. I do believe that human happiness or well-being on a hitherto unimaginably large scale, and not just for a select few, is possible. This goal could be achieved, however, only at the cost of many men, and not just a few being willing and able to tackle their personal, social, and ethical conflicts. This means having the courage and integrity to forego waging battles on false fronts, finding solutions for substitute problems—for instance, fighting the battle of stomach acid and chronic fatigue instead of facing up to a marital conflict.

Our adversaries are not demons, witches, fate, or mental illness. We have no enemy whom we can fight, exorcise, or dispel by "cure." What we do have are *problems in living*—whether these be biologic, economic, political, or sociopsychological. In this essay I was concerned only with problems belonging in the last mentioned category, and within this group mainly with those pertaining to moral values. The field to which modern psychiatry addresses itself is vast, and I made no effort to encompass it all. My argument was limited to the proposition that mental illness is a myth, whose function it is to disguise and thus render more palatable the bitter pill of moral conflicts in human relations.

NOTE

1. Freud went so far as to say that: "I consider e[illegible] to be taken for granted. Actually I have never do[illegible] mean thing" (Jones, 1957, p. 247). This surely [illegible] strange thing to say for someone who has studied [illegible] as a social being as closely as did Freud. I menti[illegible] here to show how the notion of "illness" (in the ca[illegible] psychoanalysis, "psychopathology," or "mental [illegible]ness") was used by Freud—and by most of his fol[illegible]ers—as a means for classifying certain forms of hu[illegible] behavior as falling within the scope of medicine, [illegible] hence (by *fiat*) outside that of ethics!

REFERENCES

Hollingshead, A. B., & Redlich, F. C. *Social C[illegible] and Mental Illness.* New York: Wiley, 1958.

Jones, E. *The Life and Work of Sigmund Freud.* [illegible] 3. New York: Basic Books, 1957.

Langer, S. R. *Philosophy in a New Key.* New Y[illegible] Mentor Books, 1953.

Peters, R. S. *The Concept of Motivation.* Lond[illegible] Routledge & Kegan Paul, 1958.

Szasz, T. S. "Malingering: 'Diagnosis' or So[illegible] Condemnation?" *AMA Archives of Neurology and [illegible]chiatry* 1956, 76: 432–43.

Szasz, T. S. *Pain and Pleasure: A Study of Bod[illegible] Feelings.* New York: Basic Books, 1957. (a)

Szasz, T. S. "The Problem of Psychiatric Nosol[illegible] A Contribution to a Situational Analysis of Psychia[illegible] Operations." *American Journal of Psychiatry* 1957, [illegible] 405–13. (b)

Szasz, T. S. "On the Theory of Psychoanalytic Tr[illegible]ment." *International Journal of Psycho-Analysis* 19[illegible] 38: 166–82. (c)

Szasz, T. S. "Psychiatry, Ethics and the Crimi[illegible] Law." *Columbia Law Revue* 1958, 58: 183–98.

Szasz, T. S. "Moral Conflict and Psychiatry." Y[illegible] *Revue* 49 (June), 1960: 555–66.

CHAPTER 7

The Need for a New Medical Model: A Challenge for Biomedicine

GEORGE L. ENGEL

AT A RECENT CONFERENCE on psychi-
ric education, many psychiatrists seemed to be saying to medicine, 'lease take us back and we will never again deviate from the 'medical odel.'" For, as one critical psychiatrist put it, "Psychiatry has become a odgepodge of unscientific opinions, assorted philosophies and 'schools of ought,' mixed metaphors, role diffusion, propaganda, and politicking for iental health' and other esoteric goals" (1). In contrast, the rest of medi-
ne appears neat and tidy. It has a firm base in the biological sciences, iormous technologic resources at its command, and a record of astonish-
g achievement in elucidating mechanisms of disease and devising new

treatments. It would seem that psychiatry would do well to emulate its sister medical disciplines by finally embracing once and for all the medical model of disease.

But I do not accept such a premise. Rather, I contend that all medicine is in crisis and, further, that medicine's crisis derives from the same basic fault as psychiatry's, namely, adherence to a model of disease no longer adequate for the scientific tasks and social responsibilities of either medicine or psychiatry. The importance of how physicians conceptualize disease derives from how such concepts determine what are considered the proper boundaries of professional responsibility and how they influence attitudes toward and behavior with patients. Psychiatry's crisis revolves around the question of whether the categories of human distress with which it is concerned are properly considered "disease" as currently conceptualized and whether exercise of the traditional authority of the physician is appropriate for their help functions. Medicine's crisis stems from the logical inference that since "disease" is defined in terms of somatic parameters, physicians need not be concerned with psychosocial issues which lie outside medicine's responsibility and authority. At a recent Rockefeller Foundation seminar on the concept of health, one authority urged that medicine "concentrate on the 'real' diseases and not get lost in the psychosociological underbrush. The physician should not be saddled with problems that have arisen from the abdication of the theologian and the philosopher." Another participant called for "a disentanglement of the organic elements of disease from the psychosocial elements of human malfunction," arguing that medicine should deal with the former only (2).

THE TWO POSITIONS

Psychiatrists have responded to their crisis by embracing two ostensibly opposite positions. One would simply exclude psychiatry from the field of medicine, while the other would adhere strictly to the "medical model" and limit psychia field to behavioral disorders consequent to b dysfunction. The first is exemplified in the w ings of Szasz and others who advance the p tion that "mental illness is a myth" since it c not conform with the accepted concept of dis (3). Supporters of this position advocate the moval of the functions now performed by psy atry from the conceptual and professional ju diction of medicine and their reallocation new discipline based on behavioral scie Henceforth medicine would be responsible the treatment and cure of disease, while the discipline would be concerned with the reedu tion of people with "problems of living." Imp in this argument is the premise that while medical model constitutes a sound framew within which to understand and treat disease, not relevant to the behavioral and psycholog problems classically deemed the domain of chiatry. Disorders directly ascribable to brain order would be taken care of by neurolog while psychiatry as such would disappear a medical discipline.

The contrasting posture of strict adherenc the medical model is caricatured in Ludw view of the psychiatrist as physician (1). Acc ing to Ludwig, the medical model premises "t sufficient deviation from normal represents *ease*, that disease is due to known or unkno natural causes, and that elimination of th causes will result in cure or improvement in dividual patients" (Ludwig's italics). While knowledging that most psychiatric diagno have a lower level of confirmation than m medical diagnoses, he adds that they are "quantitatively different provided that men disease is assumed to arise largely from 'natu rather than meta-psychological, interpersonal societal causes." "Natural" is defined as "biolo cal brain dysfunctions, either biochemical neurophysiological in nature." On the ot hand, "disorders such as problems of living, cial adjustment reactions, character disorde dependency syndromes, existential depressio various social deviancy conditions [would] excluded from he concept of mental illness e these disorders arise in individuals with preably intact neurophysiological functioning are produced primarily by psychosocial varies." Such "non-psychiatric disorders" are not perly the concern of the physician-psychiat and are more appropriately handled by nondical professionals.

n sum, psychiatry struggles to clarify its status hin the mainstream of medicine, if indeed it ongs in medicine at all. The criterion by ich this question is supposed to be resolved s on the degree to which the field of activity of chiatry is deemed congruent with the existing dical model of disease. But crucial to this blem is another, that of whether the contemary model is, in fact, any longer adequate for dicine, much less for psychiatry. For if it is not, n perhaps the crisis of psychiatry is part and cel of a larger crisis that has its roots in the del itself. Should that be case, then it would imprudent for psychiatry prematurely to abann models in favor of one that may also be ved.

THE BIOMEDICAL MODEL

e dominant model of disease today is biomedl, with molecular biology its basic scientific cipline. It assumes disease to be fully acunted for by deviations from the norm of meaable biological (somatic) variables. It leaves room within its framework for the social, psyological, and behavioral dimensions of illness. e biomedical model not only requires that disse be dealt with as an entity independent of sol behavior, it also demands that behavioral errations be explained on the basis of disorred somatic (biochemical or neurophysiologi) processes. Thus the biomedical model emaces both reductionism, the philosophic view at complex phenomena are ultimately derived m a single primary principle, and mind-body alism, the doctrine that separates the mental from the somatic. Here the reductionistic primary principle is physicalistic; that is, it assumes that the language of chemistry and physics will ultimately suffice to explain biological phenomena. From the reductionist viewpoint, the only conceptual tools available to characterize and experimental tools to study biological systems are physical in nature (4).

The biomedical model was devised by medical scientists for the study of disease. As such it was a scientific model; that is, it involved a shared set of assumptions and rules of conduct based on the scientific method and constituted a blueprint for research. Not all models are scientific. Indeed, broadly defined, a model is nothing more than a belief system utilized to explain natural phenomena, to make sense out of what is puzzling or disturbing. The more socially disruptive or individually upsetting the phenomenon, the more pressing the need of humans to devise explanatory systems. Such efforts at explanation constitute devices for social adaptation. Disease par excellence exemplifies a category of natural phenomena urgently demanding explanation (5). As Fabrega has pointed out, "disease" in its generic sense is a linguistic term used to refer to a certain class of phenomena that members of all social groups, at all times in the history of man, have been exposed to. "When people of various intellectual and cultural persuasions use terms analogous to 'disease,' they have in mind, among other things, that the phenomena in question involve a person-centered, harmful, and undesirable deviation or discontinuity . . . associated with impairment or discomfort" (5). Since the condition is not desired it gives rise to a need for corrective actions. The latter involve beliefs and explanations about disease as well as rules of conduct to rationalize treatment actions. These constitute socially adaptive devices to resolve, for the individual as well as for the society in which the sick person lives, the crises and uncertainties surrounding disease (6).

Such culturally derived belief systems about disease also constitute models but they are not scientific models. These may be referred to as popular or folk models. As efforts at social adaptation, they contrast with scientific models which are primarily designed to promote scientific investigation. The historical fact we have to face is that in modern Western society biomedicine not only has provided a basis for the scientific study of disease, it has also become our own culturally specific perspective about disease, that is, our folk model. Indeed the biomedical model is now the dominant folk model of disease in the Western world (5, 6).

In our culture the attitudes and belief systems of physicians are molded by this model long before they embark on their professional education, which in turn reinforces it without necessarily clarifying how its use for social adaptation contrasts with its use for scientific research. The biomedical model has thus become a cultural imperative, its limitations easily overlooked. In brief, it has now acquired the status of *dogma.* In science, a model is revised or abandoned when it fails to account adequately for all the data. A dogma on the other hand, requires that discrepant data be forced to fit the model or be excluded. Biomedical dogma requires that all disease, including "mental" disease, be conceptualized in terms of derangement of underlying physical mechanisms. This permits only two alternatives whereby behavior and disease can be reconciled: the *reductionist,* which says that all behavioral phenomena of disease must be conceptualized in terms of physicochemical principles; and the *exclusionist,* which says that whatever is not capable of being so explained must be excluded from the category of disease. The reductionists concede that some disturbances in behavior belong in the spectrum of disease. They categorize these as mental diseases and designate psychiatry as the relevant medical discipline. The exclusionists regard mental illness as a myth and would eliminate psychiatry from medicine. Among physicians and psychiatrists today the reductionists are the true believers, the exclusionists are the apostates, while both condem heretics those who dare to question the ultin truth of the biomedical model and advoca more useful model.

HISTORICAL ORIGINS OF REDUCTIONISTIC BIOMEDICAL MODEL

In considering the requirements for a more clusive scientific medical model for the stud disease, an ethnomedical perspective is hel (6). In all societies, ancient and modern, pr erate and literate, the major criteria identification of disease have always been havioral, psychological, and social in nat Classically, the onset of disease is marked changes in physical appearance that frigh puzzle, or awe, and by alterations in function in feelings, in performance, in behavior, or in lationships that are experienced or perceive threatening, harmful, unpleasant, deviant, desirable, or unwanted. Reported verbally demonstrated by the sufferer or by a witn these constitute the primary data upon which based first-order judgments as to whether or n person is sick (7). To such disturbing beha and reports all societies typically respond by d ignating individuals and evolving social inst tions whose primary function is to evaluate, terpret, and provide corrective measures (5, Medicine as an institution and as a discipli and physicians as professionals, evolved as o form of response to such social needs. In course of history, medicine became scientific physicians and other scientists developed a t onomy and applied scientific methods to the u derstanding, treatment, and prevention of dist bances which the public first had designated "disease" or "sickness."

Why did the reductionistic, dualistic biom ical model evolve in the West? Rasmuss identifies one source in the concession of est lished Christian orthodoxy to permit dissecti he human body some five centuries ago (8). :h a concession was in keeping with the Chris- view of the body as a weak and imperfect ves- for the transfer of the soul from this world to next. Not surprisingly, the Church's permis- 1 to study the human body included a tacit in- liction against corresponding scientific inves- tion of man's mind and behavior. For in the s of the Church these had more to do with re- on and the soul and hence properly remained domain. This compact may be considered ;ely responsible for the anatomical and struc- al base upon which scientific Western medi- e eventually was to be built. For at the same e, the basic principle of the science of the , as enunciated by Galileo, Newton, and scartes, was analytical, meaning that entities e investigated be resolved into isolable causal ins or units, from which it was assumed that whole could be understood, both materially 1 conceptually, by reconstituting the parts. th mind-body dualism firmly established der the imprimatur of the Church, classical ence readily fostered the notion of the body as machine, of disease as the consequence of akdown of the machine, and of the doctor's k as repair of the machine. Thus, the scientific proach to disease began by focusing in a frac- nal-analytic way on biological (somatic) pro- sses and ignoring the behavioral and psychoso- l. This was so even though in practice many ysicians, at least until the beginning of the h century, regarded emotions as important for development and course of disease. Actually, ch arbitrary exclusion is an acceptable strategy scientific research, especially when concepts d methods appropriate for the excluded areas not yet available. But it becomes counterpro- ctive when such strategy becomes policy and e area originally put aside for practical reasons permanently excluded, if not forgotten alto- ther. The greater the success of the narrow ap- oach the more likely is this to happen. The bio- edical approach to disease has been successful beyond all expectations, but at a cost. For in serving as guideline and justification for medical care policy, biomedicine has also contributed to a host of problems, which I shall consider later.

LIMITATIONS OF THE BIOMEDICAL MODEL

We are now faced with the necessity and the challenge to broaden the approach to disease to include the psychosocial without sacrificing the enormous advantages of the biomedical approach. On the importance of the latter all agree, the reductionist, the exclusionist, and the heretic. In a recent critique of the exclusionist position, Kety put the contrast between the two in such a way as to help define the issues (9). "According to the medical model, a human illness does not become a specific disease all at once and is not equivalent to it. The medical model of an illness is a process that moves from the recognition and palliation of symptoms to the characterization of a specific disease in which the etiology and pathogenesis are known and treatment is rational and specific." Thus taxonomy progresses from symptoms, to clusters of symptoms, to syndromes, and finally to diseases with specific pathogenesis and pathology. This sequence accurately describes the successful application of the scientific method to the elucidation and the classification into discrete entities of disease in its generic sense (5, 6). The merit of such an approach needs no argument. What do require scrutiny are the distortions introduced by the reductionistic tendency to regard the specific disease as adequately, if not best, characterized in terms of the smallest isolable component having causal implications, for example, the biochemical; or even more critical, is the contention that the designation "disease" does not apply in the absence of perturbations at the biochemical level.

Kety approaches this problem by comparing diabetes mellitus and schizophrenia as paradigms of somatic and mental diseases, pointing out the appropriateness of the medical model for both. "Both are symptom clusters or syndromes, one described by somatic and biochemical abnormalities, the other by psychological. Each may have many etiologies and shows a range of intensity from severe and debilitating to latent or borderline. There is also evidence that genetic and environmental influences operate in the development of both." In this description, at least in reductionistic terms, the scientific characterization of diabetes is the more advanced in that it has progressed from the behavioral framework of symptoms to that of biochemical abnormalities. Ultimately, the reductionists assume schizophrenia will achieve a similar degree of resolution. In developing his position, Kety makes clear that he does not regard the genetic factors and biological processes in schizophrenia as are now known to exist (or may be discovered in the future) as the only important influences in its etiology. He insists that equally important is elucidation of "how experiential factors and their interactions with biological vulnerability make possible or prevent the development of schizophrenia." But whether such a caveat will suffice to counteract basic reductionism is far from certain.

THE REQUIREMENTS OF A NEW MEDICAL MODEL

To explore the requirements of a medical model that would account for the reality of diabetes and schizophrenia as human experiences as well as disease abstractions, let us expand Kety's analogy by making the assumption that a specific biochemical abnormality capable of being influenced pharmacologically exists in schizophrenia as well as in diabetes, certainly a plausible possibility. By obliging ourselves to think of patients with diabetes, a "somatic disease," and with schizophrenia, a "mental disease," in exactly the same terms we will see more clearly how inclusion of somatic and psychosocial factors is indispensable for both; or more pointedly, how c centration on the biomedical and exclusio the psychosocial distorts perspectives and e interferes with patient care.

1. In the biomedical model, demonstratio the specific biochemical deviation is gene regarded as a specific diagnostic criterion for disease. Yet in terms of the human experienc illness, laboratory documentation may only i cate disease potential, not the actuality of the ease at the time. The abnormality may be p ent, yet the patient not be ill. Thus the prese of the biochemical defect of diabetes or sc ophrenia at best defines a necessary but n sufficient condition for the occurrence of human experience of the disease, the illn More accurately, the biochemical defect co tutes but one factor among many, the comp interaction of which ultimately may culmi in active disease or manifest illness (10). Nor the biochemical defect be made to acco for all of the illness, for full understanding quires additional concepts and frames of re ence. Thus, while the diagnosis of diabetes is suggested by certain core clinical manifestati for example, polyuria, polydipsia, polypha and weight loss, and is then confirmed by l oratory documentation of relative insulin d ciency, how these are experienced and how t are reported by any one individual and how t affect him, all require consideration of psyc logical, social, and cultural factors, not to m tion other concurrent or complicating biologi factors. Variability in the clinical expression of abetes as well as of schizophrenia, and in the dividual experience and expression of these nesses reflects as much these other elements a does quantitative variations in the specific b chemical defect.

2. Establishing a relationship between parti lar biochemical processes and the clinical data illness requires a scientifically rational appro to behavioral and psychosocial data, for th are the terms in which most clinical phenome

reported by patients. Without such, the relia-ty of observations and the validity of correla-s will be flawed. It serves little to be able to cify a biochemical defect in schizophrenia ne does not know how to relate this to partic-r psychological and behavioral expressions of disorder. The biomedical model gives insuf-ent heed to this requirement. Instead it en-rages bypassing the patient's verbal account placing greater reliance on technical proce-es and laboratory measurements. In actuality task is appreciably more complex than the medical model encourages one to believe. An mination of the correlations between clinical l laboratory data requires not only reliable thods of clinical data collection, specifically h-level interviewing skills, but also basic un-standing of the psychological, social, and cul-al determinants of how patients communicate nptoms of disease. For example, many verbal ressions derive from bodily experiences early life, resulting in a significant degree of ambi-ity in the language patients use to report symp-ns. Hence the same words may serve to express mary psychological as well as bodily distur-nces, both of which may coexist and overlap complex ways. Thus, virtually each of the nptoms classically associated with diabetes y also be expressions of or reactions to psycho-gical distress, just as ketoacidosis and hypo-cemia may induce psychiatric manifestations, cluding some considered characteristic of hizophrenia. The most essential skills of the ysician involve the ability to elicit accurately d then analyze correctly the patient's verbal ac-unt of his illness experience. The biomedical odel ignores both the rigor required to achieve iability in the interview process and the neces-y to analyze the meaning of the patient's report psychological, social, and cultural as well as anatomical, physiological, or biochemical rms (7).

3. Diabetes and schizophrenia have in com-on the fact that conditions of life and living constitute significant variables influencing the time of reported onset of the manifest disease as well as of variations in its course. In both conditions this results from the fact that psychophysiologic responses to life change may interact with existing somatic factors to alter susceptibility and thereby influence the time of onset, the severity, and the course of a disease. Experimental studies in animals amply document the role of early, previous, and current life experience in altering susceptibility to a wide variety of diseases even in the presence of a genetic predisposition (11). Cassel's demonstration of higher rates of ill health among populations exposed to incongruity between the demands of the social system in which they are living and working and the culture they bring with them provides another illustration among humans of the role of psychosocial variables in disease causation (12).

4. Psychological and social factors are also crucial in determining whether and when patients with the biochemical abnormality of diabetes or of schizophrenia come to view themselves or be viewed by others as sick. Still other factors of a similar nature influence whether or not and when any individual enters a health care system and becomes a patient. Thus, the biochemical defect may determine certain characteristics of the disease, but not necessarily the point in time when the person falls ill or accepts the sick role or the status of a patient.

5. "Rational treatment" (Kety's term) directed only at the biochemical abnormality does not necessarily restore the patient to health even in the face of documented correction or major alleviation of the abnormality. This is no less true for diabetes than it will be for schizophrenia when a biochemical defect is established. Other factors may combine to sustain patienthood even in the face of biochemical recovery. Conspicuously responsible for such discrepancies between correction of biological abnormalities and treatment outcome are psychological and social variables.

6. Even with the application of rational therapies, the behavior of the physician and the relationship between patient and physician powerfully influence therapeutic outcome for better or for worse. These constitute psychological effects which may directly modify the illness experience or indirectly affect underlying biochemical processes, the latter by virtue of interactions between psychophysiological reactions and biochemical processes implicated in the disease (11). Thus, insulin requirements of a diabetic patient may fluctuate significantly depending on how the patient perceives his relationship with his doctor. Furthermore, the successful application of rational therapies is limited by the physician's ability to influence and modify the patient's behavior in directions concordant with health needs. Contrary to what the exclusionists would have us believe, the physician's role is, and always has been, very much that of educator and psychotherapist. To know how to induce peace of mind in the patient and enhance his faith in the healing powers of his physician requires psychological knowledge and skills, not merely charisma. These too are outside the biomedical framework.

THE ADVANTAGES OF A BIOPSYCHOSOCIAL MODEL

This list surely is not complete but it should suffice to document that diabetes mellitus and schizophrenia as paradigms of "somatic" and "mental" disorders are entirely analogous and, as Kety argues, are appropriately conceptualized within the framework of a medical model of disease. But the existing biomedical model does not suffice. To provide a basis for understanding the determinants of disease and arriving at rational treatments and patterns of health care, a medical model must also take into account the patient, the social context in which he lives, and the complementary system devised by society to deal with the disruptive effects of illness, that is, the physician role and the health care system. This requires a biopsychosocial model. Its scop determined by the historic function of the pl cian to establish whether the person solici help is "sick" or "well"; and if sick, why sick in which ways sick; and then to develop a ratio program to treat the illness and restore and m tain health.

The boundaries between health and dise between well and sick are far from clear never will be clear, for they are diffused by tural, social, and psychological consideratio The traditional biomedical view, that biolog indices are the ultimate criteria defining dise leads to the present paradox that some peo with positive laboratory findings are told that t are in need of treatment when in fact they feeling quite well, while others feeling sick are sured that they are well, that is, they have no " ease" (5, 6). A biopsychosocial model which cludes the patient as well as the illness wo encompass both circumstances. The doctor's t is to account for the dysphoria and the dysfu tion which lead individuals to seek medical he adopt the sick role, and accept the status of tienthood. He must weight the relative contri tions of social and psychological as well as biological factors implicated in the patient's d phoria and dysfunction as well as in his decisi to accept or not accept patienthood and wit the responsibility to cooperate in his own hea care.

By evaluating all the factors contributing both illness and patienthood rather than givi primacy to biological factors alone, a b psychosocial model would make it possible to plain why some individuals experience as " ness" conditions which others regard merely "problems of living," be they emotional reactio to life circumstances or somatic symptoms. F from the individual's point of view his decisi between whether he has a "problem of living" is "sick" has basically to do with whether or not accepts the sick role and seeks entry into t health care system, not with what, in fact, is sponsible for his distress. Indeed, some peop y the unwelcome reality of illness by dismiss-as "a problem of living" symptoms which may ctuality be indicative of a serious organic pro-s. It is the doctor's, not the patient's, responsi-ty to establish the nature of the problem and lecide whether or not it is best handled in a dical framework. Clearly the dichotomy be-en "disease" and "problems of living" is by no ans a sharp one, either for patient or for doctor.

VHEN IS GRIEF A)ISEASE?

enhance our understanding of how it is that oblems of living" are experienced as illness by ne and not by others, it might be helpful to nsider grief as a paradigm of such a borderline ndition. For while grief has never been consid-d in a medical framework, a significant num-of grieving people do consult doctors because disturbing symptoms, which they do not nec-arily relate to grief. Fifteen years ago I ad-ssed this question in a paper titled "Is grief a ease? A challenge for medical research" (13). aim too was to raise questions about the ade-acy of the biomedical model. A better title ght have been, "When is grief a disease?," just one might ask when schizophrenia or when di-etes is a disease. For while there are some obvi-s analogies between grief and disease, there are o some important differences. But these very ntradictions help to clarify the psychosocial di-ensions of the biopsychosocial model.

Grief clearly exemplifies a situation in which ychological factors are primary; no preexisting emical or physiological defects or agents need invoked. Yet as with classic diseases, ordinary ief constitutes a discrete syndrome with a rel-vely predictable symptomatology which in-ıdes, incidentally, both bodily and psychologi-l disturbances. It displays the autonomy typical disease; that is, it runs its course despite the suf-rer's efforts or wish to bring it to a close. A con-tent etiologic factor can be identified, namely, significant loss. On the other hand, neither the sufferer nor society has ever dealt with ordinary grief as an illness even though such expressions as "sick with grief" would indicate some connection in people's minds. And while every culture makes provisions for the mourner, these have generally been regarded more as the responsibility of religion than of medicine.

On the face of it, the arguments against including grief in a medical model would seem to be the more persuasive. In the 1961 paper I countered these by comparing grief to a wound. Both are natural responses to environmental trauma, one psychological, the other physical. But even at the time I felt a vague uneasiness that this analogy did not quite make the case. Now 15 years later a better grasp of the cultural origins of disease concepts and medical care systems clarifies the apparent inconsistency. The critical factor underlying man's need to develop folk models of disease, and to develop social adaptations to deal with the individual and group disruptions brought about by disease, has always been the victim's ignorance of what is responsible for his dysphoric or disturbing experience (5, 6). Neither grief nor a wound fits fully into that category. In both, the reasons for the pain, suffering, and disability are only too clear. Wounds or fractures incurred in battle or by accident by and large were self-treated or ministered to with folk remedies or by individuals who had acquired certain technical skills in such matters. Surgery, developed out of the need for treatment of wounds and injuries, has different historical roots than medicine, which was always closer in origin to magic and religion. Only later in Western history did surgery and medicine merge as healing arts. But even from earliest times there were people who behaved as though grief-stricken, yet seemed not to have suffered any loss; and others who developed what for all the world looked like wounds or fractures, yet had not been subjected to any known trauma. And there were people who suffered losses whose grief deviated in one way or another from what the culture had come to accept as the normal course; and others whose wounds failed to heal or festered or who became ill even though the wound had apparently healed. Then, as now, two elements were crucial in defining the role of patient and physician and hence in determining what should be regarded as disease. For the patient it has been his not knowing why he felt or functioned badly or what to do about it, coupled with the belief or knowledge that the healer or physician did know and could provide relief. For the physician in turn it has been his commitment to his professional role as healer. From these have evolved sets of expectations which are reinforced by the culture, though these are not necessarily the same for patients as for physicians.

A biopsychosocial model would take all of these factors into account. It would acknowledge the fundamental fact that the patient comes to the physician because either he does not know what is wrong or if he does he feels incapable of helping himself. The psychobiological unity of man requires that the physician accept the responsibility to evaluate whatever problems the patient presents and recommend a course of action, including referral to other helping professions. Hence the physician's basic professional knowledge and skills must span the social, psychological, and biological, for his decisions and actions on the patient's behalf involve all three. Is the patient suffering normal grief or melancholia? Are the fatigue and weakness of the woman who recently lost her husband conversion symptoms, psychophysiological reactions, manifestations of a somatic disorder, or a combination of these? The patient soliciting the aid of a physician must have confidence that the M.D. degree has indeed rendered that physician competent to make such differentiations.

A CHALLENGE FOR BOTH MEDICINE AND PSYCHIATRY

The development of a biopsychosocial medical model is posed as a challenge for both medicine and psychiatry. For despite the enormous gains which have accrued from biomedical resea there is a growing uneasiness among the pu as well as among physicians, and especi among the younger generation, that health ne are not being met and that biomedical researc not having a sufficient impact in human ter This is usually ascribed to the all too obvi inadequacies of existing health care delivery tems. But this certainly is not a complete ex nation, for many who do have adequate acce health care also complain that physicians lacking in interest and understanding, are pre cupied with procedures, and are insensitive the personal problems of patients and their fa lies. Medical institutions are seen as cold and personal; the more prestigious they are as cen for biomedical research, the more common s complaints (14). Medicine's unrest derives fro growing awareness among many physicians the contradiction between the excellence of th biomedical background on the one hand and weakness of their qualifications in certain a butes essential for good patient care on the ot (7). Many recognize that these cannot be proved by working within the biomedical mo alone.

The present upsurge of interest in primary c and family medicine clearly reflects disencha ment among some physicians with an approa to disease that neglects the patient. They are n more ready for a medical model which wo take psychosocial issues into account. Even fr within academic circles are coming some sh challenges to biomedical dogmatism (8, 15). Th Holman ascribes directly to biomedical red tionism and to the professional dominance of adherents over the health care system such desirable practices as unnecessary hospitali tion, overuse of drugs, excessive surgery, and appropriate utilization of diagnostic tests. writes, "While reductionism is a powerful t for understanding, it also creates profound m understanding when unwisely applied. Red tionism is particularly harmful when it negle impact of nonbiological circumstances n biologic processes." And, "Some medical comes are inadequate not because appropri- technical interventions are lacking but be- se our conceptual thinking is inadequate" . How ironic it would be were psychiatry to in- on subscribing to a medical model which e leaders in medicine already are beginning uestion.

'sychiatrists, unconsciously committed to the medical model and split into the warring ps of reductionists and exclusionists, are ay so preoccupied with their own professional ntity and status in relation to medicine that y are failing to appreciate that psychiatry now he only clinical discipline within medicine cerned primarily with the study of man and human condition. While the behavioral sci- es have made some limited incursions into dical school teaching programs, it is mainly on psychiatrists, and to a lesser extent clinical chologists, that the responsibility falls to de- op approaches to the understanding of health d disease and patient care not readily accom- shed within the more narrow framework and h the specialized techniques of traditional bio- dicine. Indeed the fact is that the major for- lations of more integrated and holistic con- pts of health and disease proposed in the past years have come not from within the biomed- l establishment but from physicians who have wn upon concepts and methods which orig- ated with psychiatry, notably the psycho- namic approach of Sigmund Freud and psy- oanalysis and the reaction-to-life-stress ap- oach of Adolf Meyer and psychobiology (16). tually, one of the more lasting contributions of th Freud and Meyer has been to provide mes of reference whereby psychological ocesses could be included in a concept of dis- se. Psychosomatic medicine—the term itself vestige of dualism—became the medium ereby the gap between the two parallel, but dependent ideologies of medicine, the biological and the psychosocial, was to be bridged. Its progress has been slow and halting, not only because of the extreme complexities intrinsic to the field itself, but also because of unremitting pressures, from within as well as from without, to conform to scientific methodologies basically mechanistic and reductionistic in conception and inappropriate for many of the problems under study. Nonetheless, by now a sizable body of knowledge, based on clinical and experimental studies of man and animals has accumulated. Most, however, remains unknown to the general medical public and to the biomedical community and is largely ignored in the education of physicians. The recent solemn pronouncement by an eminent biomedical leader (2) that "the emotional content of organic medicine [has been] exaggerated" and "psychosomatic medicine is on the way out" can only be ascribed to the blinding effects of dogmatism.

The fact is that medical schools have constituted unreceptive if not hostile environments for those interested in psychosomatic research and teaching, and medical journals have all too often followed a double standard in accepting papers dealing with psychosomatic relationships (17). Further, much of the work documenting experimentally in animals the significance of life circumstances or change in altering susceptibility to disease has been done by experimental psychologists and appears in psychology journals rarely read by physicians or basic biomedical scientists (11).

GENERAL SYSTEMS THEORY PERSPECTIVE

The struggle to reconcile the psychosocial and the biological in medicine has had its parallel in biology, also dominated by the reductionistic approach of molecular biology. Among biologists too have emerged advocates of the need to develop holistic as well as reductionistic explanations of life processes, to answer the "why?"

and the "what for?" as well as the "how?" (18, 19). Von Bertalanffy, arguing the need for a more fundamental reorientation in scientific perspectives in order to open the way to holistic approaches more amenable to scientific inquiry and conceptualization, developed general systems theory (20). This approach, by treating sets of related events collectively as systems manifesting functions and properties on the specific level of the whole, has made possible recognition of isomorphies across different levels of organization, as molecules, cells, organs, the organism, the person, the family, the society, or the biosphere. From such isomorphies developed fundamental laws and principles that operate commonly at all levels of organization, as compared to those which are unique for each. Since systems theory holds that all levels of organization are linked to each other in a hierarchical relationship so that change in one affects change in the others, its adoption as a scientific approach should do much to mitigate the holist-reductionist dichotomy and improve communication across scientific disciplines. For medicine, systems-theory provides a conceptual approach suitable not only for the proposed biopsychosocial concept of disease but also for studying disease and medical care as interrelated processes (10, 21). If and when a general-systems approach becomes part of the basic scientific and philosophic education of future physicians and medical scientists, a greater readiness to encompass a biopsychosocial perspective of disease may be anticipated.

BIOMEDICINE AS SCIENCE AND AS DOGMA

In the meantime, what is being and can be done to neutralize the dogmatism of biomedicine and all the undesirable social and scientific consequences that flow therefrom? How can a proper balance be established between the fractional-analytic and the natural history approaches, both
so integral for the work of the physician and
medical scientist (22)? How can the clinicia
helped to understand the extent to which his
entific approach to patients represents a distin
"human science," one in which "reliance is
the integrative powers of the observer of a c
plex nonreplicable event and on the experim
that are provided by history and by animals
ing in particular ecological settings," as Marg
Mead puts it (23)? The history of the rise and
of scientific dogmas throughout history may
some clues. Certainly mere emergence of
findings and theories rarely suffices to overth
well-entrenched dogmas. The power of vested
terests, social, political, and economic, are for
dable deterrents to any effective assault on
medical dogmatism. The delivery of health c
is a major industry, considering that more tha
percent of our national economic product is
voted to health (2). The enormous existing
planned investment in diagnostic and therap
tic technology alone strongly favors approac
to clinical study and care of patients that emp
size the impersonal and the mechanical (24).
example, from 1967 to 1972 there was an incre
of 33 percent in the number of laboratory t
conducted per hospital admission (25). Plann
for systems of medical care and their financin
excessively influenced by the availability a
promise of technology, the application and eff
tiveness of which are often used as the criteria
which decisions are made as to what constitu
illness and who qualifies for medical care. T
frustration of those who find what they believe
be their legitimate health needs inadequat
met by too technologically oriented physician
generally misinterpreted by the biomedical
tablishment as indicating "unrealistic expec
tions" on the part of the public rather than bei
recognized as reflecting a genuine discrepan
between illness as actually experienced by t
patient and as it is conceptualized in the b
medical mode (26). The professionalization
biomedicine constitutes still another formi

barrier (8, 15). Professionalization has engen-ed a caste system among health care person- and a peck order concerning what constitute ropriate areas for medical concern and care, the most esoteric disorders at the top of the Professional dominance "has perpetuated vailing practices, deflected criticisms, and in-ated the profession from alternate views and ial relations that would illuminate and im-ve health care" (15, p. 21). Holman argues, not convincingly, that "the Medical establish-nt is not primarily engaged in the disinter-ed pursuit of knowledge and the translation of t knowledge into medical practice; rather in nificant part it is engaged in special interest ad-acy, pursuing and preserving social power" p. 11).

Jnder such conditions it is difficult to see how orms can be brought about. Certainly con-outing another critical essay is hardly likely to ng about any major changes in attitude. The blem is hardly new, for the first efforts to in-duce a more holistic approach into the under-duate medical curriculum actually date back Adolf Meyer's program at Johns Hopkins, ich was initiated before 1920 (27). At Roch-er, a program directed to medical students and physicians during and after their residency ining, and designed to inculcate psychosocial owledge and skills appropriate for their future rk as clinicians or teachers, has been in exis-ice for 30 years (28). While difficult to measure tcomes objectively, its impact, as indicated a questionnaire on how students and gradu-s view the issues involved in illness and tient care, appears to have been appreciable). In other schools, especially in the immedi- post–World War II period, similar efforts were inched, and while some flourished briefly, ost soon faded away under the competition of ore glamorous and acceptable biomedical ca-ers. Today, within many medical schools there again a revival of interest among some faculty, t they are few in number and lack the influ-ence, prestige, power, and access to funding from peer review groups that goes with conformity to the prevailing biomedical structure.

Yet today, interest among students and young physicians is high, and where learning opportu-nities exist they quickly overwhelm the available meager resources. It would appear that given the opportunity, the younger generation is very ready to accept the importance of learning more about the psychosocial dimensions of illness and health care and the need for such education to be soundly based on scientific principles. Once ex-posed to such an approach, most recognize how ephemeral and insubstantial are appeals to hu-manism and compassion when not based on ra-tional principles. They reject as simplistic the no-tion that in past generations doctors understood their patients better, a myth that has persisted for centuries (30). Clearly, the gap to be closed is be-tween teachers ready to teach and students eager to learn. But nothing will change unless or until those who control resources have the wisdom to venture off the beaten path of exclusive reliance on biomedicine as the only approach to health care. The proposed biopsychosocial model pro-vides a blueprint for research, a framework for teaching, and a design for action in the real world of health care. Whether it is useful or not remains to be seen. But the answer will not be forthcom-ing if conditions are not provided to do so. In a free society, outcome will depend upon those who have the courage to try new paths and the wisdom to provide the necessary support.

SUMMARY

The dominant model of disease today is biomed-ical, and it leaves no room within its framework for the social, psychological, and behavioral di-mensions of illness. A biopsychosocial model is proposed that provides a blueprint for research, a framework for teaching, and a design for action in the real world of health care.

George L. Engel

REFERENCES AND NOTES

This article was adapted from material presented as the Loren Stephens Memorial Lecture, University of Southern California Medical Center, 1976; the Griffith McKerracher Memorial Lecture at the University of Saskatchewan, 1976; the Annual Hutchings Society Lecture, State University of New York—Upstate Medical Center, Syracuse, 1976. Also presented during 1975 to 1976 at the University of Maryland School of Medicine, University of California—San Diego School of Medicine University of California—Los Angeles School of Medicine, Massachusetts Mental Health Center, and the 21st annual meeting of Midwest Professors of Psychiatry, Philadelphia. The author is a career research awardee in the U.S. Public Health Service.

1. A. M. Ludwig, *J Am Med Assoc* 234, 603 (1975).
2. *RF Illust*, 3, 5 (1976).
3. T. S. Szasz, *The Myth of Mental Illness* (Harper & Row, New York: 1961); E. F. Torrey, *The Death of Psychiatry* (Chilton, Radnor, Pa.: 1974).
4. R. Rosen, in *The Relevance of General Systems Theory*, E. Laszlo, ed. (Braziller, New York: 1972), p. 45.
5. H. Fabrega, *Arch Gen Psychiatry* 32, 1501 (1972).
6. H. Fabrega, *Science* 189, 969 (1975).
7. G. L. Engel, *Ann Intern Med* 78, 587 (1973).
8. H. Rasmussen, *Pharos* 38, 53 (1975).
9. S. Kety, *Am J Psychiatry* 131, 957 (1974).
10. G. L. Engel, *Perspect Biol Med* 3, 459 (1960).
11. R. Ader, in *Ethology and Development*, S. A. Barnett, ed. (Heinemann, London: 1973), p. 37; G. L. Engel, *Gastroenterology* 67, 1085 (1974).
12. J. Cassel, *Am J Public Health* 54, 1482 (1964).
13. G. L. Engel, *Psychosom Med* 23, 18 (1961).
14. R. S. Duff and A. B. Hollingshead, *Sickness and Society* (Harper & Row, New York: 1968).
15. H. R. Holman, *Hosp Pract* 11, 11 (1976).
16. K. Menninger, *Ann Intern Med* 29, 318 (1948); J. Romano, *J Am Med Assoc* 143, 409 (1950); G. L. Engel, *Midcentury Psychiatry*, R. Grinker, ed. (Thomas, Springfield, Ill.: 1953), p. 33; H. G. Wolff, ed., *An Outline of Man's Knowledge* (Doubleday, New York: 1960), p. 41; G. L. Engel, *Psychological Dev[…] ment in Health and Disease* (Saunders, Philadel[…] 1962).
17. G. L. Engel and L. Salzman, *N Engl J Med* […] 44 (1973).
18. R. Dubos, *Mirage of Health* (Harper & […] New York, 1959); *Reason Awake* (Columbia Unive[…] Press, New York: 1970); E. Mayr, in *Behavior and […] lution*, A. Roe and G. G. Simpson, eds. (Yale Unive[…] Press, New Haven, Conn.: 1958), p. 341; *Science* […] 1501 (1961); *Am Sci* 62, 650 (1974); J. T. Bonner, *On[…] velopment: The Biology of Form* (Harvard Unive[…] Press, Cambridge, Mass.: 1974); G. G. Simpson, […] *ence* 139, 81 (1963).
19. R. Dubos, *Man Adapting* (Yale University P[…] New Haven, Conn.: 1965).
20. L. von Bertalanffy, *Problems of Life* (Wiley, […] York: 1952); *General Systems Theory* (Braziller, […] York: 1968). See also E. Laszlo, *The Relevance of […] eral Systems Theory* (Braziller, New York: 1972); […] *Systems-View of the World* (Braziller, New York: 19[…] Dubos (19).
21. K. Menninger, *The Vital Balance* (Viking, […] York: 1963); A. Sheldon, in *Systems and Medical C[…]* A. Sheldon, F. Baker, C. P. McLaughlin, eds. ([…] Press, Cambridge, Mass.: 1970), p. 84; H. Brody, […] *spect Biol Med* 16, 71 (1973).
22. G. L. Engel, in *Physiology, Emotion, and […] chosomatic Illness*, R. Porter and J. Knight, eds. (E[…] vier-Excerpta Medica, Amsterdam: 1972), p. 384.
23. M. Mead, *Science* 191, 903 (1976).
24. G. L. Engel, *J Am Med Assoc* 236, 861 (1976).
25. J. M. McGinnis, *J Med Educ* 51, 602 (1976).
26. H. Fabrega and P. R. Manning, *Psychosom M[…]* 35, 223 (1973).
27. A. Meyer, *J Am Med Assoc* 69, 861 (1917).
28. A. H. Schmale, W. A. Greene, F. Reichsman, […] Kehoe, G. L. Engel, *Adv Psychosom Med* 4, 4 (19[…] G. L. Engel, *J Psychosom Res* 11, 77 (1967); L. You[…] *Ann Intern Med* 83, 728 (1975).
29. G. L. Engel, *J Nerv Ment Dis* 154, 159 (19[…] *Univ Rochester Med Rev* (winter 1971–1972), p. 10.
30. G. L. Engel, *Pharos* 39, 127 (1976).

CHAPTER 8

When Do Symptoms Become a Disease?

ROBERT A. ARONOWITZ

SYMPTOMS TO DISEASE: THE HISTORICAL CONTEXT

WHEN DOES OR SHOULD a collection of mptoms constitute a disease? The investigator or clinician who asks is question (the "symptoms-to-disease" question) usually wants to know hether there are rules or norms, currently or in the past, that say whether particular collection of largely symptom-based criteria has enough spec-city, utility, or plausibility to justify the appellation *disease*.

I answer this question by first examining how the meanings and contexts the words *symptom* and *disease* have changed over the past 200 years. I en look at examples of past and present symptom complexes that have een treated as specific entities in Western medicine, and I draw some con-usions about our norms for naming and classifying them. My goal is not to judge whether these norms are good or bad but to make the norms explicit so that we understand what is at stake in the many controversies over the definition and legitimacy of contemporary symptom-based diagnoses.

A partial answer to the symptoms-to-disease question can be found in the differences between older and modern entries for the word *symptom* (from the Greek, combining roots for "to fall" and "together") in the *Oxford English Dictionary* (1). In the dictionary's citations from the Middle Ages to the late nineteenth century, *symptoms* were generally the bodily or mental phenomena that a person experienced and that arose from, accompanied, or (often) constituted a particular illness. An 1804 citation, for example, states that "His skin was hot, and his pulse strong. These symptoms could be attributed to . . . inflammation of the brain." Changes experienced by people or observed by physicians (such as "pulse strong") could be called symptoms.

By the latter half of the nineteenth century, *symptom* had taken on other meanings. An 1869 citation in the *Oxford English Dictionary* states that "Diseases are distinguished from each other either by such alterations in the organs themselves, or their secretions, as can be ascertained by the senses of the observer (physical signs); or by changes in the functions of the parts affected (symptoms)." Symptoms had become subjective, explicitly and consciously opposed to *signs*, the objective alterations noted by the physician. Symptoms by themselves were less likely to constitute disease because they did not arise directly from the "alterations of organs" but rather from the organs' less precise *functions*. Symptoms were defined in the context of the increasingly prominent scientific, medical, and social act of distinguishing specific diseases from each other. In this act, symptoms were to play an increasingly subordinate role to signs.

This new understanding of ill health as a result of specific disease, increasingly defined more by signs than symptoms, was accompanied by a relentless push to define disease at ever "dee levels (from subjective experience to organ rangements and then to cellular derangeme As a result, many patients lost their sympt based and clinically based diagnoses and bec medical "orphans."

In the beginning of the twentieth century, example, a physician—on the basis of a his and physical examination—might offer the d nosis *peptic ulcer disease* to patients who late the century would lose or never receive this d nosis if the characteristic "objective" abnorr ity, the visualized gastric or duodenal ulcer, not detected by an upper gastrointestinal serie a specialist's endoscope. But neither these tients nor their symptoms disappeared. A c mon medical response has been to create new creasingly nonspecific symptom-based diagn for these patients, such as the negatively nan *nonulcer dyspepsia*.

Just as both lay and medical people h generally viewed the shift from symptom-ba to mechanism- or anatomy-based diagnosis progress, they have often stigmatized the res ing nonspecific diagnoses, the patients who h received them, and even the physicians who h cared for these patients. This stigma—combi with many other cultural developments, such a more widespread consumer ethos, lay advoc for specific diseases, and the power of special terests to influence specific health legislation has led to intense pressure to find mechanis for, redefine, or simply rename nonspecific di noses so that they seem more specific and im putative underlying mechanisms. (One exam is the call to replace the term *chronic fatigue s drome* with the term *postviral syndrome*.) Th developments, in turn, have contributed to medical backlash against affected patients a their symptom-based, nonspecific diagnoses, sulting in a cycle of medical and political cont versies over disease definition.

Thus, the contemporary context for the "syn toms-to-disease" question is typically a cont y over the legitimacy of a residual, negatively ned disease entity that has little clinical or ›ratory specificity. Knowing this context, we guess that these entities will have a difficult e meeting any proposed normative criteria for ›na fide specific disease.

Jnderstanding the history of symptom-based ;noses, we can make sense of what is at stake hese controversies. In the early twentieth cen-, symptom-based diagnoses were not typically hrouded in the current kinds of controversies. e medical meanings of such diagnoses were very different from those in use today, but y were put to different clinical and social uses. To take one example, some U.S. physicians in early decades of the twentieth century de-ed whether angina pectoris should be defined a freestanding, symptom-based, "functional" order—a characteristic pattern of chest pain nptoms not connected to one organic lesion—as a symptom of a specific, anatomically ined disease: coronary artery obstruction lead-; to myocardial ischemia. Although the de-es were heated, pitting generalists against cialists and clinical skills against new technol-, the underlying assumptions and the stakes fered from those in contemporary debates er "symptom-based" diagnoses, such as the ronic fatigue syndrome (2). The term *func-nal disorder* still had something of its earlier h-century meaning—physiologic, diffuse, and lden—as opposed to its more modern "ab-ice of mechanism" meaning. While "func-nal" diagnoses, such as the symptom-based gina pectoris, might have been held in lower gard than other diagnoses, they were not always ictly divided from "real" diagnoses. For the rpose of diagnosis, distinctions between mind d body, anatomic and functional, were less early demarcated.

Many aspects of medical practice in earlier as were supporting characters in this looser ›sology. The reality of limited effective treat-ents and the weak resolution of diagnostic technology contributed to less hubris about the power of diagnosis and more accommodation of uncertainty by both physician and patient. The greater relative number of general practitioners, who frequently used clinical strategies such as watchful waiting and placebo prescription (practices often derided by specialists), was also part of a less confrontational, more flexible, more individualized style of diagnosis. Economic relations between patients and physicians were different too: There were fewer middle-class "consumers" of medical care, and payment was made or bartered directly between patient and physician rather than provided by third parties on the basis of specific diagnoses and treatments. In sum, less was riding on the specificity of diagnoses, symptom-based or otherwise. Although we cannot and would not want to set back the clock, this historical overview reminds us that contemporary interest in and controversies over symptom-based diagnoses reflect the increased expectations placed on specific diseases.

PATHS TO SPECIFICITY: HISTORICAL ACCIDENT AND FALSE APPEARANCES

What paths have symptom complexes taken en route to acquiring the status of specific diseases? The history of many well-accepted rheumatologic diagnoses shows much about how symptom clusters have come to be accepted as having some specificity in clinical practice. These entities are frequently used by clinicians today, and their utility and specificity are arguably sustained by effective clinical strategies and by the later identification of specific, mediating immunologic mechanisms.

Many of these entities, such as Still disease (1897), the Reiter syndrome (1916), and the Behçet syndrome (1937), had their origins in the work of astute clinicians who carefully examined and reported on small numbers of patients seen in private practice (3–5). Although these syndromes were not immediately recognized as new entities and their names were not coined by the men after whom the syndromes were later named, these symptom clusters owe their existence as specific diseases to the norms and practices of an older era much different from our own. They have been "grandfathered" into our current nosology.

I strongly doubt whether these diagnoses could be newly coined and promoted today. Experienced clinicians have less authority with which to get such work accepted and published and to garner the grant support necessary for protected time to do and write up research. Most prestigious medical journals do not publish small, uncontrolled case series. What is new and exciting today, with few exceptions, are diseases defined by new agents and (preferably molecular) mechanisms, not by purely clinical criteria.

It is also important to recognize that many contemporary symptom-based diseases owe their existence to an initial and often erroneous suspicion of this more conventional, mechanism-based specificity. For example, what we now call the chronic fatigue syndrome began as chronic Epstein–Barr virus infection (2).

The fact that social factors largely explain which symptom clusters get accepted as diseases has direct relevance to the care of patients. To patients whose symptoms are features of a few rheumatologic diseases but do not definitively point to any single disease, I have frequently mused that they and I were born at least 50 years too late. A few such patients and I might have had my own eponymic disease, and they might be the focus of scientific interest. When I successfully convince such patients that the absence of a simple match between their symptoms and an existing disease may be due to "historical accident" and the limitations of contemporary medical knowledge and diagnostic technology, their illnesses sometimes become less frightening and seem to be less their own fault. Such patients are sometimes more willing to pursue, in a spir trial and error, treatments that work for simila agnoses.

For patients whose clinical presentations n closely fit the definitions of existing rheum logic diseases, I often use a complementary s egy to reduce the fear that may come from r ing up on the disease or from knowing about bad outcomes of others with the same diagn I open a medical text to those confusing ta displaying the consensus criteria for rheuma arthritis or systemic lupus erythematosus, which combinations of symptoms, signs, and oratory and radiologic abnormalities are mi and matched. For some patients, this visual play of the negotiated nature of medical cl fication is an eye opener, helping them acc the idiosyncrasy of their own illnesses. This i syncrasy is by itself neither reassuring nor da ing, but patients may learn that their uncerta about the future is not peculiar to them an neither their own fault (for example, it does result from their inability to accurately re their symptoms or their medical history) nor t physician's fault. Much of the problem is rather to the limitations of medical knowle and the necessarily imperfect match between dividual suffering and medical categories.

THE DURABILITY OF SYMPTOM-BASED AND CLINICALLY BASED DIAGNOSES: THE HISTORY OF ASTHMA

The existence of symptom-based and clinica based diagnoses cannot be explained by hist cal accident and false appearances alone. Ma such diseases on the contemporary scene h not only thrived but have resisted plausi redefinition on more "objective" grounds.

The history of asthma is illustrative. In ma classic Greek texts, authors used the word *asth* escribe a specific degree of abnormal breath- , somewhere in severity between orthopnea dyspnea. Until the eighteenth century, ma was more a symptom-based anything n it was a symptom. Over the nineteenth and ntieth centuries, Western physicians reformu- d asthma as a symptom-based, specific dis- e—something that was the same across dif- nt patients and could be distinguished by sicians from the many new diseases that were cribed during this period. Asthma's clinical cificity was strengthened by, but not reducible innovations in technology and diagnostic ctices. Using stethoscopes, 19th-century phy- ans could more accurately and consistently r wheezing, which became an important but pathognomonic sign of the disease.

ater in the nineteenth century, European l U.S. physicians searched for more objective ns and test results with which to define and di- nose asthma, such as specific body types, envi- nmental associations, autopsy findings, and croscopic abnormalities. Potentially most use- for an objective definition of asthma was the plication of various lung volume and other ysiologic measurements that were adapted m research and clinical practice in tuberculo- (Many of these points were illustrated in an nibit on the history of asthma at the National orary of Medicine: Breath of Life; R. Arono- tz and C. Keirns, curators. Bethesda, Mary- d, March 1999–March 2001. Available at www. m.nih.gov/hmd/breath/breathhome.html.)

Despite many new insights into the pathophys- ogic basis of asthma, asthma has remained a di- nosis based mostly on what the clinician sees d hears. The retention of a clinically based finition has been a choice, albeit an implicit e, made by researchers, clinicians, and pa- nts. There are many possible clinical reasons y physicians and others have never reached a nsensus on a singular, objective definition of thma. The inconsistent relationship between symptoms and clinical signs and results on objective tests (such as a positive response to methacholine challenge) has been recognized and frequently bemoaned. Clinicians have believed that not all asthmatic patients wheeze; some "merely" cough or have paroxysms of breathing difficulties. The popular clinical maxim that "all that wheezes is not asthma" reminded diagnosticians in different generations that asthma, like many other clinically based diagnoses, was an elusive and residual diagnostic category to be considered only after other specific causes of wheezing or related symptoms were "ruled out."

But there are also social explanations why asthma has not been redefined more objectively. A more reductionist definition of asthma would have broken the continuity with past knowledge and would necessarily have excluded many patients, past and present, whom clinicians suspect have something similar. Retention of the clinically based definition might also reflect a related concern that the biomedical knowledge and technology used to potentially redefine asthma, however well received at the moment, are likely to change. A surer long-term bet may be the retention of a clinically based definition that is continuous with the past. It is also possible that many researchers, clinicians, and patients realize that a more objective definition would result in a much smaller patient population, making asthma less of a pressing social and biomedical problem and undermining efforts to provide funding for and sustain research interest in asthma.

But even if researchers and clinicians agreed on a more "objective" definition of asthma, there would remain the problem of asthma's stubborn idiosyncrasy—clinicians have long recognized that different people have different emotional, environmental, and physiologic triggers and clinical courses. The retention of a symptom-based and clinically based definition for asthma represents in part a response to this idiosyncrasy, allowing patients and clinicians to use a great diversity of approaches to a very heterogeneous patient population under the umbrella of a single diagnosis.

EFFORTS TO LEGITIMATE SYMPTOM-BASED DIAGNOSES

Parallel to the processes by which symptom clusters gain recognition as specific entities are the equally complex strategies with which clinicians and others try to legitimize the existence of these entities. These strategies—like the symptom-based diseases they are meant to rationalize—often get blurrier and more paradoxical the more closely they are examined.

Psychiatric diseases illustrate both the important role that response to treatment has played in the legitimization of symptom-based diseases and the hazards of this strategy. The mid–twentieth century discovery that people with manic-depressive or bipolar disorder, a hitherto symptom-based entity, uniquely responded to lithium salts was a powerful argument for the specificity, unity, and biological plausibility of the diagnosis (6).

The potential hazards of this strategy for particular diagnoses as well as for the practitioners who offer them are illustrated by the contemporary history of another symptom-based psychiatric diagnosis: depression. In *Listening to Prozac*, psychiatrist Peter Kramer offers an interesting but troubling discussion of what the Food and Drug Administration would call the "off-label" uses of Prozac (7). Kramer and other clinicians have noted that Prozac has benefited many people who do not have depression or who have another diagnosable psychiatric disease. Such effects include alleviation of insomnia, improved self-esteem, decreased social inhibition, and greater mental agility.

Even if only a small fraction of these claims were true and were true only for a subset of Prozac users, this wide spectrum of response could undermine the specificity and unity of depression and the legitimacy of psychi
symptom-based diagnoses. If we take the w
ranging effects attributed to Prozac down the
pery slope, we have a system of classifying me
symptoms in which each person differs from
next person by his or her particular loca
along an unlimited number of symptom and
sonality continua, rather than by residing wi
or outside of a discrete number of bounded (
chiatric disease) circles.

These examples show the strengths and d
gers of using response to treatment as a post
argument for the specificity of symptom clus
A potentially more robust strategy, used in
chiatric nosology but also in a range of sympt
based diagnoses in primary care, has been to fi
create, or test the specificity of symptom clus
by applying quantitative methods to clinical d
to (1) see which combinations of symptoms t
to hang together or (2) understand the impl
tions of grouping symptoms in different w
The problematic epistemology of using fac
analysis to create a robust case definition of,
the Gulf War syndrome, is clear—no amoun
hanging together, in a quantitative sense, can
around the problem that the variables in su
models may have little biological plausibi
may be different ways of labeling and measur
the same thing, or may reflect social influen
and other confounders.

The last strategy commonly used to legitim
symptom clusters as diseases is probably the m
prevalent today: the use of expert consensus pa
els, such as those that have produced the di
nostic and statistical manuals for psychiatric
agnoses. As a member of an expert panel
Lyme disease, I struggled with the best diagnos
criteria for the chronic forms of the disease. T
central issue was whether symptoms alone we
specific enough to make the diagnosis. The pa
sought criteria with which to distinguish chro
Lyme disease from entities such as the chronic
tigue syndrome and fibromyalgia. The consens
was that people with chronic symptoms, ev

se with serologic evidence of previous expo- to *Borrelia burgdorferi,* should be given a gnosis of Lyme disease only if they have one of w well-defined late presentations, each of ch contains one or more threshold condi- s that is either a physician-discovered sign (for mple, frank arthritis with observable and "tap- le" fluid) or an objective test result (such as ebrospinal fluid findings consistent with asep- meningitis). This decision did not simply fol- from biological evidence that only persons o met these criteria had *B. burgdorferi* infec- or its immunologic sequelae. We did not and not have the technological means to reliably l directly apprehend the underlying patho- ic processes that presumably cause the late nptoms of Lyme disease.

How, then, was this consensus decision made? e panel inferred from the medical literature antibiotic treatment and from the clinical ex- rience of its members that the narrower, more ojective" definition of chronic Lyme disease uld be more specific. At the same time, the nel was not unaware that this definition would er the diagnosis from many patients whom me disease specialists would rather not treat, luding those who questioned medical author- , did not play by the sick role rules, had depres- n or other psychiatric conditions, had low esholds for seeking medical care, had height- ed awareness of their own bodily processes, or, rst of all, did not improve with known treat- ents. The critical appraisal of medical evidence uld not be separated from knowledge of who uld be the likely winners and losers if Lyme sease were defined one way or another. To no e's surprise, attempts such as this one to keep mptom clusters out of the Lyme disease defini- n have been controversial.

CONCLUSION

e can now return to the question that bewil- red researchers, clinicians, and patients have asked of medical history: "When does or should a collection of symptoms become a disease?" The examples of symptom-based diseases that I have discussed here —the well-accepted and the controversial, those that were redefined using objective tests and those that resisted such redefinition, symptom clusters that have never been named and those that have—all point to a sociocultural answer more than to a biological or clinical one. The situation is analogous to a long-simmering controversy in linguistics over the general criteria for distinguishing dialects from languages. Hoping to end what he thought was a futile controversy, a famous linguist reportedly said "a language is a dialect with an army." In other words, dialects were distinguished from languages primarily by social and political realities. This observation was meant not to ignore the very real and measurable differences between different speech groups but to point out that these differences, while setting some boundaries, did not ultimately determine how the groups would be classified. Similarly, although biological and clinical factors set some boundaries for which symptoms might plausibly be linked in a disease concept, social influences largely explain which symptom clusters have made it as diseases.

There are many symptom clusters whose specificity has evoked controversy, but it remains striking that concepts such as a real or legitimate disease, or even terms such as *symptom, syndrome,* and *disease,* are almost never explicitly defined in these debates. Perhaps this is to be expected and not bemoaned. As so many observers have pointed out, physiologic, psychological, and social processes are uniquely combined in any single person to constitute illness (8). It should be of no surprise that the suffering of people can be only imperfectly mapped to a set of objective disease ideal-types.

Recognition of the fact that social influences determine which symptom clusters succeed as diseases also has policy and clinical implications. At the policy level, we need to recognize the limitations of medical evidence and the importance of having balanced representation of potential winners and losers in deliberations about these diagnoses. At the clinical level, we need to recognize and accommodate the essential continuity between persons who have symptoms that have been given a name and disease-like status and persons whose suffering remains unnamed and unrecognized.

ACKNOWLEDGMENTS

The author thanks Charles E. Rosenberg, Ph.D., and Marjorie Bowman, M.D., for comments on an earlier draft of this paper.

REFERENCES

1. *Oxford English Dictionary*, 2nd ed. New York, Oxford University Press; 1992.

2. Aronowitz, R. A. *Making Sense of Illness: Scie Society and Disease*. New York, Cambridge Unive Press; 1998.

3. Keen, J. H. "George Frederic Still: Regis Great Ormond Street Children's Hospital." *Br Journal of Rheumatology* 1998: 37:1247.

4. Reiter, Hans. "Reiter's syndrome." *JAMA* 1 11:821–22.

5. Kyle, R. A., Shampo, M. A. "Hulusi Behc, et *JAMA* 1982: 247:1925.

6. Cade, J. F. "Lithium Salts in the Treatment of chotic Excitement." *Medical Journal of Australia* 1 36:349–52.

7. Kramer, P. D. *Listening to Prozac*. New Y Viking; 1993.

8. Kleinman, A. *The Illness Narratives: Suffer Healing, and the Human Condition*. New York, B Books; 1988.

PART II

Characterizing Health, Disease, and Illness

AS THE READINGS IN Part I make clear, sease-states may be created, invented, reified, and even honored for var-us social, economic, or political purposes. But do diseases exist as onto-gical entities apart from the social and normative dimensions that they ight happen to map? Are instances of disease the result of a discrete de-ur taken by an organism (or one or more of an organism's parts) en route ward a natural, universal *telos*? Is mental illness distinct from physical ill-ess and if so, why? Part II begins by answering these questions.

CHRISTOPHER BOORSE frames the notion of disease as untoward devia-on in natural functioning relative to the typical design of individuals of a ecies. Boorse's proposition that medicine uses "an autonomous framework of medical theory" and that this "theoretical corpus looks in every way continuous with theory in biology and the other natural sciences," and thus is value-free, flew in the face of his more normativist contemporaries. Boorse went on to show that to distinguish between disease and illness necessarily involves an assessment of the values implicit in the latter and also an assessment that certain conditions are met, whereas diagnoses of diseases remain independent of subjective perceptions and value-free. Further, Boorse claimed that based on his illness-criteria it is unlikely one might accurately assess most psychological conditions as "mental illnesses"—but rather they are character flaws or idiosyncrasies of personality. But note Professor Boorse's addendum. It is a crucial note that clarifies his view on the status of illness in addition to referencing later works, which develop his viewpoint.

In an interesting twist on nonnormativism, the position that holds that diseases are objective, universal, and value-free, K. Danner Clouser, Charles Culver, and Bernard Gert offer their concept of "malady." They suggest that "malady" captures objective and universal "evils" such as pain, death, and disability but accounts for norms at the same time (i.e., the norms that are shared universally by members of our species). Clouser, Culver, and Gert undercut the strong normativists by claiming that their concept, when understood and applied correctly, can even be applied to various mental states to help demarcate mental maladies from other conditions. They ground and condition the concept of "malady" using the Thomistic notion of sustaining causes (or the absence thereof) and nuance it further to account for conditions that could give rise to anhedonia (inability to experience pleasure), stigma, and loss of freedom.

Roberto Mordacci and Richard Sobel craft a comprehensive account of the meanings of "health." At base, health is more than an end that can be attained through medicine: health is a means to reaching an ultimate good—plentitude. They account for, but do not limit thei position to obstacles in human flourishing, wh may be manifested as biological variation, so institutions, cultural traditions, or any comb tion thereof. They offer examples of hea diminishing pathogens, as well as hea enhancing factors (salutogens), and contend all these are instrumental on an existential l and should also be operational in how a cult or medical institution frames its definition health.

R. E. Kendell explains how the term "me illness" is a misnomer, originating from a flaw modern medical epistemology and Cartes mind/body dualism. This dualism, in turn, wa marked transition from the premodern, holi notion that mental health was part and parce bodily health. Kendell shows us that theoreti recognition of this holism has reemerged, desp the continued practical and semantic distinct used to separate mental and physical illness

In an update to an earlier article, Arth Caplan claims that the concept of disease grounded upon the flawed distinction betwe natural and unnatural. In dissecting this disti tion, Caplan points out that inevitability and widespread prevalence of certain conditions say tooth decay or bacterial infection—do exclude them from the possibility of medical agnosis as disease and treatment. Then why physicians consider aging to be a natural proc not deserving of curative efforts? Perhaps agi has a natural purpose and perhaps attempts cure senescence run counter to what might se the greater good of the species? Perhaps there neo-Aristotelian explanation that adequately counts for the goal and function of aging?

Caplan suggests that arguments claiming agi is natural are based on theological, evolutiona and philosophical notions of goal and functic and that these are inadequate. Rather, Capl suggests that aging is a constellation of clinic symptoms and biological changes that meet t basic criteria—which he lays out in some

Characterizing Health, Disease, and Illness

—for being considered a disease. As such, ıg may be a socially neglected disease. It is a ıdition that defies medicalization not simply ause there is no cure or because it is tradi- ıally considered natural, but rather because of steep ethical obligations society must accept ɜn such a condition is granted disease status. ʒy highlighting the confusing factors that go ı a "diagnosing event," WINSTON CHIONG helps us to summarize the various characterizations of health and disease and the clinical implications of these concepts. He describes the faltering distinctions used in the day-to-day clinical work-up, which are based on the classic disease-as-entity medical model. Using clinical examples, Chiong shows how this paradigm has eroded and is now inadequate.

CHAPTER 9

On the Distinction between Disease and Illness

CHRISTOPHER BOORSE[1]

IN THIS CENTURY A STRONG tendency ıs developed to debate social issues in psychiatric terms. Whether the pic is criminal responsibility, sexual deviance, feminism, or a host of oth-'s, claims about mental health are increasingly likely to be the focus of dis-ıssion. This growing preference for medicine over morals, which might ː called the *psychiatric turn*, has an obvious appeal. In the paradigm ealth discipline, physiological medicine, judgments of health and disease 'e normally uncontroversial. The idea of reaching comparable certainty ɔout difficult ethical problems is an inviting prospect. Unfortunately our ɾasp of the issues that surround the psychiatric turn continues to be im-eded, as does psychiatric theory itself, by a fundamental misunderstanding of the concept of health. With few exceptions, clinicians and philosophers are agreed that health is an essentially evaluative notion. According to this consensus view, a value-free science of health is impossible. This thesis I believe to be entirely mistaken. I shall argue in this essay that it rests on a confusion between the theoretical and the practical senses of "health," or in other words, between disease and illness.

Two presuppositions of my whole discussion should be noted at the outset. The first is substantive: with Szasz and Flew, I shall assume that the idea of health ought to be analyzed by reference to physiological medicine alone.[2] It is a mistake to view physical and mental health as equally well-entrenched species of a single conceptual genus. In most respects, our institutions of mental health are recent offshoots from physiological medicine, and their nature and future are under continual controversy. In advance of a clear analysis of health in physiological medicine, it seems an open question whether current applications of the health vocabulary to mental conditions have any justification at all. Such applications will therefore be put on probation in the first two sections below. The other presupposition of my discussion is terminological. For convenience in distinguishing theoretical from practical uses of "health," I shall adhere to the technical usage of "disease" found in textbooks of medical theory. In such textbooks "disease" is simply synonymous with "unhealthy condition." Readers who wish to preserve the much narrower ordinary usage of "disease" should therefore substitute "theoretically unhealthy condition" throughout.

NORMATIVISM ABOUT HEALTH

It is safe to begin any discussion of health by saying that health is normality, since the terms are interchangeable in clinical contexts. But this remark provides no analysis of health until one specifies the norms involved. The most obv proposal, that they are pure statistical mean widely recognized to be erroneous. On the hand, many deviations from the average— unusual strength or vital capacity or eye colc are not unhealthy. On the other hand, practic everyone has some disease or other, and there also particular diseases such as tooth decay minor lung irritation that are nearly unive Since statistical normality is therefore nei necessary nor sufficient for clinical norma most writers take the following view about norms of health: that they must be determined whole or in part, by acts of evaluation. More cisely, the orthodox view is that all judgment health include value judgments as part of th meaning. To call a condition unhealthy is at l in part to condemn it; hence it is impossible define health in nonevaluative terms. I shall r to this orthodox view as *normativism.*

Normativism has many varieties, which often not clearly distinguished from one anot by the clinicians who espouse them. The co mon feature of healthy conditions may, for ample, be held to be either their desirability the individual or their desirability for soci The gap between these two values is a persist source of controversy in the mental-health main. One especially common variety of norm tivism combines the thesis that health judgme are value judgments with ethical relativis The resulting view that society is the final thority on what counts as disease is typical psychiatric texts, as illustrated by the followi quotation:

> While professionals have a major voice influencing the judgment of society, it is the c lective judgment of the larger social group t determines whether its members are to be view as sick or criminal, eccentric or immoral.[3]

For the most part my arguments against norm tivism will apply to all versions indiscriminate It will, however, be useful to make a minimal on of normativist positions into strong and ık. Strong normativism will be the view that lth judgments are pure evaluations without criptive meaning; weak normativism allows h judgments a descriptive as well as a norma- component.[4]

ıs an example of a virtually explicit statement trong normativism by a clinician, consider Dr. d Marmor's remark in a recent psychiatric ıposium on homosexuality:

> . to call homosexuality the result of disturbed exual development really says nothing other han that you disapprove of the outcome of that levelopment.[5]

f we may substitute "unhealthy" for "dis- bed," Marmor is claiming that to call a condi- ı unhealthy is only to express disapproval of it. other words—to collapse a few ethical distinc- ns—for a condition to be unhealthy it is nec- ary and sufficient that it be bad. Now at least f of this view, the sufficiency claim, is demon- ıbly false of physiological medicine. It is unde- ıble to be moderately ugly or, for that matter, lack the manual dexterity of Liszt, but neither these conditions is a disease. In fact, there are desirable conditions regularly corrected by ysicians which are not diseases: Jewish nose, gging breasts, adolescent fertility, and un- nted pregnancies are only a few of many ex- ıples. Thus strong normativism is an erroneous count of health judgments in their paradigm a of application, and its influence upon men- -health theorists is regrettable.

Unlike Marmor, however, many clinical writ- s take positions that can be construed as com- itting them merely to weak normativism. A od example is Dr. Marie Jahoda, who con- ıdes her survey of current criteria of psycho- gical health with these words:

> Actually, the discussion of the psychological meaning of various criteria could proceed with- out concern for value premises. Only as one calls these psychological phenomena "mental health" does the problem of values arise in full force. By this label, one asserts that these psychological at- tributes are "good." And, inevitably, the question is raised: Good for what? Good in terms of mid- dle class ethics? Good for democracy? For the continuation of the social *status quo*? For the in- dividual's happiness? For mankind? . . . For the encouragement of genius or of mediocrity and conformity? The list could be continued.[6]

Jahoda may here mean to claim only that call- ing a condition healthy *involves* calling it good. Her remarks are at least consistent with the weak normativist thesis that healthy conditions are good conditions which satisfy some further de- scriptive property as well. On this view, "healthy" is a mixed normative-descriptive term of the same sort as "honest" and "courageous." The fol- lowing passage by Dr. F. C. Redlich is likewise consistent with the weak view:

> Most propositions about normal behavior refer implicitly or explicitly to ideal behavior. Devia- tions from the ideal obviously are fraught with value judgments; actually, all propositions on normality contain value statements in various de- grees.[7]

Redlich's term "contain" suggests that he too sees the goodness of something as merely one neces- sary condition of its healthiness, and similarly for badness and unhealthiness.

Yet even weak normativism runs into coun- terexamples within physiological medicine. It is obvious that a disease may be on balance desir- able, as with the flat feet of a draftee or the mild infection produced by inoculation. It might be suggested in response that diseases must at any rate be prima facie undesirable. The trouble with this suggestion is that it is obscure. Consider the case of a disease that has infertility as its sole important effect. In what sense is infertility prima facie undesirable? Considered in abstraction from the actual effects of reproduction on

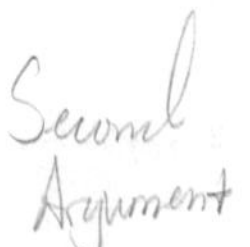

human beings, it is hard to see how infertility is either desirable or undesirable. Possibly those who see it as "prima facie" undesirable assume that most people want to be able to have more children. But the corollary of this position will be that writers of medical texts must do an empirical survey of human preferences to be sure that a condition is a disease. No such considerations seem to enter into human physiological research, any more than they do into standard biological studies of the diseases of plants and animals. Here indeed is another difficulty for any normativist, weak or strong. It seems clear that one may speak of diseases in plants and animals without judging the conditions in question undesirable. Biologists who study the diseases of fruit flies or sharks need not assume that their health is a good thing for us. On the other hand, there is not much sense in talking about the best interests of, say, a begonia. So it seems that normativists must interpret health judgments about plants and lower animals as analogical, in the same way as would be statements about the courage or considerateness of wolves and rats.

If normativism about health is at once so influential and so objectionable, one must ask what persuasive arguments there are in its support. I know of only three arguments, of which one will be treated in the next section. A germ of an argument appears in the passage by Redlich just quoted. Health judgments involve a comparison to an ideal; hence, Redlich concludes, they are "fraught with value judgments." It seems evident, however, that Redlich is thinking of ideals such as beauty and holiness rather than the chemist's ideal gas or Weber's ideal bureaucrat. The fact that a gas or a bureaucrat deviates from the ideal type is nothing against the gas or the bureaucrat. There are normative and nonnormative ideals, as there are in fact normative and nonnormative norms. The question is which sort health is, and Redlich has here provided no grounds for an answer.

A second and equally incomplete argum for normativism is suggested by the first two cl ters of Margolis' *Psychotherapy and Moral* Margolis argues in his first chapter that psyc analysts have been mistaken in holding that t therapeutic activities can "escape moral scruti (p. 13). From this he concludes that "it is reas able to view therapeutic values as forming pa a larger system of moral values" (p. 37) and plicitly endorses normativism. But this infere is a non sequitur. From the fact that *the* pro tion of health is open to moral review, it in no follows that health judgments are value ju ments. Wealth and power are also "values" in sense that people pursue them in a morally c cizable fashion; neither is a normative conc The pursuit of any descriptively definable co tion, if it has effects on persons, will be ope moral review.

These two arguments, like the health lit ture generally, do next to nothing to rule out alternative view that health is a descriptiv definable property which is usually valua Why, after all, may not health be a concep the same sort as intelligence, or deductive va ity? Though the idea of intelligence is certai vague, it does not seem to be normative. Inte gence is the ability to perform certain intellec tasks, and one would expect that these intel tual tasks could be characterized without pres posing their value.[9] Similarly, a valid argum may, for theoretical purposes, be descriptiv defined[10] roughly as one that has a form no stance of which could have true premises an false conclusion. Intelligence in people and lidity in arguments being generally valued, t statement that a person is intelligent or an arg ment valid does tend to have the force of a r ommendation. But this fact is wholly irreleva to the employment of the terms in theories of telligence or validity. To insist that evaluation still part of the very meaning of the terms wou be to make an implausible claim to which th

obvious counterexamples. Exactly the same
/ be true of the concept of health. At any rate,
have already seen some of the counterexam-
s.

ince the distinction between force and mean-
in philosophy of language is in a rather prim-
: state, it is doubtful that weak normativism
ut health can be either decisively refuted or
isively established. But I suggest that its cur-
t prevalence is largely the result of two quite
:table causes. One is the lack of a plausible de-
ptive analysis; the other is a confusion be-
en theoretical and practical uses of the health
abulary. The required descriptive analysis I
ll try to sketch in the next section. As for the
ond cause, one should always remember that
ual commitment to theory and practice is one
the features that distinguish a clinical disci-
ne. Unlike chemists or astronomers, physins and psychotherapists are professionally en-
ged in practical judgments about how certain
ople ought to be treated. It would not be sur-
sing if the terms in which such practical judg-
nts are formulated have normative content.
ne might contend, for example, that calling a
ncer "inoperable" involves the value judgment
t the results of operating will be worse than
ving the disease alone. But behind this conptual framework of medical practice stands an
tonomous framework of medical theory, a
dy of doctrine that describes the functioning of
ealthy body, classifies various deviations from
ch functioning as diseases, predicts their be-
vior under various forms of treatment, etc.
is theoretical corpus looks in every way con-
uous with theory in biology and the other nat-
al sciences, and I believe it to be value-free.
The difference between the two frameworks
nerges most clearly in the distinction between
ease and illness. It is disease, the theoretical
ncept, that applies indifferently to organisms of
species. That is because, as we shall see, it is
be analyzed in biological rather than ethical
terms. The point is that illnesses are merely a subclass of diseases, namely, those diseases that have certain normative features reflected in the institutions of medical practice. An illness must be, first, a reasonably *serious* disease with incapacitating effects that make it undesirable. A shaving cut or mild athlete's foot cannot be called an illness, nor could one call in sick on the basis of a single dental cavity, though all these conditions are diseases. Secondly, to call a disease an illness is to view its owner as deserving special treatment and diminished moral accountability. These requirements of "illness" will be discussed in some detail shortly, with particular attention to "mental illness." But they explain at once why the notion of illness does not apply to plants and animals. Where we do not make the appropriate normative judgments or activate the social institutions, no amount of disease will lead us to use the term "ill." Even if the laboratory fruit flies fly in listless circles and expire at our feet, we do not say they succumbed to an illness, and for roughly the same reasons as we decline to give them a proper funeral.

There are, then, two senses of "health." In one sense it is a theoretical notion, the opposite of "disease." In another sense it is a practical or mixed ethical notion, the opposite of "illness."[11] Let us now examine the relation between these two concepts more closely.

DISEASE AND ILLNESS

What is the theoretical notion of a disease? An admirable explanation of clinical normality was given thirty years ago by C. Daly King.

> The normal . . . is objectively, and properly, to be defined as that which functions in accordance with its design?[12]

The root idea of this account is that the normal is the natural. The state of an organism is theoretically healthy, i.e., free of disease, insofar as its mode of functioning conforms to the natural design of that kind of organism. Philosophers have, of course, grown repugnant to the idea of natural design since its cooptation by natural-purpose ethics and the so-called argument from design. It is undeniable that the term "natural" is often given an evaluative force. Shakespeare as well as Roman Catholicism is full of such usages, and they survive as well in the strictures of state legislatures against "unnatural acts." But it is no part of biological theory to assume that what is natural is desirable, still less the product of divine artifice. Contemporary biology employs a version of the idea of natural design that seems ideal for the analysis of health. The crucial element in the idea of a biological design is the notion of a natural function. I have argued elsewhere that a function in the biologist's sense is nothing but a standard causal contribution to a goal actually pursued by the organism.[13] Organisms are vast assemblages of systems and subsystems which, in most members of a species, work together harmoniously in such a way as to achieve a hierarchy of goals. Cells are goal-directed toward metabolism, elimination, and mitosis; the heart is goal-directed toward supplying the rest of the body with blood; and the whole organism is goal-directed both to particular activities like eating and moving around and to higher-level goals such as survival and reproduction. The specifically physiological functions of any component are, I think, its species-typical contributions to the apical goals of survival and reproduction. But whatever the correct analysis of function statements, there is no doubt that biological theory is deeply committed to attributing functions to processes in plants and animals. And the single unifying property of all recognized diseases of plants and animals appears to be this: that they interfere with one or more functions typically performed within members of the species.

The account of health thus suggested is in one sense thoroughly Platonic. The health of an organism consists in the performance by each part of its natural function. And as Plato also saw, of the most interesting features of the analys that it applies without alteration to mental he as long as there are standard mental function another way, however, the classical heritag misleading, for it seems clear that biolog function statements are descriptive rather t normative claims.[14] Physiologists obtain t functional doctrines without at any stage hav to answer such questions as, What is the func of a man? or to explicate "a good man" on analogy of "a good knife." Functions are no tributed in this context to the whole organisn all, but only to its parts, and the functions of a are its causal contributions to empirically gi goals. What goals a type of organism in fact p sues, and by what functions it pursues them, be decided without considering the value of p suing them. Consequently health in the theo ical sense is an equally value-free concept. T notion required for an analysis of health is that of a good man or a good shark, but that good specimen of a human being or shark.

All of this amounts to saying that the epis mology King suggested for health judgments at bottom, a statistical one. The question the fore arises how the functional account avoids earlier objections to statistical normality. K did explain how to dissolve one version of the p adox of saying that everyone is unhealthy. Clea all the members of a species can have some c ease or other as long as they do not have the sa disease. King somewhat grimly compares the j of extracting an empirical ideal of health fron set of defective specimens to the job of recc structing the Norden bombsight from assort aerial debris (p. 495). But this answer does n touch universal diseases such as tooth decay. though King nowhere considers this objectic the natural-design idea nevertheless suggests answer that I suspect is correct. If what make condition a disease is its deviation from the na ral functional organization of the species, then calling tooth decay a disease we are saying tha ɔt simply in the nature of the species—and we this because we think of it as mainly due to en- ›nmental causes. In general, deficiencies in functional efficiency of the body are diseases :n they are unnatural, and they may be unnat- l either by being atypical or by being attributa- mainly to the action of a hostile environment. ɪis explanation is accepted,[15] then the func- ɪal account simultaneously avoids the pitfalls tatistical normality and also frees the idea of oretical health of all normative content.

Theoretical health now turns out to be strictly ɪlogous to the mechanical condition of an ar- ct. Despite appearances, "perfect mechanical ɪdition" in, say, a 1965 Volkswagen is a de- ɪptive notion. Such an artifact is in perfect chanical condition when it conforms in all re- cts to the designer's detailed specifications. ›rmative interests play a crucial role, of course, the initial choice of the design. But what the lkswagen design actually *is* is an empirical tter by the time production begins. Thence- ward a car may be in perfect condition regard- s of whether the design is good or bad. If one ›laces its stock carburetor with a high-perfor- ɪnce part, one may well produce a better car, t one does not produce a Volkswagen in better :chanical condition. Similarly, an automatic nera may function perfectly and take wretched :tures; guided missiles and instruments of tor- e in perfect mechanical condition may serve :crable ends. Perfect working order is a matter ›t of the worth of the product but of the con- mity of the process to a fixed design. In the case organisms, of course, the ideal of health must determined by empirical analysis of the species ther than by the intentions of a designer. But ɪerwise the parallel seems exact. A person who mutation acquires a sixth sense, or the ability regenerate severed limbs, is not thereby :althier than we are. Sixth senses and limb re- neration are not part of the human design, ɪich at any given time, for better or worse, just what it is.

We have been arguing that health is descriptively definable within medical theory, as intelligence is in psychological theory or validity in logical theory. Nevertheless medical theory is the basis of medical practice, and medical practice unquestioningly presupposes the value of health. We must therefore ask how the functional view explains this presumption that health is desirable.

In the case of physiological health, there are at least two general reasons why the functional normality that defines it is usually worth having. In the first place, most people do want to pursue the goals with respect to which physiological functions are isolated. Not only do we want to survive and reproduce, but we also want to engage in those particular activities, such as eating and sex, by which these goals are typically achieved. In the second place—and this is surely the main reason the value of physical health seems indisputable—physiological functions tend to contribute to all manner of activities neutrally. Whether it is desirable for one's heart to pump, one's stomach to digest, or one's kidneys to eliminate hardly depends at all on what one wants to do. It follows that essentially all serious physiological diseases will satisfy the first requirement of an illness, namely, undesirability for its bearer.

This explanation of the fit between medical theory and medical practice has the virtue of reminding us that health, though an important value, is conceptually a very limited one. Health is not unconditionally worth promoting, nor is what is worth promoting necessarily health. Although mental-health writers are especially prone to ignore these points, even the constitution of the World Health Organization seems to embody a similar confusion:

> Health is a state of complete physical, mental, and social well-being, and not merely the absence of disease or infirmity.[16]

Unless one is to abandon the physiological paradigm altogether, this definition is far too wide. Health is functional normality, and as such is desirable exactly insofar as it promotes goals one can justify on independent grounds. But there is presumably no intrinsic value in having the functional organization typical of a species if the same goals can be better achieved by other means. A sixth sense, for example, would increase our goal-efficiency without increasing our health; so might the amputation of our legs at the knee and their replacement by a nuclear-powered air-cushion vehicle. Conversely, as we have seen, there is no a priori reason why ordinary diseases cannot contribute to well-being under appropriate circumstances.

In such cases, however, we will be reluctant to describe the person involved as ill, and that is because the term "ill" *does* have a negative evaluation built into it. Here again a comparison between health and other properties will be helpful. Disease and illness are related somewhat as are low intelligence and stupidity, or failure to tell the truth and speaking dishonestly. Sometimes the presumption that intelligence is desirable will fail, as in a discussion of qualifications for a menial job such as washing dishes or assembling auto parts. In such a context a person of low intelligence is unlikely to be described as stupid. Sometimes the presumption that truth should be told will fail, as when the Gestapo inquires about the Jews in your attic. Here the untruthful householder will not be described as speaking dishonestly. And sometimes the presumption that diseases are undesirable will fail, as with alcoholic intoxication or mild rubella intentionally contracted. Here the term "illness" is unlikely to appear despite the presence of disease. One concept of each pair is descriptive; the other adds to the first evaluative content, and so may be withheld where the first applies.

If we supplement this condition of undesirability with two further normative conditions, I believe we have the beginning of a plausible analysis of "illness." A disease is an *illness* only if it is serious enough to be incapacitating, therefore is

(i) undesirable for its bearer;
(ii) a title to special treatment; and
(iii) a valid excuse for normally criticizable behavior.

The motivation for condition (ii) needs no planation. As for (iii), the connection betweer ness and diminished responsibility has o been argued,[17] and I shall mention here only suggestive point. Our notion of illness belong the ordinary conceptual scheme of persons their actions, and it was developed to apply physiological diseases. Consequently the r tion between persons and their illnesses is c ceived on the model of their relation to their b ies. It has often been observed that physiologi processes, e.g., digestion or peristalsis, do usually count as actions of ours at all. By the sa token, we are not usually held responsible for results of such processes when they go wro though we may be blamed for failing to take st to prevent malfunction at some earlier time. N if this special relation between persons and th bodies is the reason for connecting disease w nonresponsibility, the connection may br down when diseases of the mind are at stake stead. I shall now argue, in fact, that conditic (i), (ii), and (iii) all present difficulties in the main of mental health.

MENTAL ILLNESS

For the sake of discussion, let us simply assu that the mental conditions usually called patl logical are in fact unhealthy by the theoreti standard sketched in the last section. That is, shall assume both that there are natural men functions and also that recognized types of p chopathology are unnatural interferences wi these functions.[18] Is it reasonable to make a p l extension of the vocabulary of medical prac- by calling these mental diseases mental ill- ses? Let us consider each condition on "ill- s."

Condition (i) was the undesirability of an ill- s for its bearer. Now there are obstacles to sferring our general arguments that physio- ical health is desirable to the psychological nain. Mental states are not nearly so neutral to choice of actions as physiological states are. In ticular, to evaluate the desirability of mental lth we can hardly avoid consulting our desires; in the mental-health context it could be those y desires that are judged unhealthy. From a oretical standpoint desires must be assigned a tivational function in producing action. Thus wants may or may not conform to the species ign. But if our wants do not conform to the cies design, it is not immediately obvious why should want them to. If there is no good reason want them to, then we have a disease which is an illness. It is conceivable that this diver- ice between the two notions is illustrated by mosexuality. It can hardly be denied that one rmal function of sexual desire is to promote re- duction. If one does not have a desire for het- sexual sex, however, the only good reason for nting to have such a desire seems to be that e would be happier if one did. But this judg- nt needs to be supported by evidence. The de- ability of having species-typical desires is not arly so obvious on inspection as the desirability having species-typical physiological functions.

One of the corollaries of this point is that ent debates over homosexuality and other putable diagnoses usually ignore at least one portant issue. Besides asking whether, say, mosexuality is a disease, one should also ask at difference it makes if it is. I have suggested at biological normality is an instrumental her than an intrinsic good. We always have the ht to ask, of normality, what is in it for us that already desire. If it were possible, then, to maximize intrinsic goods such as happiness, for ourselves and others, with a psyche full of deviant desires and unnatural acts, it is hard to see what practical significance the theoretical judgment of unhealthiness would have. I do not actually have serious doubts that disorders such as neuroses and psychoses diminish human happiness. It is also true that what is desirable for a person need not coincide with what the person wants; though an anorectic may not wish to eat, it is desirable that he or she do so. But we must be clear that requests to justify the value of health in other terms are always in order, and there are reasons to expect that such justification will require more evidence in the psychological domain than in the physiological.

We have been discussing the value of psychological normality for the individual, as dictated by condition (i) on illness, rather than its desirability for society at large. Since clinicians often assume that mental health involves social adjustment, it may be well to point out that the functional account of health shows this too to be a debatable assumption requiring empirical support. Certainly nothing in the mere statement that a person has a mental disease entails that he or she is contributing less to the social order than an arbitrary normal individual. There is no contradiction in calling van Gogh or Blake or Dostoyevsky mentally disturbed while admiring their work, even if they would have been less creative had they been healthier. Conversely, there is no a priori reason to assume that the healthy human personality will be morally worthy or socially acceptable. If Freud and Lorenz are right about the existence of an aggressive drive, there is a large component of the normal psyche that is less than admirable. Whether or not they are right, the suggestion clearly makes sense. Perhaps most psychiatrists would agree anyway that antisocial behavior is to be expected during certain developmental stages, e.g., the so-called anal-sadistic period or adolescence.

It must be conceded that *Homo sapiens* is a social species. Other organisms of this class, such as ants and bees, display elaborate fixed systems of social adaptations, and it would be remarkable if the human design included no standard functions at all promoting socialization. On the basis of the physiological paradigm, however, it is not at all clear that contributions to society can be viewed as requirements of health except when they also contribute to individual survival and reproduction. No matter how this issue is decided, the crucial point remains: the nature and extent of social functions in the human species can be discovered only empirically. Despite the contrary convictions of many clinicians, the concept of mental health itself provides no guarantee that healthy individuals will meet the standards or serve the interests of society at large. If it did, that would be one more reason to question the desirability of health for the individual.

Let us now go on to condition (ii) on a disease which is an illness: that it justify "special treatment" of its owner. It is this condition together with (iii) that gives some plausibility to the many recent attempts to explain mental illness as a "social status" or "role."[19] The idea that the "sick role" is a special one is consistent with the statistical normality of having some disease or other. Since illnesses are serious diseases that incapacitate at the level of gross behavior, everyone can be minimally diseased without being ill. In the realm of mental health, however, many psychiatrists suggest the stronger thesis that it is statistically normal to be significantly incapacitated by neurosis.[20] A similar problem may arise on Benedict's famous view that the characteristic personality type of some whole societies is clinically paranoid.[21] A statistically normal condition, according to our analysis, can be a disease only if it can be blamed on the environment. But one might plausibly claim that most or all existing *cultural* environments do injure children, filling their minds with excessive anxiety about sexual pleasure, grotesque role models, absurd prejudices about reality, etc. It is at least possible some degree of neurosis or psychosis is a ne universal environmental injury in our spec Only an empirical inquiry into the incidence etiology of neurosis can show whether this po bility is a reality. If it is, however, one can m tain the idea that serious diseases are illne only by abandoning one of the presupposition the illness concept: that not everyone can be i

The last and clearest difficulty with "me illness" concerns condition (iii), the role of ness in excusing conduct. We said that the i that serious diseases excuse conduct derives fr the model of the relation of agents to their c physiology. Unfortunately the relation of age to their own psychology is of a much more i mate kind. The puzzle about mental illnes that it seems to be an activity of the very sea responsibility—the mind and character— therefore to be beyond all hope of excuse.

This inference is hardly inescapable; ther room for considerable controversy to whic cannot do justice here. Strictly speaking, me disorders are disturbances of the personality. persons, not personalities, who are held respo ble for actions, and one central element in idea of a person is certainly consciousness. T means that there may be some sense in contr ing responsible persons with their mental eases insofar as these diseases lie outside th conscious personalities. Perhaps from a psyc analytic standpoint this condition is often me psychosis and neurosis. The unconscious p cesses that surface in these disorders seem at f sight more like things that happen within us, e peristalsis, than like things we do. But seve points make this classification look oversim fied. Unconscious ideas and wishes are still ideas and wishes in a more compelling se than movements of the gut are our movemen They may have been conscious at an earlier ti or be made conscious in therapy, whereupon becomes increasingly difficult to disclaim sponsibility for them. It seems quite unclear t are more responsible for many conscious de-s and beliefs than for these unconscious ones. ally, the hope for contrasting responsible peo- with their mental diseases grows vanishingly in the case of a character disorder, where the ealthy condition seems to be integrated into conscious personality.

n view of these points and the rest of the dis-sion, I think we must accept the following clusion. While conditions (i), (ii), and (iii) ly fairly automatically to serious physical dis-es, not one of them should be assumed to ly automatically to serious mental diseases. If term "mental illness" is to be applied at all, it uld probably be restricted to psychoses and bling neuroses. But even this decision needs re analysis than I have provided in this essay. eems doubtful that on any construal mental ess will ever be, in the mental-health move-nt's famous phrase, "just like any other ill-s."

What are the implications of our discussion for social issues to which psychiatry is so fre-ently applied? As far as the criminal law is con-ned, our results suggest that psychiatric theory ne should not be expected to define legal re-nsibility, e.g., in the insanity defense.[23] Al-ugh the notion of responsibility is a compo-nt of the notion of illness, it belongs not to dical theory but to ethics, and one can fix its undaries only by rational ethical debate. It ms certain that such a simple responsibility t as that the act of the accused not be "the prod-t of mental disease" is unsatisfactory. No doubt ny of us have antisocial tendencies that derive m underlying psychopathology of an ordinary rt. When these tendencies erupt in a parking vi-tion or negligent collision, it hardly seems in-mane or unjust to apply legal sanctions.[24] But is is not surprising, for no psychiatric concept is operly designed to answer moral questions. I n not saying that psychiatry is irrelevant to law d ethics. Anyone writing or applying a criminal de is certainly well advised to obtain the best available information about human nature, including the information about human nature that constitutes mental-health theory. The point is that one cannot expect to substitute psychiatry for moral debate, any more than moral evaluations can be substituted for psychiatric theory. Insofar as the psychiatric turn consists in such substitutions, it is fundamentally misconceived.

The other main implications of our discussion seem to me twofold. First, there is not the slightest warrant for the recurrent fantasy that what society or its professionals disapprove of is ipso facto unhealthy. This is not merely because society may disapprove of the wrong things. Even if ethical relativism were true, society still could not fix the functional organization of the members of a species. For this reason it could never be an infallible authority either on disease or on illness, which is a subclass of disease. Thus one main source of the tendency to call radical activists, bohemians, feminists, and other unpopular deviants "sick" is nothing but a conceptual confusion.

The second moral suggested by our discussion is that it is always worth asking, in any particular case, how strong the presumption is that health is desirable. When the value of health is left both unquestioned and obscure, it has a tendency to undergo inflation. The diagnosis especially of a "mental illness" is then likely to become an amorphous and peculiarly repellent stigma to be removed at any cost. The use of muscle-paralyzing drugs to compel prisoners to participate in "group therapy" is a particularly gruesome example of this sort of thinking.[25] But there are many other situations in which everyone would profit by asking what exactly is wrong with being unhealthy. In a way liberal reformers tend to make the opposite mistake: in their zeal to remove the stigma of disease from conditions such as homosexuality, they wholly discount the possibility that these conditions, like most diseases, are somewhat unideal. If the value of health, as I have argued in this essay, is nothing but the value of conformity to a generally excellent species design, then by recognizing that fact we may improve both the clarity and the humanity of our social discourse.

AUTHOR'S NOTE (1981)

Among many revisions I would make in the paper today, two are especially important. First, the view that illness is disease laden with values (i)–(iii) now seems a mistaken concession to normativism. Illness is better analyzed simply as systemically incapacitating disease, hence as no more normative than disease itself. Features (i)–(iii) are common social evaluations of illness, underlying the sick role, but they are probably no part of the meaning of "illness." On this view both a disease-illness distinction and a theory-practice distinction remain central to philosophy of medicine, without the former being a case of the latter. Second, as a terminological policy, I would avoid "disease" as a generic term for all pathological conditions. Medical usage often contrasts diseases with injuries, static defects, poisonings, and other kinds of lesion. For these reasons the essay seems mistitled. A better title would be "On the distinction between the pathological and the sick role," although (remembering *Iolanthe*) I am also tempted to suggest "Not on the distinction between disease and illness."

AUTHOR'S NOTE (2003)

For Boorse's account, see: Christopher Boorse. 1987. "Concept of Health." In Donald VanDeVeer and Tom Regan, ed., *Health Care Ethics: An Introduction.* Philadelphia: Temple University Press, pp. 351–93. Christopher Boorse. 1997. "A Rebuttal on Health." In James M. Humber and Robert F. Almeder, ed., *What Is Disease?* Totowa, N.J.: Humana Press, pp. 1–134.

NOTES

1. I thank the Delaware Institute for Medical Education and Research and the National Institute of Mental Health (Grant R03 MH 24621) for support in wr this essay.

2. Thomas S. Szasz, *The Myth of Mental Il* (New York: Hoeber-Harper, 1961); Antony Flew, *C or Disease?* (New York: Macmillan, 1973), pp. 40

3. Ian Gregory, *Fundamentals of Psych* (Philadelphia: W. B. Saunders, 1968), p. 32.

4. R. M. Hare, in *Freedom and Reason* (New Y Clarendon Press, 1963), chap. 2, argues that no te have prescriptive meaning alone. If this view is cepted, the difference between strong and weak mativism concerns the question of whether "heal is "primarily" or "secondarily" evaluative.

5. Judd Marmor, "Homosexuality and Cult Value Systems," *American Journal of Psychiatry* (1973): 1208.

6. Marie Jahoda, *Current Concepts of Positive M tal Health* (New York: Basic Books, 1958), pp. 7 See also her remark in *Interrelations Between Social Environment and Psychiatric Disorders* (N York: Milbank Memorial Fund, 1953), p. 142 : ".. evitably at some place there is a value judgment volved. I think that mental health or mental sick cannot be conceived of without reference to so basic value."

7. F.C. Redlich, "The Concept of Normali *American Journal of Psychotherapy* 6 (1952): 553.

8. Joseph Margolis, *Psychotherapy and Mora* (New York: Random House, 1966).

9. Exactly what intellectual abilities are include intelligence is, of course, unclear and may vary fr culture to culture. (See N. J. Block and Ge Dworkin, "IQ, Heritability and Inequality. Part I," *P losophy and Public Affairs* 3, no. 4 [summer 1974]: 3 But this does not show that for any particular grou speakers "intelligent" is a normative term, i.e., has p itive evaluation as part of its meaning.

10. The contrary view, which might be called n mativism about validity, is defended by J. O. Urmso "Some Questions Concerning Validity," *Revue In nationale de Philosophie* 25 (1953): 217–29.

11. Thomas Nagel has suggested that the adject "ill" may have its own special opposite "well." C

king about health might be greatly clarified if lness" had some currency.

. C. Daly King, "The Meaning of Normal," *Yale nal of Biology and Medicine* 17 (1945): 493–94. t definitions of health in medical dictionaries in- le some reference to functions. Almost exactly g's formulation also appears in Frederick C. lich and Daniel X. Freedman, *Theory and Practice sychiatry* (New York: Basic Books, 1966), p. 113.

3. C. Boorse. 1976. "Wright on Functions." *Philo- hical Review* 85: 70–78.

4. The view that function statements are normative erates the third argument for normativism. It is pre- ted most fully by Margolis in "Illness and Medical ues," *The Philosophy Forum* 8 (1959): 55–76, section t is also suggested by Ronald B. de Sousa, "The Pol- s of Mental Illness," *Inquiry* 15 (1972): 187–201, p. and possibly by Flew as well in *Crime or Disease?* 39–40. I think philosophers of science have made much progress in giving biological function state- nts a descriptive analysis for this argument to be very vincing.

5. For further discussion of environmental injuries other details of the functional account of health tched in this section, see my essay "Health as a The- tical Concept." [C. Boorse. 1977. "Health as a The- tical Concept." *Philosophy of Science*, 44: 542–73.]

6. Quoted by Flew, *Crime or Disease?*, p. 46.

7. A good discussion of this point and of the unde- bility condition (i) is provided by Flew in the ex- mely illuminating second chapter of *Crime or Dis- e?* Flew takes these conditions as part of the aning of "disease" rather than "illness"; but since he ms to be working from the ordinary usage of "dis- e," there may be no real disagreement here.

18. The plausibility of these two claims is discussed length in my essay, "What a Theory of Mental alth Should Be," in *Journal of the Theory of Social haviour.* [C. Boorse. 1976. "What a Theory of Men- Health Should Be." *Journal of the Theory of Social havior*, 6: 61–84.]

19. An example of this approach is Robert B. Edger- , "On The 'Recognition' of Mental Illness," in Stanley C. Plog and Robert B. Edgerton, *Changing Perspectives in Mental Illness* (New York, 1969), pp. 49–72.

20. Only one example of this suggestion is Dr. Reuben Fine's statement that neurosis afflicts 99 percent of the population. See Fine's "The Goals of Psychoanalysis," in *Goals of Psychotherapy*, ed. Alvin R. Mahrer (New York: Appleton-Century-Crofts, 1967), p. 95. I consider the issue of whether all neurosis can be called unhealthy in the essay cited in note 16.

21. See the descriptions of the Kwakiutl and the Dobu in Ruth Benedict, *Patterns of Culture* (Boston: Houghton Mifflin, 1934).

22. A number of clinicians have seriously suggested that people who are ill can be distinguished from those who are well by their presence in your office. One such author goes as far as to calculate an upper limit on the incidence of mental illness from the number of members in the American Psychiatric Association. On a literal reading, this patient-in-the-office test implies that one could wipe out mental illness once and for all by dissolving the APA and outlawing psychotherapy. But the whole idea seems silly anyway in the face of various studies that indicate that the population at large is, by the ordinary descriptive criteria for mental disorder, no less disturbed than the population of clinical patients.

23. The same conclusion is defended by Herbert Fingarette in "Insanity and Responsibility," *Inquiry* 15 (1972): 6–29.

24. Thus I disagree with H. L. A. Hart, among others, who writes: "...the contention that it is fair or just to punish those who have broken the law must be absurd if the crime is merely a manifestation of a disease." The quotation is from "Murder and the Principles of Punishment: England and the United States," reprinted in *Moral Problems*, ed. James Rachels (New York: Harper & Row, 1975), p. 274.

25. For this and other "therapeutic" abuses in our prison system, see Jessica Mitford, *Kind and Usual Punishment* (New York: Knopf/Random House, 1973), chap. 8.

CHAPTER 10

Malady: A New Treatment of Disea

K. DANNER CLOUSER, CHARLES M
CULVER, AND BERNARD GERT

THE DEFINITION OF CONCEPTS li disease and illness is an important problem in the philosophy of medici because of its inherent conceptual interest and because of its relationsh to many practical matters. For example, it might be claimed that differe persons, groups, and cultures define disease-concepts quite subjective and thus idiosyncratically. In this view there can be no objective guidelin to help decide, say, whether such conditions as addiction to tobacco having had a breast amputated represent diseases or maladies, and th whether smoking clinics or breast reconstruction surgery ought to covered by health insurance. On the other hand, it might be asserted th there are fairly clear and objective universal criteria for defining diseas cepts. It might then follow that the disease- or ady-status of most human conditions can be ›rmined fairly clearly and that these criteria also help explain why a few conditions are y borderline.

'here can also be disagreements, with impor- t implications, among those who believe that ective disease-criteria exist. For example, if believes that a necessary criterion for disease ıe presence of some "abnormality" in physio- ical functioning, then mental conditions such ›hobias and compulsions will probably be ex- ded at the outset. By contrast, if one claims t "abnormal" physiological functioning is not n a criterion for determining whether physi- conditions are considered diseases, then it l be an open question whether and to what ex- t various mental conditions satisfy the actual teria for disease- or malady-status.

We believe that there are objective definitional teria, and that they apply equally to mental l physical conditions. Before presenting these teria, though, we want to discuss the array of lady-terms that exist in the English language. ree of the most important words are "disease," ness," and "injury," but there are many more: ound," "disorder," "defect," "affliction," "le- n," and "disfigurement," to list a few. While se terms have distinct though partly overlap- ıg connotations, which can be identified fairly cisely, there is nevertheless an arbitrary ele- nt in the labeling. For example, most of those nditions regarded as injuries (such as broken nbs) are not called diseases and vice versa ıeasles is not an injury), but it seems impossi- e to construct any definition of disease that es not include injuries. Indeed an occasional thology textbook[1] does use the term "traumatic eases," which is easily comprehensible though t ordinarily used. As an interesting example of e arbitrary nature of this labeling, the condition perienced by deep-sea divers who return from e depths too quickly is referred to either as aisson *disease*" or "decompression *illness*," yet, essentially all the associated ill effects are due to the cellular *injury* caused by nitrogen bubbles forming in various bodily tissues.

Illness and disease are closely related, but diseases—more robust ontologically than ill- nesses—are regarded as entities having charac- teristic signs and symptoms with known or dis- coverable etiologies. Diseases can exist before the appearance of symptoms (for example, a cer- vical cancer detected by a Pap smear), though they nearly always lead to manifest symptoms. In illnesses, by contrast, symptoms are predominant and the underlying pathogenesis is almost ig- nored; for example, it seems appropriate to speak of a "disease process" but not of an "illness pro- cess." Thus diseases at a presymptomatic stage (whether cancer or tooth decay) would not gen- erally be regarded as illnesses. And someone who was poisoned (for example, by an overdose of as- pirin) would generally be regarded as being ill but not as having a disease. But this distinction seems to have no logical basis: some infections (which are prototypical examples of diseases) exert their deleterious effects chiefly through the secretion of poisons (toxins).[2]

Many important kinds of conditions do not seem to be diseases, illnesses, or injuries; for ex- ample, an ordinary tension headache or a hernia. A hernia seems more like an injury but that does not seem exactly right. Idiopathic mental retar- dation does not fit any of these three categories. Nor is it clear how to classify someone who is hav- ing an allergic reaction. Even less clear is how to describe someone who has a significant allergy but is now free of any symptoms.

We believe that all illnesses, injuries, diseases, headaches, hernias, and even asymptomatic al- lergies do have something in common, and we propose "malady" as the general term that in- cludes them all. Later we shall offer a more pre- cise definition, but for now we shall mean by mal- ady, roughly, any condition in which there is something wrong with a person.

SOME PAST DEFINITIONS OF DISEASE

There have been many attempts to set out a formal definition of disease, but physicians have only rarely recognized a distinction among disease, illness, injury, and related terms. Consequently, illness is often used interchangeably with disease, and injuries are regarded merely as a subclass of diseases. What most of the following authors have in fact intended to define is what we call a malady, so that in addition to diseases they have included injuries, illnesses, headaches, and the like in their definitions. However, by not realizing what they have done, they have often been misled by one or another particular feature of the term "disease." Some definitions are general, vague, and too inclusive. Thus a pathology textbook states: "Disease is any disturbance of the structure or function of the body or any of its parts; an imbalance between the individual and his environment; a lack of perfect health."[3]

This seems to offer three separate but equivalent definitions. Under the first definition, clipping nails and puberty would be diseases, as well as asymptomatic situs inversus (transposition of the viscera, with the liver on the left and the heart on the right) and being tied to a chair. The second definition is too vague to be of any use, and the third is circular.

A textbook on internal medicine says: "... disease may be defined as a deprivation or lack of ease, a discomfort or an annoyance, or a morbid condition of the body or of some organ or part thereof."[4] There are similar problems here. Of the two separate definitions offered, the first is too sweeping and would include inflation, quarrelsome in-laws, poor television reception, and ill-fitting shoes; while the second is circular and depends on the phrase "morbid condition," which is merely a synonym for "disease." Most books on medicine and pathology make no attempt to define disease, which is appropriate enough since the exercise is irrelevant to their purposes. H ever, it might be said in their defense that thes tempts were probably not meant to be taken seriously.

One cluster of definitions that *is* meant t taken seriously utilizes a dynamic metapho which a person is pictured as constantly inter ing and adapting to changes in the environm disease then corresponds to a failure in that a tation. An early expression is found in Will White's 1926 book, *The Meaning of Disease:*

> Disease can only be that state of the organ that for the time being, at least, is fighting a lo game whether the battle be with temperat water, microorganisms, disappointment or w not. In any instance, it may be visualized as reaction of the organism to some sort of ene impact, addition, or deprivation.[5]

Thus one wrestler held down by another is fering from a disease.

A more modern version is found in Geo Engel's *Psychological Development in Hea and Disease:*

> When adaptation or adjustment fail and the existing dynamic steady state is disrupted, the state of disease may be said to exist until a r balance is restored which may again permit effective interaction with the environment.[6]

Aside from the ambiguities and the questi begging inherent in "adaptation" and "balanc the emphasis in this definition (and the prec ing one) on the deterioration of a previous m normal state seems to rule out all congenital a hereditary diseases.

J. G. Scadding has written a series of pape concerned with the definition of disease, in most recent of which he offers the following "f mal definition":

> A disease is the sum of the abnormal phenome displayed by a group of living organisms in as ciation with a specified common characteristic

:t of characteristics by which they differ from the orm for their species in such a way as to place iem at a biological disadvantage.[8]

;cadding's definition is a step forward. He very licitly introduces the notion of deviation from orm for a species which, though it does not de- e the prominence he gives it, is necessary for lerstanding the essential elements of the con- t of malady. His "biological disadvantage" cri- on also points in the right direction, but is too ue. R. E. Kendell, in a recent paper, interprets ological disadvantage" as meaning decreased ility or longevity.[9] But even Kendell recog- es that his revision of Scadding's definition ves one with the "rather disconcerting" result t a condition such as psoriasis would not qual- as a disease.

Several recent authors have also correctly ntified aspects of disease. Robert Spitzer and n Endicott[10] include in their definition of "a dical disorder" that it is intrinsically associated h distress, disability, or certain types of disad- ıtage. We think they are on the right track. nald Goodwin and Samuel Guze[11] consider a disease "any condition associated with dis- mfort, pain, disability, death, or an increased li- lity to these states, regarded by physicians and public as properly the responsibility of the dical profession." We agree with the first part their definition but will show later the second rt ("regarded by physicians . . .") is not neces- y. Many of these points were anticipated by ster King in a fine older paper, in which he in- rporates both the notions of various evils and e deviation from a norm in his discussion of dis- se.[12]

THE DEFINITION OF MALADY

aving something wrong: maladies and evils. We e not providing an entirely new account of "dis- se" or "malady," just a more precise and systematic one than has been provided before. In a sense we are going to determine what a malady is by seeing what it is for a person to have something wrong with himself or herself. Briefly, to have something wrong with oneself is to have a condition, other than one's rational beliefs or desires,[13] such that one is suffering or has an increased probability of suffering some evil. Further, whatever its original cause, this condition must now be part of oneself, and hence cannot be removed simply by changing one's physical or social environment.

In this section we shall focus on that aspect of maladies that links them so intimately with the suffering of evils. It is important to note that as we use the term, "evil" has no moral connotations; one could substitute the term "harm" for "evil" as in "make sure no harm comes to him." Many accounts of disease have linked the concept very closely to death, pain, or disability. But in none of these accounts has there been any attempt to draw out the apparently obvious but unexplained common feature.

It may seem odd to ask the question "What do death, pain, and disability have in common?" but in fact it is an important question. Part of the problem is that it seems so obvious that death, pain, and disability go together that no attention has been paid to explaining what they have in common.

Apples, peaches, pears, and plums are all fruits, but what is the genus of which death, pain, and disability are species? The answer is: no one wants them. In fact everyone wants to avoid them. Thus what unites death, pain, and disability is the attitude that people take toward them. But there are times when persons actually seek death, and willingly endure pain or disability. Generally these times occur when something else has gone wrong; that is, persons seek death when life has become too painful, or they endure pain or disability to save their own lives or the lives of those they love. Thus a qualification must be added: all persons avoid death, pain, and disability, *unless they have some reason not to avoid them.*

As we use the term, "reasons" are conscious beliefs that can be used to justify—make rational—actions that would otherwise be irrational. We have already indicated some things that will count as reasons, for example, beliefs that someone will avoid death, pain, and disability. But beliefs that someone will avoid loss of freedom, opportunity, or pleasure also count as reasons, as do beliefs that someone will gain increased abilities, freedom, opportunity, or pleasure. Note that not all reasons are egoistic; beliefs that others will avoid death, pain, and disability also count as reasons.[14]

It now seems as if all persons will avoid death, pain, and disability, unless they have a reason not to do so. But even this is not completely accurate, for some persons sometimes act irrationally and do not avoid, indeed sometimes even seek, death, pain, or disability for no reason, for example, severely depressed persons. We do not deny that there is a psychodynamic explanation for their irrational actions, only that they have any conscious beliefs about benefiting anyone such that their harming themselves counts as acting rationally. We must say then that death, pain, and disability are always avoided by persons acting rationally unless they have a reason not to do so. Though somewhat cumbersome, this description is a sufficient account of what death, pain, and disability have in common and what distinguishes them from almost everything else—for example, books, chemistry, and love. However, we can eliminate this cumbersome description by simply defining an evil (or harm) as "that which all persons acting rationally will avoid unless they have a reason not to." We can now say, as we actually did at the beginning of this discussion, that death, pain, and disability are evils. Evils are the genus of which death, pain, and disability are species. What death, pain, and disability have in common is normative and thus "malady" is a normative term.

In so saying we mean that it is not a matt indifference whether we or someone we car has a malady; maladies are regarded as bad-th to be avoided. But we are not holding the v that what counts as a malady is culturally d mined in a parochial sense, that is, that each ture determines its own unique set of mala Malady is a universal concept. Every society gards death, pain, and disability as evils or har In no society do any rational persons seek th things; rather they all avoid them, unless t have a reason not to. In particular circumstan many societies provide reasons for seeking de pain, or disability through religious or cult beliefs about the benefit to be gained by suffer such an evil. But anthropologists studying a c ture always require some explanation for a practice that involves killing, causing pain to disabling oneself. They do not require expla tions for saving one's own life, relieving one's o pain, or preventing disabilities to oneself.

A malady is a condition that involves the s fering or the increased risk of suffering an e Different societies may not know that a partic condition is a malady because it may be so demic that they regard it as a normal feature the species; but they can be mistaken about th just as they can be mistaken about any other m ter of fact. This is why we cannot include as p of the definition of malady that the condition regarded as the responsibility of the medical p fession. Similarly some societies may consi having a given malady as a good thing, perha because they regard it as a sign of the favor of t gods. This too does not conflict with our analys Someone may have a good reason for having malady but it is still a malady. For example, it m be to a soldier's advantage to be sick when his horts are being picked for a particularly da gerous assignment. Considered simply by itsel malady is normally avoided; we do not de that there are circumstances in which it c come to be regarded as something good. To pu in classical philosophical terms, though maladi intrinsically bad, they can be instrumentally d.

)eath, pain, and disability are not the only c evils. Loss of freedom or opportunity, and of pleasure, must be added to the list. By ı we mean not only physical pain but also the ›leasant feelings of anxiety, sadness, and dis- ısure in their various manifestations. Simi- y, disabilities should not be limited to physical bilities, but should also include mental dis- ities, such as aphasia, and volitional disabili- , such as compulsions and phobias. All the ns on this list are basic evils: every person ing rationally will avoid these things unless he he has some reason not to. Thus, the list of s is not arbitrary but one in which all mem- s share a common feature. The concept of an is not one that is simply developed ad hoc to ount for the concept of a malady.[15]

Iaving something wrong with oneself: mal- es and the absence of distinct sustaining ıses. On our account, not just anything that ıses or increases the risk of suffering an evil is ıalady. One is suffering a malady if and only if evil, or increased risk thereof, one is suffering not in continuing dependence upon causes arly distinct from oneself. (We are also exclud- rational beliefs and desires, for reasons dis- ssed earlier.) We will use the notion of "sus- ning cause" (roughly as used by Aquinas in his ird Proof) to refer to a cause whose effects me and go simultaneously (or nearly so) with its pective presence and absence. Thus a wres- r's hammerlock may be painful, but it is not a lady. Similarly, though being in a runaway car nificantly increases one's risk of incurring in, disability, and death, one is clearly not suf- ing a malady—yet. A smoke-filled room can ıse labored breathing and increase the risk of ffocation; extreme cold can cause pain and the s of ability to move one's limbs easily. Never- eless, these conditions are not maladies. How- er, if these situations affect a person so that he she continues to suffer the evils, or is at increased risk of suffering them, even when these special situations are no longer present, then that person has a malady.

Thus a person suffering a malady must have a condition not sustained by something distinct from himself. The condition may well have been originally caused by factors distinct from the person, but it is not now in a state of continuing dependence on those distinct factors; rather it is present even in their absence. We could say that to be a malady the evil-producing condition must be part of the person. However, for reasons of conceptual rigor, we state it more formally in the negative: the person has a malady if and only if the evil he or she is suffering does *not* have a sustaining cause that is clearly distinct from the person.

Admittedly, distinct sustaining causes cannot be determined without some residual vagueness. Precise simultaneity of cause with its effect, and of deletion of cause with deletion of its effect, are rare. Effects often have slight time lags: a suffocating person might not immediately recover upon receiving sufficient air; or a person in a grossly overheated room might still feel overheated after leaving the room. Nevertheless, in principle the distinction can be made, and practice falls in line. If the time lag before recovery is brief, the person does not have a malady; on the other hand, if it is highly probable that a malady will develop from a current distinct sustaining cause, we may respond as though the malady already existed.

Our account of a clearly distinct sustaining cause may suggest that those causes are always external elements, that is, not inside one's body. However, an increased risk of evil may have a sustaining cause that, though "clearly distinct" from the person, is nevertheless *within* the person; for example, a poison capsule held in the mouth. What if the poison capsule is swallowed but is still undissolved? At what point does a "clearly distinct" sustaining cause become *not* so clearly distinct from the person? For example, suppose a man were dying from poison that had been dissolved, absorbed, and spread throughout his body but that the poison could be quickly removed from his body by some chelating agent which would then very rapidly return him to normal. Would that make the poison a "clearly distinct" sustaining cause and consequently poisoning not a malady? If so the next step might be to consider viruses and bacteria in the same way, namely, as sustaining causes distinct from the person, the removal of which would lead to immediate cure. But that would be absurd, since the presence of these harmful organisms in a person paradigmatically constitutes a malady. When poison, viruses, germs, and the like have become biologically integrated or cannot be removed quickly and easily, then we do not regard them as distinct sustaining causes, but as part of the person.

When the evil-causing element is within the person, two distinct factors determine whether the person has a malady. Is the element biologically integrated? Can it be removed easily and quickly without special skill or equipment? If it is either biologically integrated or not easily and quickly removable, then the person has a malady. Where integration or assimilation of a substance takes place, we always consider it a part of the person: body cells are invaded and interacted with, injury is done, biochemical exchanges take place, body defenses react. On the other hand, it may seem counter-intuitive to regard an unassimilated foreign substance (such as a small marble) as part of the person. Many such items are swallowed, do not actually penetrate the body (do not traverse the gut epithelium) and are excreted harmlessly. However, if the object is causing harm and if its total removal without subsequent detriment is not possible without special skill or equipment, the person has a malady (for example, food caught in the trachea which can only be removed by someone who knows the Heimlich maneuver).

Of course, certain vaguenesses remain because "easily and quickly removable" and "special skill or equipment" are not precise exp sions and may sometimes be subject to cult differences. Nevertheless, they give definite helpful guidance in making distinctions a otherwise confused junction. Thus a tongue pressor or a proctoscope, though causing p would be clearly distinct from the person hence not part of a malady. However a surg patient, with a clamp mistakenly left inside, c ing pain or disability, has a malady since clamp is not easily removable and thus is clearly distinct from the person.

These matters have of course always cau labeling problems. Marbles and clamps, un they are presently causing some evil, are ordi ily simply called "accidents," without refere to disease, malfunctioning, pathology, lesion any of the other malady labels. However, in amining the subtleties of what constitutes a m ady, we are making distinctions at a level ordinarily recognized or considered, so our o nary sense of the language does not give us su cient direction.

Abnormality and distinct sustaining causes is often claimed that one is suffering a malad one is abnormal in either structure or functi We believe that abnormality, though crucial relevant to the concept of malady only indirec as a necessary feature in explaining disability, creased risk, and distinct sustaining cause.[16]

When a person is suffering an evil we deci whether he or she has a malady by determ ing whether members of the species charact istically suffer a similar evil, or increased r thereof, in this environment or circumstan For example, if a woman is suffering because s has walked into a hot boiler room she does have a malady; rather the environment is abn mal and should be regarded as the cause of h suffering. However, if a woman is in modera discomfort because a cat to which she is allerg has walked into the room, then she has a mala because it is she who is, in at least this respect, a normal. Her allergy is the cause of her sufferi ɔur use of cause, which is the ordinary use er than the scientific, we regard the abnormal nent as the cause.

ɔy environment and circumstances we mean se features of the situation that are distinct n the person. It is normal for all persons who e digested a significant amount of cyanide to suffering evils and increased risk of evils, but t does not mean they do not have a malady. e cyanide is no longer distinct from them, ıce their suffering has no distinct sustaining se.

The description of a person's environment or cumstances can be complex and here too the ıcept of abnormality can play a role. Someone ıot in normal circumstances if he or she has eaten for several days. A person who is sufng in these circumstances does not necessarhave a malady. We would determine whether person is suffering from a malady by seewhether changing the circumstances would ner quickly remove the suffering. Thus if after ing a meal, a man who had not eaten for sevl days were no longer suffering any significant effects, then we would regard the evils suffered having had as their sustaining cause not the rson's state but his circumstances. However, if neal did not clear up the problems, then we uld regard the circumstances as having caused hange in the person, so that the evils suffered longer had a distinct sustaining cause, and we uld say that the person had a malady, for exıple, malnutrition.

Abnormality and disability. The concept of disility also depends on abnormality more than it ght originally seem. Is the lack of the ability to lk a disability? The obvious answer seems to be s. But if that answer is accepted, then all infants their first year of life are disabled. In order to oid this conclusion the concept of normality ıst be used to distinguish disabilities from inilities. Infants suffer from an inability to walk ther than a disability. Similarly the lack of abil- to fly is not a disability in humans but an inability. Both inabilities and disabilities involve the lack of abilities, but a lack of ability is an inability rather than a disability if either (1) it is characteristic of the species or of members of the species prior to a certain level of maturation to lack that ability; for example, the lack of ability of humans to fly without mechanical aid, or the lack of ability of infants to walk;[17] or (2) the lack of the ability is due to the lack of some specialized training not naturally provided to all or almost all members of the species; for example, instruction in tennis or chess.

The clearest case of a disability is a person who once had an ability that is characteristic of the species (such as the ability to walk) and then lost it because of a disease or injury. Children born deaf or blind are born disabled and have not lost an ability that they once had; but a woman who, through rigorous training, once had the ability to run a mile in five minutes and then lost that ability by discontinuing training would not thereby be disabled, for having this ability is not characteristic of the species.

We can also distinguish varying levels of an ability. Thus a person may have the ability to walk, but only five or six steps at a time; the ability to speak, but only five or six words; or the ability to see, but only vague shapes and colors. Persons with such very limited abilities are usually thought of as suffering from disabilities. But if a man lacks the ability to walk a mile, is he suffering from a disability? The existence of some person of the same species with no special training who can walk a mile is not sufficient reason to say the first person has a disability. For we know that some people have natural abilities that far outstrip the natural abilities of most of the species, and we would not want to be forced to the conclusion that most of us are therefore suffering from a disability.

This question shows the close connection between the concepts of disability and of normality, or of what is characteristic of the species. Though some clear cases of disability present no problems, such as someone who cannot walk at all, in many cases it is genuinely a matter of decision whether or not to call a low level of an ability a disability. However, there can still be guidelines for making that decision. We know that in the absence of widespread environmentally caused injury or disease, the fact that the vast majority of the members of the species (of the appropriate gender, if relevant) lack an ability shows that such a lack is not a disability but an inability. It is somewhat less clear what percentage of nondiseased, noninjured members of a species must have ever had a specific ability in order to make that ability characteristic of the species and hence the lack of that ability a disability. Notice that the phrase "have ever had a specific ability" is used rather than "have a specific ability": we determine whether an ability is characteristic of the species not by seeing what percentage now have the ability but by seeing what percentage had the ability in their prime.

A simple majority (55 percent) having had the ability to walk ten miles is not sufficient. An overwhelming majority of nondiseased, noninjured members of the species must have had that ability for it to be characteristic of the species. Assuming that the ability to walk is distributed along a normal curve, with the ability to walk a yard, two yards, and so on, up to 100 miles or more representing points on the curve, then clear disabilities will be present when there is some discontinuity at the lower end of the curve, and people below the discontinuity will count as disabled. If there is no discontinuity obviously there will be some arbitrariness in deciding where to draw a line so that those below the line count as disabled while those above it are thought of as simply having minimal abilities. Something like this is already done in general intelligence testing, where 100 denotes average intelligence; those having lesser scores (70–80) are not regarded as mentally disabled (retarded) but merely as having lesser abilities, while those scoring 69 and under are regarded as mentally disabled (retarded) in varying degrees.

We conclude that a person is suffering a ability when he or she lacks an ability that is c acteristic of the species, or when he or she ha extraordinarily low degree of that ability. The tribution of that ability is obtained by detern ing the presence or absence of that degree of a ity in all persons at any time during their pri in the absence of environmentally caused dis or injury. Given the presence of a distributio degrees of ability obtained in this way, some is disabled if he or she is at the extreme lower of the curve. Note that those lacks of ability are due to not having reached the appropr state of maturity must be excluded. Howe once one has reached the state of maturity th is no further relativizing of the concept of abilities. It does not matter if 100 percent of liv ninety-nine-year-old persons lack the ability run; their lack of ability is still a disability. given our decision to count only the extreme end of the curve as disabled, aging will not r mally result in disabilities until the sixties or s enties or later. This seems to us a welcome c clusion, for we do not normally regard those their forties and fifties, with obviously lesser abilities, as being disabled.

Abnormality and increased risk. We h defined malady in such a way that a person only has a malady when suffering an evil with a distinct sustaining cause, but also when at creased risk of suffering some evil without suc cause. Without "increased risk" our account malady would fail to include many conditi that almost everyone regards as maladies, for ample, high blood pressure.

As with disability, one must choose betwe interpreting "increased risk" as increase in r over the previous state of the person or over wh is characteristic of the species, even though the clearest cases they go together. A man w develops high blood pressure has an increas risk of suffering an evil in both senses. Similar a woman who has ingested dioxin, which is n stored in her fat, might not now be suffering a evil but she has significantly increased the risk ı suffering, because dieting or continued sical exertion may cause the fat to become abolized by the body, thus allowing the poi- to take its toll. The woman's risk is increased n over what it was prior to ingesting the dioxin over what is characteristic of the species. wever, if a woman has been in extraordinarily d shape due to some training regimen, in- ding both diet and exercise, and then discon- ıes this regimen, she may come to have a ıter risk of suffering some evil than she did for- rly. But though now at increased risk com- ed with her former state, she may not be at any ater risk of suffering an evil than what is char- eristic of the members of the species in their me. Clearly she does not have a malady. Fur- r, a man may be born with a genetic defect t puts him at increased risk of suffering some compared with what is characteristic of the cies, even though quite clearly it is not in- ased over what it was for him formerly. Such a n would be suffering a malady. Thus "in- ased risk," as the phrase is used in the defini- n of malady, must be understood as "increased r that which is characteristic of members of species," not as increased over what it was for- rly. "Increased risk," like disability, depends on a concept of abnormality. But again abnor- lity does not enter directly into the definition malady, but only indirectly by determining at counts as a disability or an increased risk.

Though our definition of malady makes no ex- cit mention of the severity of the evil suffered, of the significance of the increased risk, actual age does take these matters into account. We distinguish between major maladies (for ex- ıple, terminal cancer, a broken leg, or severe graine headaches), minor maladies (for exam- e, a mild case of German measles, a sprained umb, or a mild tension headache) and those nditions in which the evil is so slight and tran- ory that one may prefer not to regard it as a mal- y at all (for example, a slight reaction to a vac- ne or a slightly stiff muscle due to a hard ɔrkout). There are structural deviations that are not associated with any increased risk of evil at all, and hence are not maladies, such as the absence of one's appendix.

Similarly, there are at least two kinds of pragmatic considerations that influence where, along the continuum of increasing risk, the label "malady" should be applied. First, how severe will this evil be if it does occur? If it will be slight we tend to require a significantly increased risk before labeling the condition a malady. However, if it might be severe, we accept a much lower probability of occurrence. Second, can we help prevent the evil from occurring? If early treatment would result in lessened risk or lessen the severity of the evil if it did occur, we would be much more likely to label the condition a malady.

Abnormality and the other evils: loss of pleasure and loss of freedom or opportunity. The evils (or increased risk thereof) most commonly present in maladies are death, pain, and disability. However, as we saw earlier, there are other evils—the loss of pleasure and the loss of freedom or opportunity.

Although the loss of pleasure (anhedonia) can be a distinct symptom of schizophrenia (and is distinguishable from the negative feelings of sadness or anxiety), its presence is neither necessary nor sufficient for making the diagnosis of schizophrenia. However, were there a human condition characterized solely by the loss of pleasure (perhaps secondary to some stroke of the limbic system), it would qualify as a malady according to our definition.

Loss of freedom or opportunity is an evil not uncommonly encountered in life but most frequently it is due to a distinct sustaining cause. A man locked up in jail is suffering from a loss of freedom, but he does not thereby have a malady, for it is clear that his loss of freedom has a distinct sustaining cause. Similarly, a woman threatened with violence unless she refrains from an action is not regarded as having a malady, for her loss of freedom has a distinct sustaining cause—the threat of violence by another. However, there are interesting cases where the threat of harm is due not to the actions of another, but to something about oneself. There is no question, for instance, that when one is suffering from an allergic reaction, one has a malady. But what about those times when one is not exposed to the allergen? There may still be an increased risk of suffering an evil because of the allergy. But if it is relatively easy to avoid the allergen, it does not seem accurate to say that one is really at increased risk. However, no matter how easy it is to avoid eating fish or fava beans, one still lacks the freedom to eat these items.

The man who moves to Arizona to be free of allergic reactions has avoided the pain and discomfort usually associated with his allergy, but he still suffers from a loss of freedom or opportunity to live in certain parts of the country and therefore has a malady.[18] Even if he has no desire to leave Arizona so that he is not bothered by his loss of freedom, he still has lost that freedom, just as a prisoner with a life sentence who wants to stay in jail has still lost his freedom.

Both abnormality and the loss of freedom and opportunity play an important role in the case of serious disfigurement. Though serious disfigurement almost always causes psychological suffering, anxiety, and/or depression, we wish to regard someone suffering from such disfigurement as having a malady even in those very rare cases when he or she is not suffering psychologically. Serious disfigurement is a malady because in a normal environment one is deprived of some freedom or opportunity, even though in a special environment one may feel no actual loss. Note that simply by labeling the condition as serious disfigurement we are making a judgment that the person's appearance is significantly outside some norm. Since we count something as a serious disfigurement only if it would cause, at least initially, an unfavorable reaction in others, we regard serious disfigurement as a malady because it either causes the loss of freedom and opportunity, or increases the risk of such a loss. Thus in this case we are regarding the reactions of others as normal and hence we are not regarding thei action as the key element in the loss of free or opportunity; rather the key element is the ous disfigurement of the person and hence the cause of the loss of freedom or opportu

We realize that if serious disfigurement is garded as a malady and if there is no way to a at least some cultural differences in what is c sidered seriously disfiguring, maladies will so times differ in different cultures. But even in case of disfigurement, cultural relativity will be important in the marginal or borderline c of maladies, not in the central or core examp We do not think it culture-bound to hold there is often still something wrong with sev burn victims, even if they have recovered all th abilities and are no longer in pain. We reg treatment of their serious disfigurement as tr ment of a malady.

Another kind of difficult case is that of so one who formerly suffered a chronic mal which is now perfectly controlled by availa therapy so that he is no longer suffering o increased risk of suffering an evil. For examp consider a man with hypothyroidism. If it w possible to implant a lifetime supply of co pletely safe and effective replacement hormo should we count him as having a malady? So we have few medications or artificial organs health aids that completely eliminate all e and any increased risk. Thus at present alm everyone who depends upon continuing i planted medication or artificial implants will h a malady according to our definition. Howev as technology improves, the situation we are n only imagining may become common. Do want to say that such persons, whose evils and creased risk thereof have been eliminated by co tinuing treatment, do not have maladies? On o account, if the artificial aid were in the body would say they have no malady.[19] However, they were dependent on external medication would say they still have a malady since this e ternal source limits their freedom.

DVANTAGES OF HE DEFINITION

at are the conceptual advantages of our ac-nt of malady? One advantage is the introduc- of a general word—malady—which refers to genus of which all the related conditions h as disease, illness, dysfunction, handicap, ury, sickness) are species. The term malady, ugh more general than the commonly used ns, is nevertheless explicit, precise, and us-e.

person has a malady if and only if he or she a condition, other than a rational belief or de-, such that he or she is suffering, or at increased of suffering, an evil (death, pain, disability, of freedom or opportunity, or loss of pleasure) he absence of a distinct sustaining cause.

The concept of malady can be universal and ective and at the same time have values as an egral part, namely, those values that are uni-sal. Thus our explication shows the inade-acy of the current fashion of regarding disease being heavily determined by subjective, cul-al, and ideological factors.[20] We have also tried show the logic of cultural influences in those instances where they do occur.

One possible ambiguity about our claim to iversality and objectivity should be clarified. me might claim that diseases are simply hu-n inventions or human constructs, that "dis-se" is the way humans construe some of na-e's processes that they do not like. Nature in elf, independent of human interests, has no eases, they would say. For them "objective" d "universal" would seem to mean "in the na-re of reality," or "true of the world apart from human mind." Now, what the world is like art from the existence of humans and from a man's knowing of it, we would not venture to . But a second and more important sense of mething's being objective is that there is agree-ent about it by all rational persons. Colors are t objective in the first sense but they are in the second. It is in this second sense that the evils are objective and universal. Just as all rational persons agree on the color of most objects, they also agree that certain things are to be avoided unless one has a reason not to. Both matters are universal and objective, not based on personal or subjective influences but on features common to all rational persons.

The concept of a distinct sustaining cause allows us to limit what counts as a malady to what seems intuitively accurate: namely, to those conditions of the person that are not dependent upon a continuing environmental state. Additionally, incorporating the notion of "increased risk" in our account of a malady allows us to include as maladies such conditions as high blood pressure,

Our explication is also meant to clarify the role of abnormality. Abnormality is often taken as central to the concept of malady but it actually plays a less direct role, that is, it helps us decide what counts as a disability, an increased risk, or a distinct sustaining cause. There has been a general tendency in the medical-scientific world to establish a normal range for this or that (some element of the human body), and ipso facto to have "discovered" two new maladies—hyper-this or that and hypo-this or that.[21] Our account makes it clear that this use of abnormality represents a misunderstanding of the concept of malady.

Our account of malady is based on elucidating the common elements in such conditions as disease, and so on, illness, injury, and so on. Using pain, death, and disability, along with the absence of a distinct sustaining cause as necessary features of any malady, considerably lessens the influence of ideologies, politics, and self-serving goals in manipulating malady labels. We do not mean to suggest that our concept of a malady is without vagueness. Indeed we have discussed some of the difficult cases. But now we know more precisely where those gray areas are, why they exist, and what variables would have to be decided to resolve the question in particular cases.

A more subtle benefit of this new technical sense of malady is that it is the first explicit term in any language with the appropriately high level of generality. No language that we have investigated (English, French, German, Russian, Chinese, or Hebrew) contains a clearly recognized genus term of which disease and injury are species terms. Each term in the usual cluster of malady terms has specific connotations that guide and significantly narrow its use. Of course, that is as it should be if specificity is what is desired and justified. Disease, injury, illness, dysfunction, and other such terms overlap somewhat, yet each has its own distinct connotations.

A final advantage of our explication is that its basic elements, concepts, principles, and arguments are the same when applied to mental maladies as to physical ones. Pain, disability, and the absence of distinct sustaining causes are applicable to the psychological domain as well as to the physical. We expect that our analysis will help draw critical distinctions in the realm of "mental illness" labeling, but this must remain a promissory note to be redeemed later.[22]

NOTES

1. Thomas M. Peery and Frank N. Miller, *Pathology*. 2nd ed. (Boston: Little, Brown, 1971).

2. A number of philosophers have distinguished illness from disease but we do not think this distinction is relevant to the point that concerns us here. See, however, Christopher Boorse, "On the Distinction Between Disease and Illness," *Philosophy and Public Affairs* 5 (1975): 49–68; H. Tristram Engelhardt, Jr., "Ideology and Etiology," *Journal of Medicine and Philosophy* 1 (1976): 256–68; and Joseph Margolis, "The Concept of Disease," *Journal of Medicine and Philosophy* 1 (1976): 238–55.

3. Peery and Miller, *Pathology*, p. 1.

4. Peter J. Talso and Alexander P. Remenchik, *Internal Medicine* (St. Louis: C. V. Mosby, 1968).

5. William A. White, *The Meaning of Disease* (Baltimore: Williams and Wilkins, 1926).

6. George L. Engel, *Psychological Developme[nt in] Health and Disease* (Philadelphia: Saunders, 1[…]

7. J. G. Scadding, "Principles of Definition in M[edi]cine with Special Reference to Chronic Bronchitis [and] Emphysema," *Lancet* 1 (1959): 323–25; "Meaning o[f Di]agnostic Terms in Bronchopulmonary Disease," *Br[itish] Medical Journal* 2 (1963): 1425–30; "Diagnosis: [The] Clinician and the Computer," *Lancet* 2 (1967): 877[…]

8. Scadding, "Diagnosis," p. 877.

9. R. E. Kendell, "The Concept of Disease an[d …] Implications for Psychiatry," *British Journal of Psyc[hia]try* 127 (1975): 305–15.

10. Robert L. Spitzer and Jean Endicott, "Med[ical] and Mental Disorder: Proposed Definition and C[rite]ria," in Robert L. Spitzer and Donald F. Klein (e[ds.]) *Critical Issues in Psychiatric Diagnosis* (New Y[ork:] Raven, 1978), pp. 15–39.

11. Donald W. Goodwin and Samuel B. Guze, *[Psy]chiatric Diagnosis*. 2nd ed. (New York: Oxford Uni[ver]sity Press. 1979).

12. Lester S. King, "What Is Disease?" *Philosoph[y of] Science* 21 (1954): 193–203.

13. We exclude rational beliefs and desires from evil-causing conditions that count as maladies beca[use] we do not think a man has something wrong with h[im]self if he has a rational belief, e.g., that his wife is dy[ing] of cancer, that causes him pain, or if he has a ratio[nal] desire, e.g., to go mountain climbing, that increases [the] risk of death and disability.

14. See Bernard Gert, *The Moral Rules*. 2nd [ed.] (New York: Harper & Row, 1975), chapter 2, for a fu[ller] discussion of reasons and rational action.

15. For a fuller account of evils, see Gert, chap[…]

16. Thus we disagree significantly with Boorse w[ho] makes abnormality the central feature of disease. S[ee] Christopher Boorse, "Health as a Theoretical C[on]cept," *Philosophy of Science* 44 (1977): 542–73.

17. There are also sexual differences which are ch[ar]acteristic of the species so that it is an inability that m[…] cannot bear children. See also Boorse, "Health a[s a] Theoretical Concept."

18. Thus we disagree with Spitzer and Endicott w[ho] explicitly regard such a person as not having a medi[cal] disorder (malady).

). Metal plates surgically implanted to cover bony cts in the skull do seem to constitute the elimina-of a malady. Suppose a pacemaker were developed resulted in no increased risk. Then a defective emaker would be part of a malady if its malfunc-ing were directly causing evils or increased risk of s. Though this may seem at first counter-intuitive, suspect it is because the use of synthetic or man-le materials integrated into the human body is rel-ely novel, and our language has not yet adjusted. It 1 advantage of our concept of malady that it will er the malfunctioning, breaking, decomposition, or clogging of pacemakers, artificial hips, synthetic materials, or trans-species arteries.

20. Cf. Peter Sedgwick, "Illness—Mental or Otherwise," *Hastings Center Studies* 1 (1973): 19–40.

21. Edmond A. Murphy, *The Logic of Medicine* (Baltimore: Johns Hopkins University Press, 1976); Alan Bailey, David Robinson, and A. M. Dawson, "Does Gilbert's Disease Exist?" *Lancet* 1 (1977): 931–33.

22. Preparation of this paper was aided by NEH grant 21041-75-79 (Prof. Clouser), and NEH NSF grant OSS-8018088 sustained development award (Prof. Gert).

CHAPTER 11

Health: A Comprehensive Concept

ROBERTO MORDACCI AND
RICHARD SOBEL

"IF WE DEVOTE OURSELVES to findi holes exactly shaped to house such great words as Freedom, Honour, Bl we shall spend a lifetime slipping, and sliding and searching and all in va They are words without a home, wanderers like the planets, and that is t end of it."[1]

One might assume that just as grocers know what they mean by groceri so health care providers surely must have a clear concept of health in mi when they use this great word. *Health* is one of those everyday slippery- mercury words, the meaning of which seems so obvious and self-evide that we seldom take a few moments to define the term consciously for ou selves. This is unfortunate because we cannot: (1) recognize which of o ents' expectations are authentically medical, identify the appropriate role of physicians n increasingly technological profession, and understand the interrelationships of health, dicine, and the good life. Along with our pa- ts, we share an amorphous idea of what it is to healthy beyond simply being "well-function- "[2]: a clear concept of health could add some n and substance to this vague awareness.

Descriptions of health based on physiological asurements ignore the idea of health as a le. What they offer in precision, they lack in oth; for, surely, being healthy is much more n having all your organs quietly functioning hin plus or minus two standard deviations of mal. Value-free descriptivist definitions of lth cannot be more than a component of a nprehensive concept of health, for health is ued. Health is a value beyond formalizable owledge. However, value-based definitions of lth lack universality; they depend on the indi- ual's (or a culture's) determination of what o be valued. Descriptivist definitions ignore subjective dimension, whereas normativist finitions exalt it.

The World Health Organization defined alth as "a state of complete physical, mental d social well-being and not merely the absence disease or infirmity."[3] This definition, if taken erally, is meaningless. However, we believe that normativist definitions of health, including s hopelessly utopian WHO vision, derive from common ground, a core meaning or experi- ce of health that requires interpretation.[4]

HEALTH

y experienced clinician can recall a terminally patient who objectively seemed the same the y he died as the day before except for having ften quite explicitly) lost his will to live. Im- cit in this will to live, and of special impor- nce to the secular individual, is a sense of life being worth living despite all the suffering one may encounter in life and despite the awareness of the certainty of death and nothingness.

> How admirable!
> to see lightning and not think life
> is fleeting (Basho)[5]

The healthy individual is well-functioning as a whole, in harmony physically and mentally with himself and with his surroundings. A clue to this wholeness characteristic of health can be found in words related to health. The question, *ma shlomcha*—how are you?— in Hebrew literally asks if you are whole, intact, complete, at peace. The Old English *hal*, the Old High German *heil*, and the Greek *hygeia* and *euexia* connect health and hygiene to fullness and to the good life. Other words, the Italian *salute*, the French *santé*, the Spanish *salud*, introduce another characteristic of health—salvation. To be healthy is to be "saved" from death. The Hebrew word for health uses the same root, *het*, *resh*, *aleph*, as the word for create, the opposite of death. Health thus is a good in itself, an end—something whole, harmonious, good—a fragile salvation.

LIFE NARRATIVE

But health is more than an end. The same words that hint at salvation also refer to the Judeo-Christian idea of plenitude: a hoped for full life as the ultimate good. Health can be seen as a means, a foundation for achievement,[6] as a first achievement itself (and thus a promise of further achievement), and as a necessary premise for further achievement. Health offers the possibility of blossoming.

Although we tend to speak of health as though it were a commodity—something to be lost or regained—it is not detached from the person it belongs to. It is part of the person's life story. Health is dynamic; it has a past, and a present, and it is a precondition for a future. Desire, without which there is no story, belongs to the future—there lies the hoped for full blossoming of life. Thus there seems to be a sort of inevitable metaphysics embedded in the experience and language of health and illness, which calls for awareness and for careful analysis in the light of an adequate characterization of the concepts we use. It is extremely important for medicine to be conscious of the depth of our desire for health and our fear of illness: they are not only physical or biopsychological conditions that can be faced in a reductionistic approach. The existential, moral, and symbolic dimensions of the experience of illness must be addressed as challenges the patient is required to face with his cultural, personal, and religious resources, and in which the physician is asked to help him not only as a physician but as a person. No technical answer can help the patient to understand and face the existential dimensions of health and illness: in this respect, the education physicians now receive in many countries around the world (and especially in the West) seriously limits their ability to care for their patients.

Current dogma holds that health is silent or, as Renée Leriche put it, health is the "life in the silence of the organs."[7] Italo Svevo expressed the same thought in Zeno's paradox: "health does not analyze itself, neither it looks at itself in the mirror. Only we sick people do know something about ourselves."[8] Is health transparent, not something of which we are consciously aware, whereas disease is visible, palpable, self-conscious? Certainly, to become ill is to become aware of life's limitations and of one's vulnerability.

We wonder though whether health, as such, is ever experienced, even if at an inarticulate level. Surely the fetus is in a state of near plenitude—desire is absent and all needs are met. Might this state be wordlessly sensed and imprinted in the fetal nervous system and then recalled in an inchoate way in one of those brief moments when life seems perfect?

MALADY

The totality of health is encroached upon crushed by "malady," causing the loss of he and threatening the will to live.[9] We use *ma* as an umbrella term to cover both illness, the dividual's suffering described in the first per and disease, the third-person medically codi translation of suffering. One can be ill with being diseased, diseased without feeling ill both ill and diseased. Maladies are obstacles, c ing off the opening to the possibility of plenitu A flower does not bloom and wither at the sa time; death and plenitude are incompatible p opposites *if taken simultaneously at the same l of meaning;* in some religious traditions, eter death is not just the absence of biological l but rather the loss of any contact with the sou of meaning and, therefore, of real, eternal (which is another way of characterizing ple tude). Thus one can be said to be dead while ing, and to live while dead.

However, health is not an ideal absolute one either has in its entirety or does not have all. Health and malady are mutually compati one can have a sickness yet be otherwise healt It can be remarkably difficult to answer the see ingly simple question, Is so and so healthy? deed, one can think of acquaintances with jor congenital defects, for example, who are whole and well-functioning despite their disa ity, that one does not see the defect but only th health. And one can equally easily think of a p son who feels well and appears contented ev though dementia has erased time, place, frien and family, and reduced a life narrative to r dom words amidst ellipses.

To speak of health and death in the sa breath—to suggest that by this concept of hea a dying patient could be described as healt except for his terminal illness—would be obscene joke. Yet what is meant by dying peace? Have you not seen a patient, reconciled death, experience at least moments of seren- There is a wholeness akin, in a transcenden- sense, to healing in these moments. Is this it the dying poet-surgeon George Bascom ex- ssed in his poem "Nocturne"?

Jnderstand
'm running out of time for
Triviality and cleverness.
Dying takes some thought.
At night, lying behind closed lid
And the soft safe comfort
Of the bed and God,
find a peace that seems
To lead toward timelessness;
Toward—can it be so?—a state
Where space and eons do not matter,
Where the beginning and the end
Are close as near
Are part of it.[10]

One's life narrative is now a story of illness. e core experience of illness threatens the sense iving because the promise of life in all its full- ss is seen as an illusion—the desire for pleni- le is recognized as unattainable.[11] The sick in- idual suffers isolation, loss of wholeness, loss certainty, loss of freedom to act, loss of the fa- liar world; the future is in doubt and all atten- n is concentrated on the present. When ill, we longer trust our bodies and, at an existential el, we no longer trust life.

There is a whole genre of literature, the illness rrative[12] or pathography,[13] that can be inter- eted as an archetypical "regeneration para- gm," seventeenth century spiritual autobiogra- y updated to twentieth century pathography. "I ned" (smoked), "was punished" (suffered a art attack), "was saved" (had a coronary bypass) d now I am a new and better person; I am aled even if not cured. A person, having sur- ved a dangerous journey through sickness, often gins a quest for explanation, meaning, and en reward. In an illness narrative titled "My Old and My New Lives" the author tells us he has become a new and better person in a world "more precious than ever" since his stroke.[14] He is no longer a "monster"[15]—he has been reborn as a changed individual. Something beyond the mere restitution of health has happened; there is now "the promise of a new, a more abundant, life."[16] The powerful desire for plenitude has been transfigured; it is now the fulfillment of the reflective life and not the rewards of the "type A" person that is desired. Even when health is not re- stored, and especially when the illness becomes a serious threat to life itself, the question that ill- ness poses is one about the proportion of reality to reason and desire. What we need is the material to create a meaningful texture for our mortality, and the cultural premises to engage in the task of making sense of the excruciating experience we are living.[17] The possibility for us to tell a story about our illness rests on the availability of com- municable meanings that can give an acceptable sense to our frailty, to which we can give our as- sent. We cannot be storytellers of our illness if our culture is deprived of any useful contents for that purpose; this is the tragedy of an exclusively tech- nological culture. The patient is left alone, as Arthur Frank says, just at the moment "when our capacity for telling one's own story is re- claimed."[18]

PATHOGENS

Pathogenic factors may cause or worsen maladies or may affect health independently of any influence on malady. Pathogenic factors may be biological, genetic, family related, social, eco- nomic, educational, or environmental. Abusive parents, the wrong peer pressure, the wrong neighborhood to grow up in, poor schooling, lead fumes in the environment, hatefulness, guilt—anything that closes off the possibility of life as a good, any obstacle to the achievements that one could have fulfilled can be considered a pathogenic factor. Few of these factors have anything to do with disease, physicians, or the territory of medicine. Pathogenic viruses, or bacteria, a diet high in saturated fat, smoking, excessive alcohol, a defective immune system cause maladies that disable individuals. Many of these maladies are effectively treated or prevented by physicians, but disease may be the least important of an individual's global health problems. A hoped for good life may be foreclosed not by disability but by a lack of ability or by some other obstacle quite unrelated to medical problems. The province of physicians is disability, not ability; we prevent and treat disease, we don't build better housing, arrange for piano lessons, or tutor in calculus. This does not excuse us from being very much aware of, and attentive to, the many nonmedical pathogens. On the contrary, to the extent that we ignore these factors because they are not our responsibility, we are diminished as physicians and as human beings. There is an enormous gap between saying "that is not my problem" and "that is not my problem but. . . ."

SALUTOGENS

Just as there are factors that destroy health, so there are factors that support, enhance, and produce health. Aaron Antonovsky labeled these factors "salutogens."[19] Freedom of choice is salutogenic. If one's basic needs are met, this is salutogenic. Certain personality characteristics are salutogens: curiosity, optimism, adaptability, a sense of humor, the capacity to love and to establish a durable intimate relationship with a fellow creature, whether human being or animal. Mortality in secular kibbutzim is considerably higher than in religious kibbutzim. Among the proposed explanations is the possibly stronger sense of coherence—a major salutogenic factor—in religious kibbutzim. There may be a greater tendency to see life as comprehensible, problems as manageable, life as meaningful, and to feel a greater sense of belonging. Of course, many secular individuals have no less coherent a w
view and sense of belonging—a certain (o
difficult to justify) confidence that things
work out. All this enhances health, strength
the will to live, and nourishes the sense in liv

A good world—
the dew drops fall
by one, by two (Issa)[20]

Few, if any of the salutogenic factors have a
thing directly to do with medicine or physici
When we treat or prevent a disease, we are sa
togenic; but the list of salutogenic factors has
prisingly little to do with physicians.

Health as wholeness, harmony, and well-fu
tioning, and as salvation from death is a desira
end in itself. However, the crux of a concep
health, and its greater meaning or value, is he
as a means. Health is viewed as *the experienc
life as a promise of good*; the ultimate good th
hoped for is the full life—this we refer to as pl
itude. Although this is similar to Seedhou
concept of health as a foundation for achie
ment, the idea of plenitude avoids the necessa
materialistic nuance of the term achieveme

Cultures that understand health and illn
almost exclusively in biopsychological te
prevent the deepest levels of understanding
what illness means to us. Such a culture's me
cine loses its capacity to understand the patien
a person. Having excluded the moral and sy
bolic meanings from sight, the obvious attitu
will be to medicalize the desire for health. T
recent crisis of modern medicine, notwithsta
ing all its success, should make us aware of t
urgent need to understand our relation to illn
as something other than the technological fi
against it, and our relations to health as som
thing other than the attempt to produce perf
human beings. Thus not only a redefinition
the goals of medicine is in order, but an atten
to analyze our different traditions to regain th
forgotten dimensions of health and illness
which our languages still bear traces) and to s

t a postmodern culture can retain or even e as a starting point for a new understanding. o hold a relativistic position, in this respect, ld only beg the question. We do not want just e aware that there are so many constitutions ense in which health and illness could be inbed; rather we want to construe *a sense that an believe to be true* and that we can commuate to others as something *believable*, reasone enough, and proportionate to our will for senting to it.

Vhat a strange thing!
o be alive
eneath cherry blossoms (Issa)[21]

NOTES

. J. M. Coetzee, *Foe* (New York: Penguin Books, 6), p. 145.

. Leon Kass, "Regarding the End of Medicine and Pursuit of Health," *Public Interest* 40, no. 1 (1975): 42.

. World Health Organization, "1946 Preamble to Constitution Adopted by the International Health nference, New York 1946," in *The First Ten Years of WHO* (Geneva: World Health Organization, 1958).

4. Roberto Mordacci, "Health as an Analogical Cont," *Journal of Medical Philosophy* 20, no. 5 (1995): –97.

5. Robert Hass, ed., *The Essential Haiku* (Hopewell, .: Ecco Press, 1994), p. 24.

6. David Seedhouse, *Health: The Foundation for hievement* (Chichester: J. Wiley & Sons, 1986).

7. Renée Leriche, *Philosophie de la chiurgie* (Paris: Flammarion, 1951).

8. Italo Svevo, *The Confessions of Zeno* (New York: Vintage Books, 1958).

9. K. Danner Clouser, Charles M. Culver, and Bernard Gert, "Malady: New Treatment of Disease," *Hastings Center Report* 11, no. 3 (1981): 29–37.

10. George S. Bascom, "Nocturne," in *Medicine Circle* (Kansas: Sunflower University Press, 1993).

11. S. Kay Toombs, "The Meaning of Illness: A Phenomenological Approach to the Patient-Physician Relationship," *Journal of Medicine and Philosophy* 12 (1987): 219–40.

12. Arthur W. Frank, "Reclaiming an Orphan Genre: The First-Person Narrative of Illness," *Literature and Medicine* 13, no. 1 (1994): 1–21.

13. Ann Hawkins, "A Change of Heart: The Paradigm of Regeneration in Medical and Religious Narrative," *Perspectives on Biology and Medicine* 33, no. 4 (1990): 547–59.

14. Robert McCrum, "My Old and My New Lives," *New Yorker* (May 27, 1996): 112–19.

15. Hawkins, "A Change of Heart."

16. Toombs, "The Meaning of Illness."

17. Daniel Callahan, *The Troubled Dream of Life: Living with Mortality* (New York: Simon & Schuster, 1993).

18. Arthur W. Frank, *The Wounded Storyteller* (Chicago: University of Chicago Press, 1995).

19. Aaron Antonovsky, *Unraveling the Mystery of Health* (San Francisco: Jossey-Bass, 1987).

20. Hass, *The Essential Haiku*, p. 156.

21. Ibid., p. 178.

CHAPTER 12

The Distinction between Mental an Physical Illness

R. E. KENDELL

CONDITIONS THAT NOW WOULD be garded as "mental illnesses," such as mania, melancholia and hyster have figured in classifications of disease since the time of Hippocrates, a for over 2000 years were treated by physicians with much the same range potions, medicaments and attempts to correct humoral imbalance as th employed for other more obviously medical disorders. Although Plato tributed some forms of madness to the Gods, and medieval theologians li Thomas Aquinas attributed hallucinations and insanity to demons a other supernatural influences, from the Renaissance to the second half the 18th century melancholia and other forms of insanity were generally garded as bodily illnesses, not differing in any fundamental way from oth ases. When the mid-18th century belle let-e Lady Mary Wortley Montagu commented "madness is as much a corporeal distemper ıe gout or asthma," she was simply expressing "commonplace of high and low, lay and med-opinion alike" (Porter 1987, 39).

)RIGINS OF THE)ISTINCTION

e idea that insanity was fundamentally differ-from other illnesses, that it was a disease of the ıd rather than the body, only developed to-rds the end of the 18th century. The scene was by Cartesian dualism, the dominant philo-hical influence of the time, but medical opin-ı and medical impotence also played crucial es. The development first of private mad-ıses and later of large, purpose-built lunatic lums took the management of the insane out he hands of the general run of physicians; and cause the managers of these new institutions re concerned only with insanity it was rela-ely easy for them to regard it as different from er illnesses that did not concern them. At the ne time it was becoming clear that insanity s not accompanied by the obvious pathologi-ı changes that post-mortem examination was ealing in other diseases. It was increasingly parent also that although the armamentarium 18th century medicine—special diets, bleed-g, purging, emetics and blistering—was as ef-tive in the management of hypochondriasis d hysteria as it was in other disorders, it had le effect on madness itself. In England the ccess of the clergyman Francis Willis in curing e King (George III) of his madness after the nspicuous failure of his physicians to do so, d the remarkable success of the York Retreat pened by the Quaker William Tuke in 1796) calming and curing its inmates despite using w medicaments or restraints, both had a con-lerable influence on public opinion. It was in this climate that the terms "disease of the mind," "disorder of the mind," and "mental illness" first began to be widely used. Indeed, the York Retreat was explicitly for "persons afflicted with disorders of the mind" (Hunter & Macalpine 1963).

The implication of these new terms was that madness was a disease of the mind, not of the body, and there was some debate whether diseased minds might not be better treated by philosophers than by physicians. "Moral treatment"—a benevolent, ordered regime based on moderation and religious observance rather than medication—became the mainstay of the new asylums that were built in the early years of the 19th century, and initially several of them had no physician. It was not long, though, before the medical profession reasserted itself. In Philadelphia, Benjamin Rush (1812) insisted that the fundamental pathology of what he himself referred to as "disease of the mind" was somatic (he suggested that it lay "primarily in the blood vessels of the brain") and in 1845 Wilhelm Griesinger, the first professor of psychiatry, convinced most of his German contemporaries when he argued in his influential textbook that "Psychische Krankheiten sind Erkrankungen des Gehirns" (mental illnesses are diseases of the brain). By the middle of the 19th century it was also generally accepted that the superintendent of any properly run lunatic asylum should be a physician. But the terms mental illness and mental disease survived, partly because they clearly implied that what had previously been called madness or insanity was medical territory. The doubts about causation also survived, even within the medical profession itself. Indeed, the school of psychoanalysis that emerged at the end of the 19th century regarded all mental illnesses as entirely psychogenic disorders to be treated by psychotherapy; and until the 1930s mental disease remained largely uninfluenced by the physician's pharmacopoeia and, apart from general paresis, could not be shown to be accompanied by any cerebral pathology, macroscopic or microscopic.

The failure to find any somatic pathology underlying many of the disorders that they treated affected neurologists as well as psychiatrists. Reynolds (1855) responded to this problem by distinguishing between "organic" and "functional" disorders. The former possessed a somatic pathology and the latter did not, and Reynolds assumed that the symptoms of functional disorders were due either to a decrease or an inappropriate increase in functional activity. Subsequently, the terms organic and functional came to be used by his successors simply to distinguish between conditions in which somatic pathology had and had not been demonstrated. Gowers' textbook, for example, classified Parkinson's disease, chorea, torticollis, epilepsy and narcolepsy as functional simply because at the time there was no visible lesion to justify regarding them as organic (Gowers 1970 [1893]). The terms were then adopted by psychiatrists, mainly as a convenient way of distinguishing dementias and confusional states in which a somatic pathology was apparent from affective, schizophrenic and paranoid psychoses in which no such pathology could be demonstrated. Unfortunately, the ambiguity inherent in the term functional was also taken over, with the result that some psychiatrists assumed that it implied simply that no somatic pathology had yet been demonstrated whereas others assumed that the disorders so labelled were purely mental and that they had no somatic pathology. (Contemporary neurologists still use the term functional, usually informally and nearly always to imply their conviction that the patient's symptoms are "psychogenic.")

MENTAL AND PHYSICAL ILLNESS IN CONTEMPORARY MEDICINE

A distinction between mental and physical illness is still made, both by the lay public and by many doctors, and the terms "mental disor and "mental and behavioural disorder" are used in the two most widely used official nom clatures, the World Health Organization's In national Classification of Diseases (ICD) the American Psychiatric Association's *D nostic and Statistical Manual* (DSM). This the unfortunate effect of helping to perpet two assumptions that have long since been ab doned by all thinking physicians, namely mental disorders are disorders of the mind rat than the body, and that they are fundament different from other illnesses.

In reality, neither minds nor bodies develop nesses. Only people (or, in a wider context, ganisms) do so, and when they do both mind body, psyche and soma, are usually invol Pain, the most characteristic feature of so-cal bodily illness, is a purely psychological phen enon, and the first manifestation of most inf tions, from influenza to plague, is also a subj tive change—a vague general malaise (Car 1972). Fear and other emotions play an import role in the genesis of myocardial infarction, pertension, asthma and other bodily illness and bodily changes such as fatigue, anorexia a weight loss are commonplace in psychiatric orders. That most characteristic of all psychia disorders, depressive illness, illustrates the possibility of distinguishing between physi and mental illnesses.

There is good evidence from both family a twin studies (Andreasen et al. 1986; Kendler et 1992) that genetic factors make an important co tribution to the aetiology of the whole range depressive disorders, from the mildest to the m severe. This necessarily implies that there m be innate biological differences between th who are and are not prone to depression, and t is confirmed by the fact that drugs that have effect on mood in normal people relieve depr sion in those who are ill, and the observation th a depressed mood can be precipitated in peop who are prone to depressive illnesses simply ıipulating the tryptophan content of their diet ·lgado et al. 1990). There is unassailable evi- ıce, therefore, of somatic abnormalities in this st typical and common of mental illnesses. ılogous evidence could be presented for izophrenia, obsessional disorder and panic ›rder. Indeed, in the case of schizophrenia re is extensive evidence of widespread, albeit ›tle, brain pathology as well as strong evidence genetic transmission.

The fact is, it is not possible to identify any ıracteristic features of either the symptomatol- or the aetiology of so-called mental illnesses t consistently distinguish them from physical ıesses. Nor do so-called physical illnesses have characteristics that distinguish them reliably m mental illnesses. If pathological changes l dysfunctions are restricted to organs other n the brain, as is often the case, effects on ntation and behaviour are relatively re- cted, but this is an inconstant and purely ıntitative difference, and in any case does not ›ly to diseases of the brain or situations in ich there is a secondary disturbance of cerebral ıction. There are many differences between ental" and "physical" disorders, of course. Hal- inations, delusions and grossly irrational be- viour, for example, are a conspicuous feature the former. But they occur only in a small pro- rtion of mental disorders, and also feature in confusional states that may complicate many ysical disorders. The mechanisms underlying sterical amnesia or paraplegia are very differ- t from those underlying the amnesia of de- ɜntia or the paraplegia of spinal injury and are mmonly described as "psychogenic." But a ocardial infarction precipitated by fear or ger is equally "psychogenic," and in both cases ere are good grounds for assuming that the ıotional predicament generates neuronal or docrine changes that play a critical role in pro- ıcing the loss of access to memories, loss of vol- ıtary movement or inadequate oxygenation of e myocardium. In reality, the differences between mental and physical illnesses, striking though some of them are, are quantitative rather than qualitative, differences of emphasis rather than fundamental differences, and no more profound than the differences between diseases of the circulatory system and those of the digestive system, or between kidney diseases and skin diseases.

Why then do we still talk of "mental" illnesses, or indeed of "physical" illnesses? The answer is provided in the introduction to the current (1994) edition of the *Diagnostic and Statistical Manual of Mental Disorders* (DSM-IV): "The term mental disorder unfortunately implies a distinction between 'mental' disorders and 'physical' disorders that is a reductionistic anachronism of mind/body dualism. A compelling literature documents that there is much 'physical' in 'mental' disorders and much 'mental' in 'physical' disorders. The problem raised by the term 'mental disorders' has been much clearer than its solution, and, unfortunately, the term persists in the title of DSM-IV because we have not found an appropriate substitute."

MENTAL AND PHYSICAL DISORDERS IN CONTEMPORARY CLASSIFICATIONS

Against this background it is instructive to examine the status of mental and physical disorders, and the allocation of individual syndromes to broad groupings of disease, in contemporary classifications of disease.

The International Classification of Diseases is by far the most widely used comprehensive classification. It is important to appreciate, though, that it is not a textbook of medicine, sanctified by international approval. Its status and role are more modest; it is essentially "a statistical classification of diseases and other health problems, to serve a wide variety of needs for mortality and health-care data" (World Health Organization

1992). Like its predecessors, the current revision, ICD-10, does not draw a fundamental distinction between mental and physical diseases. "Mental and behavioural disorders" (F00-99) are simply the fifth of seventeen categories of disease (World Health Organization 1992). Several of these seventeen broad groupings (e.g., infectious and parasitic diseases; neoplasms; and congenital malformations, deformations and chromosomal abnormalities) are based on aetiology. Others (e.g., diseases of the circulatory system; diseases of the respiratory system) are based on the organ system primarily affected. Some (e.g., conditions originating in pregnancy, childbirth and the puerperium; and possibly mental and behavioural disorders as well) are heterogeneous and determined mainly by the medical speciality primarily responsible for treatment. None of the three underlying principles consistently takes precedence over the other two. Carcinoma of the bronchus (C34), for example, is classified by its aetiology—as a neoplasm—rather than as a disease of the respiratory system. Vascular dementia (F01), on the other hand, is classified as a mental disorder, despite the fact that in aetiological terms it is explicitly a vascular disorder. The distinction between diseases of the nervous system (G00-99) and mental and behavioural disorders (F00-99) is particularly illuminating. Most diseases of the brain, such as encephalitis and epilepsy, are classified as diseases of the nervous system. Others, like the postencephalitic and postconcussional syndromes, are classified as mental disorders. Some, like Alzheimer's and Parkinson's diseases, are listed as diseases of the nervous system and also, if they lead to dementia (as Alzheimer's disease, of course, invariably does), as mental diseases.

The American Psychiatric Association's *Diagnostic and Statistical Manual*, like other classifications produced by professional bodies, is essentially a classification of the disorders seen and treated by contemporary American psychiatrists and clinical psychologists. If, for exam child psychiatrists are asked to treat defiant, obedient adolescents, as they are, the Manual to contain a category—oppositional defiant order—for such patients. The same reasor applies to substance-related disorders, som form disorders and sleep disorders, and woulc so even without the statement quoted abc making it clear that the Association regards distinction between mental and physical di ders as a meaningless anachronism.

Overall, it seems clear that in both ICD-10 a DSM-IV, the two most widely used classif tions of so-called mental disorders, the allocat of individual disorders to broad categories disease or disorder is determined to a consic able extent by practical considerations—mai which kind of medical specialist usually treats tients presenting with the syndrome in qu tion—rather than by fundamental aetiologi considerations. This is particularly true of the tinction between mental diseases and disease the (central) nervous system in ICD-10, wh reflects little more than a pragmatic distinct between conditions generally treated by psych trists and cerebral disorders usually treated neurologists.

PUBLIC ATTITUDES

Unfortunately, the linguistic distinction betwe mental and physical illnesses, and the min body distinction from which this was origina derived, still encourages many lay people, a some doctors and other health professionals, assume that the two are fundamentally differe Both are apt to assume that developing a "men illness" is evidence of a certain lack of moral fi and that, if they really tried, people with illnes of this kind ought to be able to control their an ieties, their despondency and their strange prec cupations and "snap out of it." It is true, of cour that most of us believe in "free will"; we belie we ourselves and other people can exercise a ain amount of control over our feelings behaviour. But there is no reason, justified ei- r by logic or by medical understanding, why ple suffering from, say, phobic anxiety or de- ssion should be able to exert more control r their symptoms than those suffering from xoedema or migraine. There is a further and ally damaging assumption that the symptoms nental disorders are in some sense less "real" n those of physical disorders with a tangible al pathology. As a result, people experiencing nse fatigue, or pain that is not accompanied ny obvious local lesion, are often dismayed or onted by being told that they are suffering n neurasthenia, the chronic fatigue syndrome "psychogenic" pain, and interpret such diag- ses as implying that their doctor does not be- e that they are really in pain or exhausted by slightest effort, and is dismissing their com- ints as "all in the mind."

ONCLUSIONS

sunderstandings of this kind are important l frequent. They undermine the relationship tween doctor and patient and often result in a usal to consult a psychiatrist or clinical psy- ologist, or to countenance a potentially effec- e treatment. The answer to such problems lies painstaking explanation and gentle persua- n, and in the longer run in better education of th the general public and doctors themselves, t in conniving with patients' convictions that eir symptoms are caused by "real" or "physical" nesses. It may be sensible sometimes to do s as a holding tactic in an individual patient. It never appropriate in other contexts. Not only the distinction between mental and physical ness ill-founded and incompatible with con- mporary understanding of disease, it is also maging to the long-term interests of patients emselves. It invites both them and their doctors to ignore what may be important causal factors and potentially effective therapies; and by implying that illnesses so described are fundamentally different from all other types of ill-health, it helps to perpetuate the stigma associated with "mental" illness. We should talk of psychiatric illnesses or disorders rather than of mental illnesses; and if we do continue to refer to "mental" and "physical" illnesses we should preface both with "so-called," to remind ourselves and our audience that these are archaic and deeply misleading terms.

REFERENCES

American Psychiatric Association (APA). 1994. *Diagnostic and Statistical Manual of Mental Disorders* (4th ed.) (DSM-IV). Washington, D.C.: APA.

Andreasen, N. C., Scheftner, W., Reich, T., et al. 1986. "The Validation of the Concept of Endogenous Depression: A Family Study Approach." *Archives of General Psychiatry*, 43, 246–51.

Canter, A. 1972. "Changes in Mood during Incubation of Acute Febrile Disease and the Effects of Pre-exposure Psychologic Status." *Psychosomatic Medicine*, 34, 424–30.

Delgado, P. L., Charney, D. S., Price, L. H., et al. 1990. "Serotonin Function and the Mechanism of Antidepressant Action: Reversal of Antidepressant-Induced Remission by Rapid Depletion of Plasma Tryptophan." *Archives of General Psychiatry*, 47, 411–18.

Gowers, W. R. 1970 (1893). *A Manual of Diseases of the Nervous System*, vol. 1. New York: Hafner.

Griesinger, W. 1845. *Pathologie und Therapie der Psychischen Krankheiten*. Reprinted (1867) as *Mental Pathology and Therapeutics*, trans. C. L. Robertson and J. Rutherford. London: New Sydenham Society.

Hunter, R., & Macalpine, I. 1963. *Three Hundred Years of Psychiatry, 1535–1860*. London: Oxford University Press.

Kendler, K. S., Neale, M. C., Kessler, R. C., et al. 1992. "A Population-Based Twin Study of Major Depression in Women: The Impact of Varying Definitions of Illness." *Archives of General Psychiatry*, 49, 257–66.

Porter, R. 1987. *Mind-forg'd Manacles*. London: Athlone Press.

Reynolds, J. R. 1855. *The Diagnosis of Diseases of the Brain, Spinal Cord, Nerves and their Appendages*. London: Churchill.

Rush, B. 1812. *Medical Inquiries and Observa[illegible] upon the Diseases of the Mind*. Philadelphia: Ki[illegible] & Richardson.

World Health Organization (WHO). 1992. *Inte[illegible] tional Statistical Classification of Diseases and Rel[illegible] Health Problems*. Geneva: WHO.

CHAPTER 13

The "Unnaturalness" of Aging—Give Me Reason to Live!

ARTHUR L. CAPLAN

NOT EVERYONE THINKS IT IS a good ea to live longer lives. Some writers, perhaps, most notably Daniel allahan, the co-founder of the Hastings Center, argue that the quest to tend life is not a self-evident good.[1] A longer life, Callahan contends, is ot necessarily a better life. Other writers, such as the philosopher/physi-an Leon Kass[2] and the political theorist Francis Fukuyama,[3] argue that e extension of life should not be pursued because lengthening life is ot consistent with human nature. It is "unnatural" to extend human lives eyond the proverbial three score and ten that the demographers assure s is what the average citizen of an economically developed nation can xpect.

Still scientists are eagerly pursuing research in many species that might lead to life extension in human beings. French scientists have produced mice that live 26% longer through genetic engineering.[4] Other scientists have produced longer-lived mice, rats and primates by placing them early in life on low calorie diets. Are these scientists and others working on techniques that might lead to significantly longer life spans for human beings engaged in unethical activities?

Callahan and those who worry about the social and economic consequences of life extension must show that our culture or other cultures are not clever enough or flexible enough to figure out how to cope with more life. But those such as Kass and Fukuyama who maintain that it is unnatural to live much longer than we now do must show why the extension of life is unnatural. Or to put the point another way they must be able to show that aging and senescence are both natural processes and as such good things. Can that case be made?

NORMALITY, NATURALNESS, AND DISEASE

It may seem somewhat odd to question the "naturalness" of a process as familiar and as universal as aging. After all, if aging is not a natural process, what is? While the prospect of aging may be greeted with mixed feelings, there would seem to be little reason to doubt the fact that aging is understood to be a normal and inevitable feature of human existence. The belief that aging is a normal and natural part of human existence is reflected in the practice of medicine. For example, no mention is made in most textbooks in the areas of medicine and pathology of aging as abnormal, unnatural, or indicative of disease. It is true that such texts often contain a chapter or two on the related subject of diseases commonly associated with aging or found in the elderly. But it is the diseases of the elderly, such as pneumo cancer, or atherosclerosis, rather than the ag process itself, that serve as the focus of desc tion and analysis.

Why should this situation exist? What i different about the physiological changes and teriorations concurrent with the aging pro that these events are considered to be unrem able natural processes, while other debilita changes are deemed to be diseases constitu health crises of the first order? Surely it can simply be the life-threatening aspects of disea such as cancer or atherosclerosis, that distingu these processes from aging. For while it may true that hardly anyone manages to avoid c tracting a terminal disease at some point in aging itself produces the same ultimate co quence as these diseases. Nor can it be the fa iarity and universality of aging that inure medi science to its unnatural aspects. Malignant n plasms, viral infections, and hypertension are ubiquitous phenomena. Yet medicine mainta a radically different stance toward these physi processes from that which it holds toward the called "natural" changes that occur during agi

It might be argued that the processes deno by the term "aging" do not fit the standard c ception of disease operative in clinical medici However, in medical dictionaries disease is most always defined as any pathological char in the body. Pathological change is inevita defined as constituting any morbid process in body. And morbid processes are usually defin in terms of disease states of the body.[5] Regard of the circularity surrounding this explication the concept of somatic disease, aging would se to have a *prima facie* claim to being counted a disease. Pathological or morbid changes often the sole criteria by which age is assessed organic tissues.

What seems to differentiate aging from otl processes or states traditionally classified as c eases is the fact that aging is perceived as a na or normal process. Medicine has traditionally ved its role as that of ameliorating or combat- the abnormal, either through therapeutic in- entions or preventive, prophylactic regimens. natural and the normal, while not outside sphere of medicine, are concepts that play roles in licensing the intervention of the med- practitioner. For it is in response to or in an- pation of abnormality that physicians' activi- are legitimated. And as E. A. Murphy, among ers, has noted, "the clinician has tended to re- d disease as that state in which the limits of the mal have been transgressed."[6] Naturalness normality have, historically, been used as e lines to determine the presence of disease the necessity of medical activity. In light of powerful belief that the abnormal and unnat- l are indicative of medicine's range of interest, s easy to see why many biological processes not thought to be the proper subject of med- intervention or therapy. Puberty, growth, maturation *as processes in themselves* all ap- r to stand outside the sphere of medical con- n since they are normal and natural occur- ces among human beings. Similarly, it seems d to think of sexuality or fertilization as possi- disease states precisely because these states commonly thought to be natural and normal mponents of the human condition.

Nonetheless, it is true that certain biological ocesses, such as contraception, pregnancy, and tility, have been the subject in recent years of ated debates as to their standing as possible dis- se states. The notions that it is natural and nor- al for only men and women to have sexual in- course or for women to undergo menopause ve been challenged in many quarters. The estion arises as to whether the process of aging and of itself can be classified as abnormal and natural in a way that will open the door for the classification of aging as a disease process and, us, a proper subject of medical attention, con- rn, and control.

AGING AND MEDICAL INTERVENTION

The past few years have seen the rise of a powerful movement for the "right to die." Some have even gone so far as to claim that physicians and health professionals have a moral obligation to play an active role in allowing patients to die under certain circumstances. To a great extent, the status of aging and dying as natural processes looms large in discussions about the "right to die" and "death with dignity." Often those who debate the degree to which the medical profession should intervene in the process of dying disagree about the naturalness of the phenomena of aging and dying. If the alleged right to die is to be built on a conception of the naturalness of aging and dying, then the conceptual status of these terms vis-à-vis "naturalness" must be thoroughly examined. The question of the naturalness of aging, senescence, and death must not be permitted to become lost in complex debates concerning the rights and obligations of patients and health professionals.

The perception of biological events or processes as natural or unnatural is frequently decisive in determining whether physicians treat states or processes as diseases.[7] One need only think of the controversies that swirl around allegations concerning the biological naturalness of homosexuality or schizophrenia to see that this is so. This claim is further borne out by an argument that is frequently made by older physicians to new medical students. Medical students often find it difficult to interact with or examine elderly patients. They may feel powerless when confronted with the seemingly irreversible debilities of old age. To overcome this reluctance, older physicians are likely to point out that aging and senescence are processes that happen to everyone, even young medical students. Aging is simply part of the human condition; it should hold no terror for a young doctor. Students are told that aging is natural and that, while there may be nothing they can do to alter the inevitable course of this process, they must learn to help patients cope with their aging as best they can. It is as if teaching physicians feel obligated to label the obviously debilitative and disease-like states of old age as natural in order to discourage the students' inclination to treat the elderly as sick or diseased.

WHAT IS AGING?

What are the grounds on which this label is applied? Why do we think of aging as a natural process? The reason that comes immediately to mind is that aging is a common and normal process. It occurs with a statistical frequency of 100%. Inevitably and uniformly bones become brittle, vision dims, joints stiffen, and muscles lose their tone. The obvious question that arises is whether commonality, familiarity, and inevitability are sufficient conditions for referring to certain biological states as natural. To answer this question, it is necessary to first draw a distinction between aging and chronological age.

In a trivial sense, given the existence of a chronological device, all bodies that exist can be said to age relative to the measurements provided by that device. But since physicians have little practical interest in making philosophical statements about the time-bound nature of existence, or empirical claims about the relativity of space and time, it is evident that they do not have this chronological sense in mind in speaking about the familiarity and inevitability of aging. In speaking of aging, physicians are interested in a particular set of biological changes that occur with respect to time. In the aged individual, cells manifest a high frequency of visible chromosomal aberrations. The nuclei of nerve cells become distorted by clumps of chromatin and the surrounding cytoplasm contains fewer organelles, such as mitochondria. Collagen fibers become increasingly rigid and inflexible, as manifest in the familiar phenomenon of skin wrinkling. The aorta becomes wider and more tortuous. The munological system weakens and the elderly son becomes more susceptible to infecti Melanin pigment formation decreases and, c sequently, hair begins to whiten.[8]

NATURALNESS, DESIGN, AND FUNCTION

Changes of this kind, in association with ag are universal and inevitable. Universality anc evitability do not, however, seem to be suffic conditions for referring to a process as natu Coronary atherosclerosis, neoplasms, high bl pressure, sore throats, colds, tooth decay, and pression are all nearly universal in their distri tion and seemingly inevitable phenomena yet we would hardly agree to calling any of th things natural processes or states. The inevita ity of infection by microorganisms among humans does not cause the physician to dism these infections as natural occurrences of no p ticular medical interest. The physician may intervene, nor even attempt to prevent such eases, but such behavior is a result of a decis concerning an unnatural disease, not a natu process.

So, if universality and inevitability are not a quate conditions for naturalness, are any ot criteria available by which naturalness can be sessed and used to drive a wedge between ag and disease? There is a further sense of "natura that may prove helpful in trying to understa why physicians are reluctant to label aging a ease, preferring to think of it as a natural proce

This sense of naturalness is rooted in the tions of design, purpose, and function. Axes designed to serve as tools for cutting trees. Sc pels are meant to be used in cutting human sue. It would seem most unnatural to use axes surgery and scalpels for lumberjacking. In so sense, although a skillful surgeon might in f be able to perform surgery with an axe, it wou be unnatural to do so. Similarly, many bodily s—the liver, spleen, blood vessels, kidneys, many glands—can perform compensatory ctions when certain other organic tissues are naged or removed. But these are not the pures or functions they were "designed" to pern. While the arteries of many organisms are able of constricting to maintain blood pres- and reduce the flow of blood during hemnage-induced shock, the function of arteries not to constrict in response to such circumnces. The presence of vasoconstriction in ares is in fact an unnatural state that signals the sician that something has gone seriously awry he body. It would seem that much of our willness to accept aging as a natural process is paric upon this sense of natural function.

Two answers are commonly given to the quesn: What is the function of aging? The first is eological explanation. God, as a punishment the sins of our ancestors in the (proverbial) den of Eden, caused humans to age and die. this view, people age because the Creator saw to design them that way for retribution or punment. Aging serves as a reminder of our moral ibility and weakness.

The second view, which is particularly wideead in scientific circles, is that the purpose or ction of aging is to clear away the old to make y for the new for evolutionary reasons. This ory was first advanced by the German cytolot and evolutionary biologist August Weisman the turn of the century.[10] Weisman argued that ing and debilitation must be viewed as adapional responses on the part of organisms to alv for new mutational and adaptive responses fluctuating environments. Aging benefits the pulation by removing the superannuated to ake room for the young. The function of aging to ensure the death of organisms to allow evotionary change and new adaptation to occur.

On both of these views aging has an intended rpose or function. And it is from this quasiistotelian attribution of a design that the "natuness" of aging is often thought to arise.

THE CONCEPT OF BIOLOGICAL FUNCTION

If the naturalness of aging resides in a functional interpretation, the philosopher can tap a rich and abundant literature on the subjects of function and purpose. However, rooting the source of the naturalness of biological processes in ideas of function or purpose also has its drawbacks, the primary problem being that philosophers have by no means reached anything even vaguely resembling a consensus about the meaning of such terms as function or purpose.[11]

Fortunately, it is possible to avoid becoming bogged down in an analysis of functional or purposive statements in analyzing the function of aging. The only distinction required for understanding the function of aging is that between the aim of explaining the existence of a particular state, organ, or process, and that of explaining how a state, organ, or process works in a particular system or organism. Functional or purposive statements are sometimes used to explain the existence of a trait or process, historically. At other times such statements are used mechanistically to explain how something works or operates. If we ask what is the function, or role, or purpose of the spleen in the human body, the question can be interpreted in two ways: How does the spleen work—what does it do in the body? Or, why does the spleen exist in its present state in the human body—what is the historical story that explains why persons have spleens?[12]

It is this latter sense of function, the historical sense, that is relevant to the determination of the naturalness or unnaturalness of aging as a biological process. For while there is no shortage of theories purporting to explain how aging works or functions, these theories are not relevant to the historically motivated question about the function of aging. The determination of the naturalness of aging, if it is to be rooted in biology, will depend not on how the process of aging actually operates, but rather on the explanation one gives for the existence or presence of aging humans.[13] This is the sense of naturalness that Kass and Fukuyama and others must rely upon to make their case against extending life through conquering aging.

DOES AGING HAVE A FUNCTION?

Two purported explanations—one theological, one scientific—of the function or purpose of aging have been given. Both are flawed. While the theological explanation of aging may carry great weight for numerous individuals, it will simply not do as a scientific explanation of why aging occurs in humans. Medical professionals may have to cope with their patients' advocacy of this explanation and their own religious feelings on the subject. But, from a scientific perspective, it will hardly do to claim that aging, as a result of God's vindictiveness, is a natural biological process, and hence not a disease worthy of treatment.

More surprisingly, the scientific explanation of aging as serving an evolutionary role or purpose is also inadequate. It is simply not true that aging exists to serve any sort of evolutionary purpose or function. The claim that aging exists or occurs in individuals because it has a wider role or function in the evolutionary scheme of things rests on a faulty evolutionary analysis. The analysis incorrectly assumes that it is possible for biological processes to exist that directly benefit or advance the evolutionary success of a species or population. In other words, it supposes that processes such as aging exist because they serve a function or purpose in the life history of a species—in this case, that of removing the old to make way for the new. However, evolutionary selection rarely acts to advance the prospects of an entire species or population. Selection acts on individual organisms and their phenotypic traits and properties. Some traits or properties confer advantages in certain environments on the organisms that possess them and this fact increases the likelihood that the genes responsible for producing th traits will be passed on to future organisms.

Given that selective forces act on individ and their genotypes and not species, it make sense to speak of aging as serving an evolutio function or purpose to benefit the species. H then do evolutionary biologists explain the e tence of aging?[14] Briefly, the explanation is features, traits, or properties in individual org isms will be selected for if they confer a rela reproductive advantage on the individual, or or her close kin. Any variation that increases clusive reproductive fitness has a very high p ability of being selected and maintained in gene pool of a species. Selection, however, c not look ahead to foresee the possible con quences of favoring certain traits at a given ti the environment selects for those traits and tures that give an immediate return. An increa metabolic rate, for example, may prove adva geous early in life, in that it may provide more ergy for seeking mates and avoiding predator may also result in early deterioration of the ganism due to an increased accumulation toxic wastes in the body of an individual thus dowed. Natural selection cannot foresee such layed debilitating consequences.

Aging exists, then, as a consequence of lack evolutionary foresight; it is simply a by-produc selective forces working to increase the chan of reproductive success in the life of an organis Senescence has no function; it is simply the advertent subversion of organic function, late life, in favor of maximizing reproductive adv tage early in life.

The common belief that aging serves a fu tion or purpose, if this belief is based on a mis prehension of evolutionary theory, is mistak And, if this is so, it would seem that the comm belief that aging is a natural process, as a co sequence of the function or purpose it serves the life of the species, is also mistaken. Con quently, unless it is possible to motivate the c scription on other grounds, it would seem th g cannot be understood as a natural process. if that is true, and if it is actually the case that at goes on during the aging process closely allels the changes that occur during paradigtic examples of disease,[15] then it would be unsonable not to consider aging a disease.

HEORIES OF AGING AND HE CONCEPT OF DISEASE

onsideration of the changes that constitute ng in human beings reinforces the similarities sting between aging and other clear-cut exams of somatic diseases. There is a set of exter- manifestations or symptoms: graying hair, reased susceptibility to infection, wrinkling n, loss of muscular tone, and frequently, loss of ntal ability. These manifestations seem to be isally linked to a series of internal cellular and ocellular changes. The presence of symptoms l an underlying etiology closely parallels the ndard paradigmatic examples of disease. If the logy is pushed a bit further, the cause for conering aging a disease appears to become even onger.

There are many theories as to what causes anges at the cellular and subcellular level that oduce the signs and symptoms associated with ng.[16] One view argues that aging is caused an increase in the number of cross-linkages at exist in protein and nucleic acid molecules. oss-linkages lower the biochemical efficiency d dependability of certain macromolecules inlved in metabolism and other chemical reacns. Free radical byproducts of metabolism are ought to accumulate in cells, thus allowing for increase in available linkage sites for replicatg nucleic acid strands and activating histone elnents. This sort of cross-linkage is thought to be rticularly important in the aging of collagen, e substance responsible for most of the overt mptoms we commonly associate with aging, ch as wrinkled skin and loss of muscular flexility.

Another view holds that aging results from an accumulation of genetic mutations in the chromosomes of cells in the body. The idea underlying this theory is that chromosomes are exposed over time to a steady stream of radiation and other mutagenic agents. The accumulation of mutational hits on the genes lying on the chromosomes results in the progressive inactivation of these genes. The evidence of a higher incidence of chromosomal breaks and aberrations in the aged is consistent with this mutational theory of aging.

Along with the cross-linkage and mutational theories, there is one other important hypothesis concerning the cause of aging. The autoimmune theory holds that, as time passes and the chromosomes of cells in the human body accumulate more mutations, certain key tissues begin to synthesize antibodies that can no longer distinguish between self and foreign material. Thus, a number of autoimmune reactions occur in the body as the immunological system begins to turn against the individual it was "designed" to protect. Arthritis and pernicious anemia are symptomatic of the sorts of debilities resulting from the malfunction of the immunological system. While this theory is closely allied to the mutation theory, the autoimmune view of aging holds that accumulated mutations do not simply result in deterioration of cellular activity, but, rather, produce lethal cellular end products that consume and destroy healthy tissue.

It would be rash to hold that any of the three hypotheses cited—the cross-linkage, mutational, or autoimmune hypotheses—will, in the end, turn out to be the correct explanation of aging. All three views are, in fact, closely related in that cross-linkages can result from periodic exposure to mutagenic agents and can, in turn, produce genetic aberrations that eventuate in cellular dysfunction or even autoimmunological reactions. What is important, however, is not whether one of these theories or *any* of them is in fact the correct theory of aging, but that all of them postulate mechanisms that are closely analogous to those mechanisms cited by clinicians in describing disease processes in the body.

The concept of disease is, without doubt, a slippery and evasive notion in medicine.[17] Once one moves away from what can be termed "paradigmatic" examples of disease, such as tuberculosis or diphtheria, toward more nebulous examples, such as acne or jittery nerves, it becomes difficult to say exactly what are the criteria requisite for labeling a condition a somatic disease. However, even though it is notoriously difficult to concoct a set of necessary and sufficient conditions for employing the term "organic disease," it is possible to cite a list of general criteria that seem relevant in attempting to decide whether a bodily state or process is appropriately labeled a disease.

One criterion is that the state or process produces discomfort or suffering. A second is that the process or state can be traced back to a specific cause, event, or circumstance. A third is that there is a set of clear-cut structural changes, both macroscopic and microscopic, that follow in a uniform, sequential manner subsequent to the initial precipitating or causal event. A fourth is that there is a set of clinical symptoms or manifestations (headache, pain in the chest, rapid pulse, shortness of breath) commonly associated with the observed physiological alterations in structure. Finally, there is usually some sort of functional impairment in the functions, behavior, or activity of a person thought to be diseased.[18] Not all diseases will satisfy all or any of the criteria I have suggested. One need only consider the arguments surrounding the classification of astigmatism, alcoholism, drug-addiction, gambling, and hyperactivity to realize the inadequacy of these criteria as necessary and sufficient conditions for the determination of disease. But that the suggested criteria are relevant to such determination is shown by the fact that advocates of all persuasions regarding controversial states and processes commonly resort to considerations of causation, clinical manifestations, etiology, functional impairment, and suffering in arguing merits of their various views concerning the tus of controversial cases.

With respect to the conceptual ambiguity rounding the notion of disease, it is importar remember that medicine is by no means uni in being saddled with what might be terr "fuzzy-edged" concepts. One need only consi the status of terms such as "species," "ada tion," and "mutation" in biology, or "stimul "behavior," and "instinct" in psychology, to r ize that medicine is not alone in the ambiguit its key terms. It is also true that, just as the bi gist is able to use biological theory to aid in determination of relevant criteria for a conc the physician is able to use his or her knowle of the structure and function of the body to cide on relevant criteria for the determinat of disease. If one accepts the relevance of five suggested criteria, aging, as a biologi process, is seen to possess all the key propertie a disease. Unlike astigmatism or nervousn aging possesses a definitive group of clinical m ifestations or symptoms; a clear-cut etiology structural changes at both the macroscopic a microscopic levels; a significant measure of i pairment discomfort, and suffering, and, if we willing to grant the same tolerance to current t ories of aging as we grant to theories in other mains of medicine, an explicit set of precipitati factors. Aging has all the relevant markings c disease process. And if my earlier argumen sound, even if an additional criterion of unna ralness were appended, aging would still m all the requirements thought relevant to t classification of a process or state as indicative disease.

SOME ETHICAL ARGUMENT AGAINST TREATING AGING AS A DISEASE

What hinges on the decision to refer to a proc or state such as aging by the word "disease" rath than by some other term? Obviously, a great de dical attention, medical support, medical tment, and medical research are devoted to treatment, care, amelioration, and preven- of disease. While it is possible to view the ac-tion of this vast professional machine either as sitive good or as a serious evil, an array of con-ations and implications surrounds the med- profession's decision to consider a phenome- worthy of its attention. Some groups have vely proselytized for the acceptance of cer- conditions, such as alcoholism or gambling, iseases. Other groups have worked to remove label of disease from behavior such as homo-uality, masturbation, and schizophrenia. A nber of motives and concerns underlie these uments. The question is, what kinds of con-erations should be considered relevant to the ermination of whether a particular state, pro-s, or condition is a disease?

do not propose to try to answer the difficult estion of what are the relevant nonorganic cri-ia affecting the choice of the disease label. her, I want to consider three specific argu-nts that might be raised against calling aging a ease—a classification that, of necessity, keeps aged in touch with the medical profession. The first counter-argument is that the decision call aging a disease would be pointless, since ctors cannot at present intervene to treat or re aging. This argument does not stand up to tical scrutiny. There are many diseases in exis-nce today for which no cure is known, but no e proposes that these disorders are any less dis-ses as a consequence. Furthermore, the em-asis on treatment and cure implicit in this ar-ment ignores the equally vital components of edical care involving understanding, educa-n, and support. The profession's and the pa-nt's interest in the healing function of medi-ne might make it difficult for physicians to cept aging as a disease, but the difficulty in hieving such acceptance does not provide a ason for rejecting the view.

The second argument is that to call aging a dis-se would involve the stigmatization of a large segment of the population; to view the aged as sick or diseased would only increase the burdens already borne by this much abused segment of society. The problem with this argument is that it tends to blend public perceptions of disease in general with the particular problem of whether seeing aging as a disease ought to carry negative and undesirable connotations. To deny that aging is a disease may be simply an easy way to avoid the more difficult problem of educating the medical profession and the lay public toward a better understanding of the threatening and nonthreatening aspects of disease. Contagiousness, death, disability, and neglect may be the real objects of concern in speaking of disease, not disease in itself.

Finally, it might be claimed, as Callahan and others do, that there would be a tremendous social and economic cost to calling aging a disease. The claim is perhaps the most unconvincing of the three that I have offered. One factor especially relevant to the determination or diagnosis of disease would seem to be that the physician confine his or her concerns to the physical and mental state of the individual patient; social and economic considerations would appear to be quite out of place. Genetic and psychological diseases place a large burden on society: dialysis machines and tomography units are enormously expensive. But these facts do not in any way change the disease status of Downs, schizophrenia, kidney failure or cancer. It may be the case that the government may decide not to spend one cent on research into aging or the treatment of aging. But such a decision should be consequent on, not prior to, a diagnosis of disease. This argument simply blurs the value questions relevant to a decision as to whether something is a disease, with value questions relevant to deciding what to do about something after it has been decided that it is a disease.

I have suggested a number of possible value issues and social problems that may enter into the decision of the medical profession to label a state or process a disease. I have also suggested that none of these issues and problems would seem to rule out a consideration of aging as a disease. The determination of disease status and the question of how physicians and society should react to disease are distinct issues. Considerations of the latter variety ought not to be allowed to color our decisions about what does and what does not constitute a disease.

Most persons in our society would be loath to see aging classified and treated as a disease. Much of the resistance to such a classification derives from the view that aging is a natural process and that, like other natural processes, it ought not, in itself, be the subject of medical intervention and therapeutic control. I have tried to show that much of the reasoning that tacitly underlies the categorization of aging as a natural or normal process rests on faulty biological analysis. Aging is not the goal or aim of the evolutionary process. Rather it is an accidental byproduct of that process. Accordingly, it is incorrect to root a belief in the naturalness of aging in some sort of perceived biological design or purpose since aging serves no such end. It may be that good arguments can be adduced for excluding aging from the purview of medicine. However, if such arguments can be made, they must draw on considerations other than that of the naturalness of aging.

NOTES

1. R. Barlow, "Ethicist Questions Quest to Extend Life." *Boston Globe.* November 14, 2002: 2; Daniel Callahan, *What Price Better Health?* (Berkeley: University of California Press, 2003)

2. Corinne Bensimon, *Libération,* December 6, 2002: 19; President's Council on Bioethics, "Beyond Therapy," Washington, D.C.: October 2003.

3. Francis Fukuyama, "Our Posthuman Future," in *The Future Is Now: America Confronts the New Genetics,* ed. William Kristol and Eric Cohen (Lanham, Md.: Rowman & Littlefield, 2002); Fukuyama, "Biotechnology and the Threat of a Posthuman Future," *Chronicle of Higher Education,* March 22, 2002: B7–B10.

4. See, for example, *Dorland's Illustrated Me[illegible] Dictionary,* 25th ed. (Philadelphia: W. B. San[illegible] 1974).

5. Ibid.

6. E. A. Murphy, *The Logic of Medicine* (Baltim[illegible] Johns Hopkins University Press, 1976), p. 122. See E. A. Murphy, "A Scientific Viewpoint on Norma[illegible] *Perspectives in Biology and Medicine* 9, no. 3 (sp[illegible] 1966): 338–48; and G. B. Risse, "Health and Dise[illegible] History of the Concepts," in *Encyclopedia of Bioeth[illegible]* ed. W. T. Reich (New York: Free Press, 1978), 579–85.

7. S. Goldberg, "What Is 'Normal'? Logical Asp[illegible] of the Question of Homosexual Behavior," *Psychi[illegible]* 38 (1975): 227–42; Charles Socarides, "Homosexu[illegible] and Medicine," *Journal of the American Medical A[illegible] ciation* 212 (1970): 1199–1202; and I. Illich, "The Po[illegible] cal Uses of Natural Death," *Hastings Center Stud[illegible]* (1974): 3–20.

8. Leonard Hayflick, "The Strategy of Senescen[illegible] *Gerontologist* 14 (1974):37–45.

9. Cf. D. B. Hausman, "What Is Natural?" *Pers[illegible] tives in Biology and Medicine* 19 (1975): 92–101, fo[illegible] illuminating discussion of the concept.

10. August Weisman, *Essays upon Heredity and [illegible] dred Biological Problems,* 2nd ed. (Oxford: Claren[illegible] Press, 1891).

11. For a sample of the extant explications of [illegible] concept of function see L. Wright, "Functions," *[illegible] losophical Review* 82 (1973): 139–68; R. Cumm[illegible] "Functional Analysis," *Journal of Philosophy* 72 (19[illegible] 741–65; and M. A. Boden, *Purposive Explanation[illegible] Psychology* (Cambridge, Mass.: Harvard Univer[illegible] Press, 1972). See also E. Nagel, *Teleology Revis[illegible]* (New York: Columbia University Press, 1979).

12. Further discussion of the distinction between [illegible] plaining the operation of a trait or feature and expla[illegible] ing the origin and presence of a trait or feature can [illegible] found in A. L. Caplan, "Evolution, Ethics and the M[illegible] of Human Kindness," *Hastings Center Report* 6, n[illegible] (1976): 20–26.

13. A. L. Caplan, "An Unnatural Process: Why I[illegible] Not Inherently Wrong to Seek a Cure for Aging," [illegible] *Fountain of Youth,* ed. S. Post (New York: Oxfo[illegible] 2004), 114–24.

4. G. C. Williams, *Adaptation and Natural Selec-* (Princeton, N.J.: Princeton University Press,); and M. T. Ghiselin, *The Economy of Nature and* *Evolution of Sex* (Berkeley: University of California s, 1974).

5. For an interesting attempt to analyze the con- ts of illness and disease, see C. Boorse, "On the Dis- tion between Illness and Disease," *Philosophy and* *lic Affairs* 5, no. 1 (1975): 49–68.

6. A. Comfort, "Biological Theories of Aging," *Human Development* 13 (1970): 127–39; L. Hayflick, "The Biology of Human Aging," *American Journal of Medical Sciences* 265, no. 6 (1973): 433–45; A. Comfort, *Aging: The Biology of Senescence* (New York: Holt, Rinehart and Winston, 1964).

17. R. M. Veatch, "The Medical Model: Its Nature and Problems," *Hastings Center Studies* 1 (1973): 59–76.

18. See Boorse, "On the Distinction between Illness and Disease."

CHAPTER 14

Diagnosing and Defining Disease

WINSTON CHIONG

THE PATIENT AND HIS WIFE are seat
when the doctor enters the room. They are holding hands, the heel of l
foot taps erratically against the leg of his chair. The doctor closes the do
behind him while glancing at his chart.

"Mr. Richardson, Mrs. Richardson, how do you do? Sorry to keep you wa ing, it's been a busy morning."

"No, no, it's no problem, doctor." The patient laughs nervously. "I've bee waiting two years to find out what's wrong with me. A couple of minutes. . he trails off and shrugs.

"I know what you mean." Pages rustle as the doctor flips through the cha "Well, you know, when you first came in to see me, I was as confused abo

r symptoms as you. Maybe more." He looks up smiles ironically—patient and wife nod po-y but do not smile back. "But with these test re-s and the changes you've been noticing over the few months, I think we have a better idea of t's going on. Mr. Richardson, I think that you e a condition that we call..."

The patient and his wife lean forward slightly, s wide: an image of pregnant anticipation.

---

at happens when a patient is given a diagno- A diagnosis is, first of all, a description of patient as a sufferer of a particular disease cess. A diagnosis can also be an explanation patients who have had symptoms but do not w their cause. Giving a name to the problem y seem to resolve the mystery, such that even ients with intractable, chronic diseases may l relief when diagnosed. And of course, a diag-sis often offers a prediction about the future rse of illness, or about the genetic or infec-s risk to others.

All of the above belong to what might be con-ered the "science" of medicine—but diagnos- disease has more subtle implications as well. ntifying a disease can confer social legitimacy a patient's symptoms, relieving patients of suspicion that they are malingering or exag-rating their woes;[1, 2] conversely, it may be seen imply that the patient is somehow abnormal requires intervention. Having a disease might rk the patient as a member of a community of fferers, as demonstrated by the many patient d family associations that exist for various ill-sses. Finally, diagnosing a disease can have im-rtant legal and economic consequences, such conferring eligibility for disability benefits or en (in the case of the insanity defense) exempt-g patients from responsibility for their actions. Thus, while disease is commonly taken to be purely scientific matter, the naming and diag-sis of diseases is also a social practice with im-ications that extend beyond the clinic doors. iven such pressures, there is reason to wonder if "disease" is truly a unified concept. Some dis-eases, such as tuberculosis or embolic stroke, pick out a highly specific etiologic agent or pro-cess; others, like Alzheimer disease or sclero-derma, indicate pathologic changes of unclear cause; while syndromes and functional disorders simply represent collections of symptoms and signs that frequently occur together. What do these labels all have in common?

This question is complicated because there is a tension in medical concepts of health and dis-ease. On one hand, they are meant to represent objective, scientific facts—this patient is healthy, this patient has disease. But on the other hand, they also involve evaluative judgments about good and bad—a healthy state is better than a diseased state, a diseased state is in some way ab-normal or dysfunctional—that are more than matters of straightforward, scientific fact. To il-lustrate: when patients are diagnosed with coro-nary artery disease, part of what is implied is that accumulations of lipids and macrophages are present in their coronary arteries, increasing the likelihood of coronary ischemia, and these are more or less objective descriptions. But another part of what is implied is that such patients have a disease, an abnormality that results in impair-ment of their quality of life, and this is an evalua-tive judgment.

"Quality of life" is a telling phrase, because it reveals how concepts like health and disease, function and dysfunction, are interwoven with conceptions of the good life. As Caplan et al. note, "What will count as minimal standards of function or as special levels of excellence will de-pend on value judgments concerning what is im-portant to be able to do as a human being."[3] In-deed, ideas about what counts as health and disease have changed over time to fit changes in value judgments and therapeutic options. For in-stance, birth control is now thought of as part of medical care because the medical community considers it important for people to plan and con-trol reproduction, while physicians of an earlier time would likely have considered reproduction to be the necessary physiologic function of sex. Impotence was once considered by most people to be just an unfortunate occurrence, but with the advent of less problematic therapies it is now considered a treatable medical condition. Both of these changes reflect changed cultural attitudes about the role of sex and sexuality in human life.

Thus, the concept of health involves a descriptive component (what someone is able to do) as well as an evaluative component (what it is important to be able to do, in order to be able to live a good life). Similarly, the concept of disease involves a duality between a description (a physiological or functional difference between the patient and the healthy norm) and an evaluation (the judgment that this difference is abnormal or dysfunctional, and not just different). However, this duality is obscured in everyday practice, in part due to the scientific aspirations of medicine and scientific assumptions built into the medical model.

For instance, consider the standard "SOAP" progress note, in which the patient's report of symptoms is termed "subjective," while physical findings and laboratory results are termed "objective." This subjective/objective distinction is based on a standard understanding of scientific observation, in which the subjective corresponds to how things seem from a particular perspective (in this instance, the patient's experience) while the objective corresponds to states of affairs that are not tied to any particular point of view (such as temperature or the concentration of ions in the blood). In Western science, the subjective and objective are often reconciled by a "reduction," in which the subjective appearance is explained by reference to the objective account of how things "really are."[4] The classic example is the Copernican heliocentric model of the cosmos, in which the subjective appearance that the sun travels around the earth is explained in terms of an objective description of the earth rota and orbiting the sun.

Medical practice employs a related mode the notion of a "disease entity," inherited in l part from the scientific aspirations of ea physicians such as Koch and Virchow.[5] On model, diseases are conceptualized as disti objective entities that are common to afflic patients. While the patient often cannot dire perceive the presence of the disease entity i (such as a microorganism or histologic chan the patient does perceive the subjective sy toms that are caused by its presence. Thus, subjective symptoms are explained by refere to objective changes in the body, in much same way that subjective appearances in the p ical world are explained by reference to objec concepts such as matter, energy and force.

The disease entity model has had great succ in explaining the symptoms associated with fectious diseases, certain cancers, and poisc which are understood as distinct entities a which often produce a "classic" set of sympto and signs in the afflicted patient. These are wid taken as ideal examples of disease processes, a they influence a paradigm in which physici are seen (or see themselves) as disease-hunt scientists or detectives collecting data to id tify the etiologic agent. (For instance, it is surprising that the overwhelming majority the vivid accounts in Berton Roueché's clas *The Medical Detectives* turn out to involve bac ria, parasites and poisons.[6]) This paradigm th structures the expectations of patients and ph cians. Both may see the physician as someo who can or should provide "answers" to the tient's problems, and both can be frustrated wh this expectation is not met.

This paradigm is less well suited to multifac rial conditions, such as type 2 diabetes melli and coronary artery disease, which are thought result from the overlap of various contributi factors rather than a single etiologic agent. St hese diseases there are objective findings that confirm and explain the patient's subjec- feelings of illness, and in this way the sub- ive/objective distinction is preserved. More blematic are functional disorders, syndromes nclear etiology (such as chronic fatigue syn- me and fibromyalgia), and complaints that do fit any recognized symptom complex. In se cases, there may be no objective findings to firm and explain the patient's subjective feel- s of illness—the subjective feeling of illness is here is. Physicians may then feel pressured by seriousness of the patient's complaints to give iagnosis that they privately regard as scientifi- ly unsubstantiated; and some have worried t giving names that pretend to explain poorly- derstood complaints may have the unin- ded effect of creating new illnesses, as with "transient mental illnesses" studied by the ilosopher Ian Hacking. For the patients' part, y may feel that without the legitimacy con- red by a recognized medical diagnosis, the erity of their symptoms and even their own sin- ity will be doubted.

What these concerns suggest is that rather than bating whether or not these syndromes and ictional disorders are "real" or "legitimate" dical conditions, scrutiny should instead focus conventional models of disease and the stan- rd assumptions that patients and physicians ng to the medical encounter. The presump- n that disabilities and functional limitations less real in the absence of an independently servable disease entity reflects an assumption at all real medical conditions must follow the me paradigm. Yet the possibility remains that e modes of explanation appropriate to illnesses like infections and poisons may not be applicable to more complex complaints, such as those involving interactions between mind, body and culture. The tensions felt by many physicians and patients suggest that new modes of characterizing medical problems are needed.

NOTES

1. Charles E. Rosenberg, "Framing Disease: Illness, Society and History," in *Framing Disease: Studies of Cultural History*, ed. Charles E. Rosenberg and Janet Golden (New Brunswick, N.J.: Rutgers University Press, 1992), pp. xiii–xxvi.

2. Jerome Groopman, "Hurting All Over," *New Yorker*, November 13, 2000, pp. 78–92.

3. Arthur L. Caplan, H. Tristram Engelhardt, Jr., and James J. McCartney, "Introduction," in *Concepts of Health and Disease: Interdisciplinary Perspectives*, ed. Arthur L. Caplan, H. Tristram Engelhardt, Jr., and James J. McCartney (Reading, Mass.: Addison-Wesley, 1981), pp. xxiii–xxxi.

4. For an influential philosophical examination and qualified critique of the pursuit of objectivity see Thomas Nagel, *The View from Nowhere* (New York: Oxford University Press, 1986).

5. H. Tristram Engelhardt, "The Concepts of Health and Disease," reprinted in *Concepts of Health and Disease: Interdisciplinary Perspectives*, ed. Arthur L. Caplan, H. Tristram Engelhardt, Jr., and James J. McCartney (Reading, Mass.: Addison-Wesley, 1981), pp. 31–46.

6. Berton Roueché, *The Medical Detectives* (New York: Truman Talley Books/Plume, 1991).

7. Ian Hacking, *Mad Travelers* (Charlottesville: University Press of Virginia, 1998).

PART III

Clinical Applications of the Concepts of Health and Disease: Controversies/ Consensus

ACCOUNTS OF ILLNESS experiences, inical cases, and social reactions to illness point to the values implicit in sease legitimating or delegitimating and the values underlying the con- pts of illness, health, and normality. Part III is a sampling of these ac- ounts. The selections follow a more or less loose continuum of life, from discussion of "correcting" ambiguous sexual nature in infants to under- anding the conceptual framework affecting social perceptions of Alzhei- ıer's disease and dementia.

ALICE DOMURAT DREGER describes the medical procedures that are rou- nely performed to "normalize" intersexed babies. She challenges the assumption that clear and distinct natural sex lines exist. To claim that there is a clear line between the genders is to claim that intersexed children are diseased. Dreger claims that intersex, while a result of some biological condition, is not a disease. To claim the intersexed are diseased imparts a value judgment onto their condition; this judgment is grounded upon what physicians may deem to be unacceptable genitalia. Thus, Dreger claims sexual identity has been reduced to the presence and form of gonadal tissue, and, as such, sexual identity has been medicalized.

Of course, it is easier to snip than to reconstruct, so even genetically male intersex children can be feminized if their phallus is clinically "inadequate." When gonadal tissue is somehow outside the statistical norms, it is to be treated like a clinical ailment: reconstructive surgery, hormone cocktails, and psychological counseling may all become part of the intersex child's long-term medical treatment regimen. Clearly, Dreger claims that the notion of "normal," which motivates aggressive treatment of intersex children, falls within a (limited) heterosexual experience that reduces the sex organs to either a receptacle or a delivery device. And this notion of "normal" assumes further that proper gonads are necessary for proper development into broadly defined gender roles. How intersexed children are treated and who determines these roles are interrelated concerns that again illustrate the relationship between values, power structures, and the concept of disease.

The basic claim that social problems are medicalized and diseases (and their corresponding sick role) are embedded in a social context has been central to the medical sociology of the latter half of the twentieth century. Early works by medical sociologists emphasized how social structures, "moral entrepreneurs," and political groups and advocacy movements shaped the concept of disease. In his seminal paper from 1975, PETER CONRAD began the discussion about the discovery of hyperkinesis as illustrative of the medicalization of deviance behavior. Conrad sur how pharmaceutical companies and gov ment contributed to the construction of a "hyperactivity disorder." Hyperkinesis, am other psychosocial conditions, was a direct re of the advances in psychopharmacology child psychology that began to incorporate havior into its clinical domain.

Conrad shows how the motives of less po ful "claimsmakers" in tandem with a strong porate stakeholder (e.g., Ciba-Geigy, the for maker of Ritalin) coalesced to create wide ceptance of a disease state, medication regim and ultimately diagnosis of hyperkinesis. T greater upshot: expert control over sociobeh ioral patterns and the shift away from individ responsibility to the "netherworld" of biologi functioning or genetics. By medicalizing w some argue to be simple underachievem laziness, and counterproductive spontaneit new form of disease (not altogether different fr Cartwright's *Dysaesthesia Aethiopis*) emerges its more recent transformation into attent deficit hyperactivity disorder (ADHD), the perkinesis diagnosis may be a new grown-up fo of childhood "rascality," created to maintai certain social order and buttressed by the ph macological tools to maintain that order. T elasticity of disease categories gives hyperkine attention deficit disorder (ADD), and ADH the potential to expand and contract with winds of social and political change.

While social structures may prop up a partic lar condition as a disease, they may also deleg mate other conditions. In addition to describi how fatigue-related illnesses wax and wane in halls of medicine, NORMA WARE presents anth pological data that are helpful in understandi how patients who suffer from these undefin maladies understand their conditions. She sho that sufferers of chronic fatigue syndrome a subject to self-doubt, stigma, psychosocial iso tion, and shame as a result of the ambiguit of their illness. Fundamentally, Ware claims th delegitimation of chronic fatigue syndrome disease is an example of how diseases are ned within the context of Western cultural as-ptions that are rooted in a dualism between d and body as well as biomedical reduction-. Consequently, these assumptions defy at-pts to understand certain psychological con-ons despite their manifestation as physical ditions.

Similar themes are echoed in the next two ers that address the significance of medical-d conditions of women. In the first, JOHN CHARDSON presents the historical and social struction of premenstrual syndrome (PMS). erging out of its original humoral construc-, clinical signs and symptoms of PMS, such hormonal and psychiatric changes, were pack-d together to form a syndrome. The author cludes that PMS is more a result of sociocul-al influences and the role of women in partic-r cultures than of biological evidence.

Richardson's conclusion primes the reader for more radical claims offered by FRANCES MC-REA, who describes the political milieu out which menopause became a disease. McCrea a normativist, stating that she believes "that finitions of health and disease are socially con-ucted and inherently political." She traces the ots of medicalized menopause to the synthesis estrogen, the advent of the pill, and estrogen placement therapy (ERT). But the risks and nefits of ERT to treat the symptoms of meno-use remain unclear. In light of these uncer-nties, could menopause (as a deficiency dis-se) be an insidious form of social control crafted by patriarchal scientific medicine? Is menopause a disease simply because women's procreative potential, physical appeal, and "pleasant" disposition and expected female pleasantries are perceived by physicians (read men) to decline? McCrea thinks so. She goes further to describe the impact of the feminist reaction to the medicalization of menopause. McCrea illustrates how disease definitions are created in an environment closer to a battlefield than an objective biomedical framework, where imperialists driven by power and greed exploit the vulnerable as part of a stigma contest.

And so, too, various manifestations of aging and the concept of normalcy take on new meaning as the modern concept of Alzheimer disease emerged. MARTHA HOLSTEIN describes the transition from the diagnosis of senile dementia (and general senility) to a more inclusive and definitive concept that captures the behavior patterns associated with this disease. The idea that Alzheimer disease was part of aging morphed through the mid-twentieth century into the idea that it is abnormally pathological and may be ameliorated through various social and medical interventions. While arguing that aging is not a disease, a new nosology (as laid out, for example, in the *Diagnostic and Statistical Manual*) pointed to Alzheimer disease as a medical condition that existed as an ontological entity apart from the illness experience. The selections in this part present some of the many clinical examples reminding us that normality, disease, and health are slippery.

CHAPTER 15

"Ambiguous Sex"—or Ambivalent Medicine?

ALICE DOMURAT DREGER

WHAT MAKES US "FEMALE" or "male," irls" or "boys," "women" or "men"—our chromosomes, our genitalia, ow we (and others) are brought up to think about ourselves, or all of the oove? One of the first responses to the birth of a child of ambiguous sex by inicians, and parents, is to seek to "disambiguate" the situation: to assign e newborn's identity as either female or male, surgically modify the iild's genitalia to conform believably to that sex identity, and provide her medical treatment (such as hormones) to reinforce the gender deded upon. The assumptions that underlie efforts to "normalize" interxual individuals and the ethics of "treatment" for intersexuality merit loser examination than they generally receive.

Alice Domurat Dreger

A number of events have lately aroused substantial public interest in intersexuality (congenital "ambiguous sex") and "reconstructive" genital surgery. Perhaps the most sensational of these is the recent publication of unexpected long-term outcomes in the classic and well-known "John/Joan" case.[1] "John" was born a typical XY male with a twin brother, but a doctor accidentally ablated John's penis during a circumcision at age eight months. Upon consultation with a team of physicians and sexologists at the Johns Hopkins Hospital (circa 1963) it was decided that given the unfortunate loss of a normal penis John should be medically reconstructed and raised as a girl—"Joan." Surgeons therefore removed John/Joan's testes and subsequently subjected Joan to further surgical and hormonal treatments in an attempt to make her body look more like a girl's. The team of medical professionals involved also employed substantial psychological counseling to help Joan and the family feel comfortable with Joan's female gender. They believed that Joan and the family would need help adjusting to her new gender, but that full (or near-full) adjustment could be achieved.

For decades, the alleged success of this particular sex reassignment had been widely reported by Hopkins sexologist John Money and others as proof that physicians could essentially create any gender out of any child, so long as the cosmetic alteration was performed early. Money and others repeatedly asserted that "Johns" could be made into "Joans" and "Joans" into "Johns" so long as the genitals looked "right" and everyone agreed to agree on the child's assigned gender. The postulates of this approach are summarized succinctly by Milton Diamond and Keith Sigmundson: "(1) individuals are psychosexually neutral at birth and (2) healthy psychosexual development is dependent on the appearance of the genitals" (p. 298). While not a case of congenital intersexuality, the John/Joan case was nevertheless used by many clinicians who treat intersexuality as proof that in intersex cases the same postulates should hold. The keys seemed to be su cal creation of a believable sexual anatomy assurances all around that the child was "rea the assigned gender.

But reports of the success of John/Joan w premature—indeed, they were wrong. Diam and Sigmundson recently interviewed the pe in question, now an adult, and report that J had in fact chosen to resume life as John at fourteen. John, now an adult, is married woman and, via adoption, is the father of her c dren. John and his mother report that in the Jo years, John was never fully comfortable wi female gender identity. Indeed, Joan actively tempted to resist some of the treatment desig to ensure her female identity; for instance, wh prescribed estrogens at age twelve, Joan secr discarded the feminizing hormones. Depres and unhappy at fourteen, Joan finally asked father for the truth, and upon hearing it, "All sudden everything clicked. For the first ti things made sense, and I understood who what I was" (p. 300). At his request, John recei a mastectomy at age fourteen, and for the n two years underwent several plastic surgery op ations aimed at making his genitals look m masculine.[2]

Diamond and Sigmundson are chiefly in ested in using this new data to conclude that " evidence seems overwhelming that normal mans are not psychosocially neutral at birth are, in keeping with their mammalian herita predisposed and biased to interact with envir mental, familial, and social forces in eithe male or female mode."[3] In other words, sex nature is not infinitely pliable; biology matte

In their report, Diamond and Sigmunds also take the opportunity of publication to co ment on the problem of the lack of long-term f low-up of cases like these. But what is also tro bling is the lack of ethical analysis around ca like this—particularly around cases of the me ical treatment of intersexuality, a phenomen many orders of magnitude more common th matic loss of the penis. While there have n some brief discussions of the ethics of de-ing intersex patients (that discussion is re-ved below), the medical treatment of people n intersexed has remained largely ignored by cists. Indeed, I can find little discussion in the ature of any of the ethical issues involved in rmalizing" children with allegedly "cosmeti-y offensive" anatomies. The underlying as-iption grounding this silence appears to be t "normalizing" procedures are necessarily oughly beneficent and that they present no ndaries. This article seeks to challenge that imption and to encourage interested parties reconsider, from an ethical standpoint, the ninant treatment protocols for children and lts with unusual genital anatomy.

REQUENCY OF NTERSEXUALITY

de from the apparent presumption that "nor-lizing" surgeries are necessarily good, I sus-t that ethicists have ignored the question of in-sex treatment because like most people they ume the phenomenon of intersexuality to be eedingly rare. It is not. But how common is it? e answer depends, of course, on how one ines it. Broadly speaking, intersexuality con-utes a range of anatomical conditions in ich an individual's anatomy mixes key mascu-e anatomy with key feminine anatomy. One ickly runs into a problem, however, when try-to define "key" or "essential" feminine and isculine anatomy. In fact, any close study of ual anatomy results in a loss of faith that there a simple, "natural" sex distinction that will not eak down in the face of certain anatomical, be-vioral, or philosophical challenges.[4]

Sometimes the phrase "ambiguous genitalia" substituted for "intersexuality," but this does t solve the problem of frequency, because we ll are left struggling with the question of what ould count as "ambiguous." (How small must a baby's penis be before it counts as "ambiguous"?) For our purposes, it is simplest to put the question of frequency pragmatically: How often do physicians find themselves unsure which gender to assign at birth? One 1993 gynecology text estimates that "in approximately 1 in 500 births, the sex is doubtful because of the external genitalia."[5] I am persuaded by more recent, well-documented literature that estimates the number to be roughly 1 in 1,500 live births.[6]

The frequency estimate goes up dramatically, however, if we include all children born with what some physicians consider cosmetically "unacceptable" genitalia. Many technically nonintersexed girls are born with "big" clitorises, and many technically nonintersexed boys are born with hypospadic penises in which the urethral opening is found somewhere other than the very tip of the penis.

HISTORICAL BACKGROUND

I came to this topic as an historian and philosopher of science. My initial interest was actually in learning how British and French medical and scientific men of the late nineteenth century dealt with human hermaphroditism. The late nineteenth century was a time when the alleged naturalness of European social sex borders was under serious challenge by feminists and homosexuals and by anthropological reports of sex roles in other cultures. I wanted to know what biomedical professionals did, at such a politically charged time, with those who *inadvertently* challenged anatomical sex borders.

The answer is that biomedical men tried their best to shore up the borders between masculinity and femininity.[7] Specifically, the experts honed in on the ovarian and testicular tissues and decided that these were the key to any body's sexual identity. The "true sex" of most individuals thus by definition settled nicely into one of the two great and preferred camps, no matter how confusing the rest of their sexual anatomies. People with testicular tissue but with some otherwise "ambiguous" anatomy were now labeled "male pseudo-hermaphrodites"—that is, "true" males. People with ovarian tissue but with some otherwise ambiguous anatomy were labeled "female pseudo-hermaphrodites"—"true" females.

By equating sex identity simply with gonadal tissue, almost every body could be shown really to be a "true male" or a "true female" in spite of mounting numbers of doubtful cases. Additionally, given that biopsies of gonads were not done until the 1910s and that Victorian medical men insisted upon histological proof of ovarian and testicular tissue for claims of "true hermaphroditism," the only "true hermaphrodites" tended to be dead and autopsied hermaphrodites.

Nevertheless, new technologies—specifically laparotomies and biopsies—in the 1910s made this approach untenable. It now became possible (and, by the standing rules, necessary) to label some living people as "true" hermaphrodites via biopsies, and disturbed physicians noted that no one knew what to do with such people. There was no place, socially or legally, for true hermaphrodites. Moreover, physicians found case after case of extremely feminine-looking and feminine-acting women who were shown upon careful analysis to have testes and no ovaries. The latter were cases of what today is called androgen-insensitivity syndrome (AIS), also known as testicular feminization syndrome. We now know that individuals with AIS (roughly 1/60,000)[8] have an XY ("male") chromosomal complement and testes, but their androgen receptors cannot "read" the masculinizing hormones their testes produce. Consequently, in utero and throughout their lives, their anatomy develops along apparently "feminine" pathways. AIS is often not discovered until puberty, when these girls do not menstruate and a gynecological examination reveals AIS. Women with AIS look and feel very much like "typical" women, and in a practical, social, legal, and everyday sense they are women, even though congenitally they have testes XY chromosome.

In the 1910s, physicians working with inte uality realized that assigning these wome the male sex (because of their testes) or admit living "true hermaphrodites" (because of t ovotestes) would only wreak social havoc. Co quently, in practice the medical profession mo away from a strict notion of gonadal "true sex ward a pragmatic concept of "gender" and ph cians began to focus their attentions on ger "reconstruction." Elaborate surgical and monal treatments have now been develope make the sexual anatomy more believable, is, more "typical" of the gender assigned by physician.

DOMINANT TREATMENT PROTOCOLS

Thus the late twentieth century medical proach to intersexuality is based essentially on anatomically strict psychosocial theory of gen identity. Contemporary theory, established disseminated largely via the work of John Mon and endorsed by the American Academy of Pe atrics,[10] holds that gender identity arises prim ily from psychosocial rearing (nurture), and directly from biology (nature); that all child must have their gender identity fixed very early life for a consistent, "successful" gender iden to form; that from very early in life the chil anatomy must match the "standard" anatomy her or his gender; and that for gender identity form psychosocially boys primarily require "ad quate" penises with no vagina, and girls primar require a vagina with no easily noticeable ph lus.[11]

Note that this theory presumes that these ru must be followed if intersexual children are achieve successful psychosocial adjustment a propriate to their assigned gender—that is, if th are to act like girls, boys, men, and women a

›posed" to act. The theory also by implication ›umes that there are definite acceptable and ›cceptable roles for boys, girls, men, and ›nen, and that this approach will achieve suc›ful psychosocial adjustment, at least far more n than any other approach.

/Iany parents, especially those unfamiliar 1 sex development, are bothered by their chil›n's intersexed genitals and receptive to offers normalizing" medical treatments. Many also ›vely seek guidance about gender assignment parenting practices. In the United States ay, therefore, typically upon the identification ›n "ambiguous" or intersexed baby, teams of ›cialists (geneticists, pediatric endocrinolo›s, pediatric urologists, and so on) are immedi›y assembled, and these teams of doctors de›e to which sex/gender a given child will be ›gned. A plethora of technologies are then used ›reate and maintain that sex in as believable a ›n as possible, including, typically, surgery on genitals, and sometimes later also on other ›omalous" parts like breasts in an assigned ›le; hormone monitoring and treatments to get ›cocktail" that will help and not contradict the ›ided sex (and that will avoid metabolic dan›s); and fostering the conviction among the ›ld's family and community that the child is in›ed the sex decided—"psychosocial" rearing of › child according to the norms of the chosen ›. Doctors typically take charge of the first two ›ds of activities and hope that the child's family ›d community will successfully manage the all›tical third.

Clinicians treating intersexuality worry that y confusion about the sexual identity of the ›ild on the part of relatives will be conveyed to e child and result in enormous psychological ›oblems, including potential "dysphoric" states adolescence and adulthood. In an effort to ›restall or end any confusion about the child's ›xual identity, clinicians try to see to it that an ›tersexual's sex/gender identity is permanently decided by specialist doctors within forty-eight hours of birth. With the same goals in mind, many clinicians insist that parents of intersexed newborns be told that their ambiguous child does really have a male or female sex, but that the sex of their child has just not yet "finished" developing, and that the doctors will quickly figure out the "correct" sex and then help "finish" the sexual development. As the sociologist Suzanne Kessler noted in her ground-breaking sociological analysis of the current treatment of intersexuality, "the message [conveyed to these parents] . . . is that the trouble lies in the doctor's ability to determine the gender, not in the baby's gender per se."[12] In intersex cases, Ellen Hyun-Ju Lee concludes, "physicians present a picture of the 'natural sex,' either male or female, despite their role in actually constructing sex."[13]

Because of widespread acceptance of the anatomically strict psychosocial theory of treatment, the practical rules now adopted by most specialists in intersexuality are these: genetic males (children with Y chromosomes) must have "adequate" penises if they are to be assigned the male gender. When a genetic male is judged to have an "adequate" phallus size, surgeons may operate, sometimes repeatedly, to try to make the penis look more "normal." If their penises are determined to be "inadequate" for successful adjustment as males, they are assigned the female gender and reconstructed to look female. (Hence John to Joan.) In cases of intersexed children assigned the female sex/gender, surgeons may "carve a large phallus down into a clitoris" (primarily attempting to make the phallus invisible when standing), "create a vagina using a piece of colon" or other body parts, "mold labia out of what was a penis," remove any testes, and so on.[14]

Meanwhile, genetic females (that is, babies lacking a Y chromosome) born with ambiguous genitalia are declared girls—no matter how masculine their genitalia look. This is done chiefly in the interest of preserving these children's potential feminine reproductive capabilities and in bringing their anatomical appearance and physiological capabilities into line with that reproductive role. Consequently, these children are reconstructed to look female using the same general techniques as those used on genetically male children assigned a female role. Surgeons reduce "enlarged" clitorises so that they will not look "masculine." Vaginas are built or lengthened if necessary, in order to make them big enough to accept average-sized penises. Joined labia are separated, and various other surgical and hormonal treatments are directed at producing a believable and, it is hoped, fertile girl.

What are the limits of acceptability in terms of phalluses? Clitorises—meaning simply phalluses in children labeled female—are frequently considered too big if they exceed one centimeter in length.[15] Pediatric surgeons specializing in treating intersexuality consider "enlarged" clitorises to be "cosmetically offensive" in girls and therefore they subject these clitorises to surgical reduction meant to leave the organs looking more "feminine" and "delicate."[16] Penises—meaning simply phalluses in children labeled male—are often considered too small if the stretched length is less than 2.5 centimeters (about an inch). Consequently, genetically male children born at term "with a stretched penile length less than 2.5 [centimeters] are usually given a female sex assignment."[17]

Roughly the same protocols are applied to cases of "true" hermaphroditism (in which babies are born with testicular and ovarian tissue). Whereas the anatomico-materialist metaphysics of sex in the late nineteenth century made true hermaphrodites an enormous problem for doctors and scientists of that time, clinicians today believe that "true hermaphrodites" (like "pseudohermaphrodites") can be fairly easily retrofitted with surgery and other treatment to either an acceptable male or acceptable female sex/gender.

One of the troubling aspects of these protocols are the asymmetric ways they treat femininity and masculinity. For example, physicians appea do far more to preserve the reproductive po tial of children born with ovaries than that of c dren born with testes. While genetically male tersexuals often have infertile testes, some r with micropenis may be able to father childre allowed to retain their testes.[18]

Similarly, surgeons seem to demand far m for a penis to count as "successful" than f vagina to count as such. Indeed, the logic beh the tendency to assign the female gender in ca of intersexuality rests not only on the belief boys need "adequate" penises, but also upon opinion among surgeons that "a functional vag can be constructed in virtually everyone [wh a functional penis is a much more diffic goal."[19] This is true because much is expecte penises, especially by pediatric urologists, very little of vaginas. For a penis to count acceptable—"functional"—it must be or h the potential to be big enough to be readily r ognizable as a "real" penis. In addition, the "fu tional" penis is generally expected to have capability to become erect and flaccid at app priate times, and to act as the conduit throu which urine and semen are expelled, also appropriate times. The urethral opening is pected to appear at the very tip of the penis. T ically, surgeons also hope to see penises that "believably" shaped and colored.

Meanwhile, very little is needed for a su cally constructed vagina to count among s geons as "functional." For a constructed vagina be considered acceptable by surgeons special ing in intersexuality, it basically just has to be hole big enough to fit a typical-sized penis. I not required to be self-lubricating or even to be all sensitive, and certainly does not need change shape the way vaginas often do wh women are sexually stimulated. So, for examp in a panel discussion of surgeons who treat int sexuality, when one was asked, "How do y define successful intercourse? How many these girls actually have an orgasm, for example ember of the panel responded, "Adequate in-ourse was defined as successful vaginal pene-ion."[20] All that is required is a receptive hole. ndeed, clinicians treating intersex children n talk about vaginas in these children as the ence of a thing, as a space, a "hole," a place to something. That is precisely why opinion ds that "a functional vagina can be con-cted in virtually everyone" because it is rela-ly easy to construct an insensitive hole surgi-y. (It is not always easy to keep them open and nfected.) The decision to "make" a female is refore considered relatively foolproof, while e assignment of male sex of rearing is in-tably difficult and should only be undertaken an experienced team" who can determine if enis will be adequate for "successful" male-od.[21]

HE PROBLEM OF "NORMALITY"

e strict conception of "normal" sexual atomy and "normal" sex behavior that under-s prevailing treatment protocols is arguably ist in its asymmetrical treatment of reproduc-e potential and definitions of anatomical "ade-acy." Additionally, as Lee and other critics of ersex treatment have noted, "[d]ecisions of nder assignment and subsequent surgical re-nstruction are inseparable from the heterosex-l matrix, which does not allow for other sexual actices or sexualities. Even within heterosexu-ty, a rich array of sexual practices is reduced vaginal penetration."[22] Not surprisingly, femi-sts and intersexuals have invariably objected to ese presumptions that there is a "right" way to a male and a "right" way to be a female, and at children who challenge these categories ould be reconstructed to fit into (and thereby inforce) them.

Indeed, beside the important (and too often sregarded) philosophical-political issue of gen-r roles, there is a more practical one: how does one decide where to put the boundaries on acceptable levels of anatomical variation? Not surprisingly, the definition of genital "normality" in practice appears to vary among physicians. For example, at least one physician has set the minimum length of an "acceptable" penis at 1.5 centimeters.[23]

Indeed, at least two physicians are convinced (and have evidence) that any penis is a big enough penis for male adjustment, if the other cards are played right. Almost a decade ago Justine Schober (neé Reilly), a pediatric urologist now based at the Hamot Medical Center in Erie, Pennsylvania, and Christopher Woodhouse, a physician based at the Institute of Urology and St. George's Hospital in London, "interviewed and examined 20 patients with the primary diagnosis of micropenis in infancy" who were labeled and raised as boys. Of the post-pubertal (adult) subjects, "All patients were heterosexual and they had erections and orgasms. Eleven patients had ejaculations, 9 were sexually active and reported vaginal penetration, 7 were married or cohabitating and 1 had fathered a child."[24]

Schober and Woodhouse concluded that "a small penis does not preclude normal male role" and should not dictate female gender reassignment. They found that when parents "were well counseled about diagnosis they reflected an attitude of concern but not anxiety about the problem, and they did not convey anxiety to their children. They were honest and explained problems to the child and encouraged normality in behavior. We believe that this is the attitude that allows these children to approach their peers with confidence" (p. 571).

Ultimately, Schober and Woodhouse agreed with the tenet of the psychosocial theory that assumes that "the strongest influence for all patients [is] the parental attitude." But rather than making these children into girls and trying to convince the parents and children about their "real" feminine identity, Schober and Woodhouse found that "the well informed and open parents . . . produced more confident and better adjusted boys." We should note that these boys were not considered "typical" in their sex lives: "The group was characterized by an experimental attitude to [sexual] positions and methods. . . . The group appears to form close and long-lasting relationships. They often attribute partner sexual satisfaction and the stability of their relationships [with women partners] to their need to make extra effort including nonpenetrating techniques" (p. 571).

"Ambiguous" genitalia do not constitute a disease. They simply constitute a failure to fit a particular (and, at present, a particularly demanding) definition of normality. It is true that whenever a baby is born with "ambiguous" genitalia, doctors need to consider the situation a potential medical emergency because intersexuality may signal a potentially serious metabolic problem, namely congenital adrenal hyperplasia (CAH), which primarily involves an electrolyte imbalance and can result in "masculinization" of genetically female fetuses. Treatment of CAH may save a child's life and fertility. At the birth of an intersex child, therefore, adrenogenital syndrome must be quickly diagnosed and treated, or ruled out. Nonetheless, as medical texts advise, "of all the conditions responsible for ambiguous genitalia, congenital adrenal hyperplasia is the only one that is life-threatening in the newborn period," and even in cases of CAH the "ambiguous" genitalia themselves are not deadly.[25]

As with CAH's clear medical issue, doctors now also know that the testes of AIS patients have a relatively high rate of becoming cancerous, and therefore AIS needs to be diagnosed as early as possible so that the testes can be carefully watched or removed. However, the genitalia of an androgen-insensitive person are not diseased. Again, while unusual genitalia may signal a present or potential threat to health, in themselves they just look different. As we have seen, because of the perception of a "social emergency" around an intersex birth, clinicians take license to [illegible] nonstandard genitalia as a medical problem [illegible] quiring prompt correction. But as Suza[illegible] Kessler sums up the situation, intersexuality [illegible] not threaten the patient's life; it threatens the [illegible] tient's culture.

PSYCHOLOGICAL HEALTH AND THE PROBLEM OF DECEPTION

Clearly, in our often unforgiving culture in[illegible] sexuality can also threaten the patient's psyc[illegible] that recognition is behind the whole treatm[illegible] approach. Nevertheless, there are two m[illegible] problems here. First, clinicians treating inte[illegible] individuals may be far more concerned w[illegible] strict definitions of genital normality than in[illegible] sexuals, their parents, and their acquaintan[illegible] (including lovers). This is evidenced time a[illegible] again, for example, in the John/Joan case:

> John recalls thinking, from preschool through [illegible] ementary school, that physicians were more c[illegible] cerned with the appearance of Joan's geni[illegible] than was Joan. Her genitals were inspected [illegible] each visit to the Johns Hopkins Hospital. [illegible] thought they were making a big issue out of no[illegible] ing, and they gave her no reason to think oth[illegible] wise. John recalls thinking: "Leave me be a[illegible] then I'll be fine. . . . It's bizarre. My genitals [illegible] not bothering me; I don't know why it is both[illegible] ing you guys so much."[26]

Second, and more basically, it is not self-evid[illegible] that a psychosocial problem should be handl[illegible] medically or surgically. We do not attempt [illegible] solve the problems many dark-skinned child[illegible] will face in our nation by lightening their ski[illegible] Similarly, Cheryl Chase has posed this intere[illegible] ing question: when a baby is born with a sever[illegible] disfigured but largely functional arm, oug[illegible] we quickly remove the arm and replace it wi[illegible] a possibly functional prosthetic, so that the pa[illegible]

; and child experience less psychological ma?[27] While it is true that genitals are more :hically charged than arms, genitals are also re easily and more often kept private, whatr their state. Quoting the ideas of Suzanne sler, the pediatric urologist Schober argues in rthcoming work that "Surgery makes parents doctors more comfortable, but counseling kes people comfortable too, and [it] is not irersible." She continues: "Simply understand- and performing good surgeries is not ficient. We must also know when to appropriy perform or withhold surgery. Our ethical y as surgeons is to do no harm and to serve best interests of our patient. Sometimes, this ans admitting that a 'perfect' solution may not attainable."[28]

ronically, rather than alleviating feelings of akishness, in practice the way intersexuality is ically handled may actually produce or conoute to many intersexuals' feelings of freakishs. Many intersexuals look at these two facts: (1) y are subject, out of "compassion," to "norlizing" surgeries on an emergency basis witht their personal consent, and (2) they are often t told the whole truth about their anatomical nditions and anatomical histories. Understandably, they conclude that their doctors see m as profound freaks and that they must really freaks. H. Martin Malin, a professor in clinical ology and a therapist at the Child and Family stitute in Sacramento, California, has found s to be a persistent theme running through insexuals' medical experience:

> As I listened to [intersexuals'] stories, certain leit motifs began to emerge from the bits of their histories. They or their parents had little, if any, counseling. They thought they were the only ones who felt as they did. Many had asked to meet other patients whose medical histories were similar to their own, but they were stonewalled. They recognized themselves in published case histories, but when they sought medical records, were told they could not be located....
>
> The patients I was encountering were not those whose surgeries resulted from life-threatening or seriously debilitating medical conditions. Rather, they had such diagnoses as "micropenis" or "clitoral hypertrophy." These were patients who were told—when they were told anything—that they had vaginoplasties or clitorectomies because of the serious psychological consequences they would have suffered if surgery had not been done. But the surgeries *had* been performed—and they were reporting longstanding psychological distress. They were certain that they would rather have had the "abnormal" genitals they [had] had than the "mutilated" genitals they were given. They were hostile and often vengeful towards the professionals who had been responsible for their care and sometimes, by transference, towards me. They were furious that they had been lied to.[29]

Given the lack of long-term follow-up studies it is unclear whether a majority of intersexuals wind up feeling this way, but even if only a small number do we must ask whether the practice of deception and "stonewalling" is essentially unethical.

Why would a physician ever withhold medical and personal historical information from an intersexed patient? Because she or he believes that the truth is too horrible or too complicated for the patient to handle. In a 1988 commentary in the *Hastings Center Report*, Brendan Minogue and Robert Tarszewski argued, for example, that a physician could justifiably withhold information from a sixteen-year-old AIS patient and/or her parents if he believed that the patient and/or family was likely to be incapable of handling the fact that she has testes and an XY chromosomal complement.[30] Indeed, this reasoning appears typical among clinicians treating intersexuality; many continue to believe that talking truthfully with intersexuals and their families will undo all the "positive" effects of the technological efforts aimed at covering up doubts. Thus despite intersexuals' and ethicists' published, repeated objections to deception, in 1995 a medical student was given a cash prize in medical ethics by the Canadian Medical Association for an article specifically advocating deceiving AIS patients (including adults) about the biological facts of their conditions. The prize-winner argued that "physicians who withhold information from AIS patients are not actually lying; they are only deceiving" because they *selectively withhold* facts about patients' bodies.[31]

But what this reasoning fails to appreciate is that hiding the facts of the condition will not necessarily prevent a patient and family from thinking about it. Indeed, the failure on the part of the doctor and family to talk honestly about the condition is likely only to add to feelings of shame and confusion. One woman with AIS in Britain writes, "Mine was a dark secret kept from all outside the medical profession (family included), but this [should] not [be] an option because it both increases the feelings of freakishness and reinforces the isolation."[32] Similarly, Martha Coventry, a woman who had her "enlarged" clitoris removed by surgeons when she was six, insists that "to be lied to as a child about your own body, to have your life as a sexual being so ignored that you are not even given the decency of an answer to your questions, is to have your heart and soul relentlessly undermined."[33]

Lying to a patient about his or her biological condition can also lead to a patient unintentionally taking unnecessary risks. As a young woman, Sherri Groveman, who has AIS, was told by her doctor that she had "twisted ovaries" and that they had to be removed; in fact, her testes were removed. At the age of twenty, "alone and scared in the stacks of a [medical] library," she discovered the truth of her condition. Then "the pieces finally fit together. But what fell apart was my relationship with both my family and physicians. It was not learning about chromosomes or te that caused enduring trauma, it was discove that I had been told lies. I avoided all med care for the next 18 years. I have severe os porosis as a result of a lack of medical attent This is what lies produce."[34]

Similarly, as B. Diane Kemp—"a social wo with more than 35 years' experience and a wor who has borne androgen insensitivity syndro for 63 years"—notes, "secrecy as a method of h dling troubling information is primitive, deg ing, and often ineffective. Even when a secre kept, its existence carries an aura of unease most people can sense.... Secrets crippled life."[35]

Clearly, the notion that deception or selec truthtelling will protect the child, the family even the adult intersexual is extraordinarily ternalistic and naive, and, while perhaps w intentioned, it goes against the dominant tre in medical ethics as those ethics guidelines applied to other, similar situations. In what ot realms are patients regularly not told the medi names for their conditions, even when they a As for the idea that physicians should not tell tients what they probably "can't handle," woul physician be justified in using this reasoning avoid telling a patient she has cancer or AID

In their commentary in the *Hastings Cen Report* Sherman Elias and George Annas poin out that a physician who starts playing with facts of a patient's condition may well find hi self forced to lie or admit prior deception. "Pr tically," Elias and Annas wrote, "it is unrealistic believe that [the AIS patient] will not ultimat learn the details of her having testicular sy drome. From the onset it will be difficult to ma tain the charade."[36] They also note that witho being told the name and details of her conditi any consent the AIS patient gives will not truly "informed." As an attorney Groveman too argu "that informed consent laws mandate that the p tient know the truth before physicians remo her testes or reconstruct her vagina."[37]

NFORMED CONSENT ND RISK ASSUMPTION

not at all clear if all or even most of the inter- surgeries done today involve what would lly and ethically constitute informed con- t. It appears that few intersexuals or their par- s are educated, before they give consent, ut the anatomically strict psychosocial model ployed. The model probably ought to be de- bed to parents as essentially unproven insofar the theory remains unconfirmed by broad- ed, long-term follow-up studies, and is directly llenged by cases like the John/Joan case as l as by ever mounting "anecdotal" reports n former patients who, disenfranchised and eled "lost to follow-up" by clinicians, have ned to the popular press and to public protest order to be heard. Of course, as long as inter- patients are not consistently told the truth of ir conditions, there is some question about ether satisfaction can be assessed with integrity long-term studies.

At a finer level, many of the latest particular smetic surgeries being used on intersexed ba- s and children today remain basically un- oven as well, and need to be described as such consent agreements. For example, a team of rgeons from the Children's Medical Center d George Washington University Medical hool has reported that in their preferred form clitoral "recession" (done to make "big" clit- ses look "right"), "the cosmetic effect is excel- nt" but "late studies with assessment of sexual atification, orgasm, and general psychological justment are unavailable ... and remain in estion."[38] In fact the procedure may result in oblems like stenosis, increased risk of infec- ns, loss of feeling, and psychological trauma. hese risks characterize all genital surgeries.)

This lack of long-term follow-up is the case not ly for clitoral surgeries; David Thomas, a pedi- ric urologist who practices at St. James's Uni- rsity Hospital and Infirmary in Leeds, England, recently noted the same problem with regard to early vaginal reconstructions: "So many of these patients are lost to follow-up. If we do this surgery in infancy and childhood, we have an obligation to follow these children up, to assess what we're doing."[39] There is a serious ethical problem here: risky surgeries are being performed as standard care and are not being adequately followed-up.[40]

The growing community of open adult intersexuals understandably question whether anyone should have either her ability to enjoy sex or her physical health risked without personal consent just because she has a clitoris, penis, or vagina that falls outside the standard deviation. Even if we did have statistics that showed that particular procedures "worked" a majority of the time we would have to face the fact that part of the time they would not work, and we need to ask whether that risk ought to be assumed on behalf of another person.

BEYOND "MONSTER ETHICS"

In a 1987 article on the ethics of killing one conjoined twin to save the other, George Annas suggested (but did not advocate) that one way to justify such a procedure would be to take "the monster approach." This approach would hold that conjoined twins are so grotesque, so pathetic, any medical procedure aimed at normalizing them would be morally justified.[41] Unfortunately, the present treatment of intersexuality in the U.S. seems to be deeply informed by the monster approach; ethical guidelines that would be applied in nearly any other medical situation are, in cases of intersexuality, ignored. Patients are lied to; risky procedures are performed without follow-up; consent is not fully informed; autonomy and health are risked because of unproven (and even disproven) fears that atypical anatomy will lead to psychological disaster. Why? Perhaps because sexual anatomy is not treated like the rest of human anatomy, or perhaps because we simply assume that any procedure which "normalizes" an "abnormal" child is merciful. Whatever the reason, the medical treatment of intersexuality and other metabolically benign, cosmetically unusual anatomies needs deep and immediate attention.

We can readily use the tools of narrative ethics to gain insight into practices surrounding intersexuality. There are now available many autobiographies of adult intersexuals.[42] Like that of John/Joan, whether or not they are characteristic of long-term outcomes these autobiographies raise serious questions about the dominant treatment protocols.

Narrative ethics also suggests that we use our imaginations to think through the story of the intersexual, to ask ourselves, if we were born intersexed, what treatment we would wish to have received. Curious about what adult nonintersexuals would have chosen for themselves, Suzanne Kessler polled a group of college students regarding their feelings on the matter. The women were asked, "Suppose you had been born with a larger than normal clitoris and it would remain larger than normal as you grew to adulthood. Assuming that the physicians recommended surgically reducing your clitoris, under what circumstances would you have wanted your parents to give them permission to do it?" In response,

> About a fourth of the women indicated they would not have wanted a clitoral reduction under any circumstance. About half would have wanted their clitoris reduced only if the larger than normal clitoris caused health problems. Size, for them, was not a factor. The remaining fourth of the sample could imagine wanting their clitoris reduced if it were larger than normal, but only if having the surgery would not have resulted in a reduction in pleasurable sensitivity.[43]

Meanwhile, in this study, "the men were asked to imagine being born with a smaller than normal penis and told that physicians recommen phallic reduction and a female gender ass ment." In response,

> All but one man indicated they would not h wanted surgery under any circumstance. Th maining man indicated that if his penis we cm. or less and he were going to be sterile would have wanted his parents to give the doc permission to operate and make him a female 36)

Kessler is cautious to note that we need m information to assess this data fully, but it d begin to suggest that given the choice most p ple would reject genital cosmetic surgery themselves.

As an historian, I also think we need to c sider the historical and cultural bases for gen conformity practices, and realize that most p ple in the U.S. demonstrate little tolerance practices in other cultures that might well considered similar. I am, of course, talking ab the recent passage of federal legislation prohi ing physicians from performing "circumcisi on the genitalia of girls under the age of eighte whether or not the girls consent or personally quest the procedure. African female genital "c ting" typically involves, in part, excision of the c oral tissue so that most or all clitoral sensati will be lost. While proponents of this traditio female genital "cutting" have insisted this pr tice is an important cultural tradition—ana gous to male circumcision culturally—advoca of the U.S. law insist it is barbaric and viola human rights. Specifically, in the federal legis tion passed in October 1996 Congress declar that: "Except as provided in subsection (b), wh ever knowingly circumcises, excises, or infil lates the whole or any part of the labia majora labia minora or clitoris of another person who h not attained the age of 18 years shall be fin under this title or imprisoned not more than years, or both."[44]

ubsection (b) specifies that: "A surgical opern is not a violation of this section if the operaı is (1) necessary to the health of the person on om it is performed, and is performed by a perlicensed in the place of its performance as a dical practitioner; or (2) performed on a perin labor or who has just given birth and is perned for medical purposes connected with that or or birth."

Surgeons treating intersexuality presumably uld argue that the procedures they perform on genitals of girls (which clearly include excin of parts of the clitoris) are indeed "necessary the health of the person on whom it is permed." While it is easy to condemn the African ctice of female genital mutilation as a baric custom that violates human rights, we uld recognize that in the United States medne's prevailing response to intersexuality is gely about genital conformity and the "proper" es of the sexes. Just as we find it necessary to tect the rights and well-being of African girls, must now consider the hard questions of the hts and well-being of children born intersexed the United States.

As this paper was in process, the attention paid the popular media and by physicians to the blems with the dominant clinical protocols reased dramatically, and many more physins and ethicists have recently come forward question those protocols. Diamond and Sigundson have helpfully proposed tentative new uidelines for dealing with persons with amguous genitalia."[45]

As new guidelines are further developed, it will critical to take seriously two tasks. First, as I ve argued above, intersexuals must not be subcted to different ethical standards from other ople simply because they are intersexed. Second, the experiences and advice of adult interxuals must be solicited and taken into considation. It is incorrect to claim, as I have heard veral clinicians do, that the complaints of adult intersexuals are irrelevant because they were subjected to "old, unperfected" surgeries. Clinicians have too often retreated to the mistaken belief that improved treatment technologies (for example, better surgical techniques) will eliminate ethical dilemmas surrounding intersex treatment. There is far more at issue than scar tissue and loss of sensation from unperfected surgeries.

ACKNOWLEDGMENTS

The author wishes to thank Aron Sousa, Cheryl Chase, Michael Fisher, Elizabeth Gretz, Daniel Federman, the members of the Enhancement Technologies and Human Identity Working Group, and Howard Brody, Libby Bogdan-Lovis, and other associates of the Center for Ethics and Humanities in the Life Sciences at Michigan State University for their comments on this work.

This article is adapted from *Hermaphrodites and the Medical Invention of Sex*, by Alice Domurat Dreger, published by Harvard University Press.

NOTES

1. Milton Diamond and H. Keith Sigmundson, "Sex Reassignment at Birth: Long-Term Review and Clinical Implications," *Archives of Pediatrics and Adolescent Medicine* 15 (1997): 298–304. Available from www.afn.org/~sfcommed/mdfnl.htm.

2. For a more in-depth biography, see John Colapinto, "The True Story of John/Joan," *Rolling Stone*, December 11, 1997, pp. 55ff.

3. Diamond and Sigmundson, "Sex Reassignment," p. 303.

4. I discuss this at length in Dreger, *Hermaphrodites and the Medical Invention of Sex* (Cambridge, Mass.: Harvard University Press, 1998); see especially prologue and chap. 1.

5. See Ethel Sloane, *Biology of Women*, 3rd ed. (Albany, N.Y.: Delmar Publishers, 1993), p. 168. According to Denis Grady, a study of over 6,500 women ath-

letes competing in seven different international sports competitions showed an incidence of intersexuality of one in 500 women, but unfortunately Grady does not provide a reference to the published data from that study (Denise Grady, "Sex Test," *Discover*, June 1992, pp. 78–82). That sampled population should not simply be taken as representative of the whole population, but this number is certainly higher than most people would expect.

6. Anne Fausto-Sterling, *Sexing the Body: Gender Politics and the Construction of Sexuality* (New York: Basic Books, 2000), chap. 2; [M. Blackless, A. Charuvastra, A. Derryck, A. Fausto-Sterling, K. Lauzanne, and E. Lee, "How Sexually Dimophic Are We? Review and Synthesis. *American Journal of Human Biology* 12, no. 2 (2000): 151–66.]; and personal communication. The highest modern-day estimate for frequency of sexually ambiguous births comes from John Money, who has posited that as many as 4 percent of live births today are of "intersexed" individuals (cited in Anne Fausto-Sterling, "The Five Sexes," *Sciences* 33 [1993]: 20–25). Money's categories tend to be exceptionally broad and poorly defined, and not representative of what most medical professionals today would consider to be "intersexuality."

7. Dreger, *Hermaphrodites*, chaps. 1–5; for a summary of the scene in Britain in the late-nineteenth century, see Dreger, "Doubtful Sex: The Fate of the Hermaphrodite in Victorian Medicine," *Victorian Studies* 38 (1995): 335–69.

8. Stuart R. Kupfer, Charmain A. Quigley, and Frank S. French, "Male Pseudohermaphroditism," *Seminars in Perinatology* 16 (1992): 319–31, at 325.

9. For summaries and critiques of Money's work on intersexuality, see especially: Cheryl Chase, "Affronting Reason," in *Looking Queer: Image and Identity in Lesbian, Bisexual, Gay, and Transgendered Communities*, ed. D. Atkins (Binghamton, N.Y.: Haworth, 1998); "Hermaphrodities with Attitude: Mapping the Emergence of Intersex Political Activism," *GLQ* 4, no. 2 (1998): 189–211; Anne Fausto-Sterling, "How to Build a Man," in *Science and Homosexualities*, ed. Vernon A. Rosario (New York: Routledge, 1997), pp. 219–25; and Ellen Hyun-Ju Lee, "Producing Sex: A[n In]terdisciplinary Perspective on Sex Assignment D[eci]sions for Intersexuals" (senior thesis, Brown Unive[rsity,] 1994).

10. American Academy of Pediatrics (Section [on] Urology), "Timing of Elective Surgery on the G[eni]talia of Male Children with Particular Referenc[e to] the Risks, Benefits, and Psychological Effect[s of] Surgery and Anesthesia," *Pediatrics* 97, no. 4 (19[96]): 590–94.

11. For example, see Patricia K. Donahoe, "The [Di]agnosis and Treatment of Infants with Intersex Ab[nor]malities," *Pediatric Clinics of North America* 34 (19[87]): 1333–48.

12. Suzanne J. Kessler, "The Medical Construc[tion] of Gender: Case Management of Intersexed Infa[nts,"] *Signs* 16 (1990): 3–26; compare the advice given [by] Cynthia H. Meyers-Seifer and Nancy J. Cha[rest,] "Diagnosis and Management of Patients with Amb[igu]ous Genitalia," *Seminars in Perinatology* 16 (19[92]): 332–39.

13. Lee, "Producing Sex," p. 45.

14. Melissa Hendricks, "Is It a Boy or a Girl?" *Jo[hns] Hopkins Magazine* (November, 1993): 10–16, p. 10.

15. Barbara C. McGillivray, "The Newborn w[ith] Ambiguous Genitalia," *Seminars in Perinatology* (1991): 365–68, p. 366.

16. Kurt Newman, Judson Randolph, and Kath[leen] Anderson, "The Surgical Management of Infants a[nd] Children with Ambiguous Genitalia," *Annals [of] Surgery* 215 (1992): 644–53, pp. 651 and 647.

17. Meyers-Seifer and Charest, "Diagnosis a[nd] Management," p. 337. See also Kupfer, Quigley, a[nd] French, "Male Pseudohermaphroditism," p. 328; R[aj]kumar Shah, Morton M. Woolley, and Gertrude C[os]tin, "Testicular Feminization: The Androgen Insen[si]tivity Syndrome," *Journal of Pediatric Surgery* 27 (199[2]): 757–60, p. 757.

18. Justine Schober, personal communication; [for] data on this, see Justine M. Reilly and C. R. J. Wo[od]house, "Small Penis and the Male Sexual Role," *Jo[ur]nal of Urology* 142 (1989): 569–71.

19. Robin J. O. Catlin, *Appleton & Lange Review*

USMILE Step 2 (East Norwalk, Conn.: Appleton ange, 1993), p. 49.

ɔ. See the comments of John P. Gearhart in M. M. ez, John P. Gearhart, Claude Migeon, and John k, "Vaginal Reconstruction after Initial Construc- of the External Genitalia in Girls with Salt-Wast- Adrenal Hyperplasia," *Journal of Urology* 148 2): 680–84, p. 684.

1. Kupfer, Quigley, and French, "Male Pseudoher- hroditism," p. 328.

2. Lee, "Producing Sex," p. 27.

3. See Donahoe, "The Diagnosis and Treatment of nts with Intersex Abnormalities."

4. Reilly and Woodhouse, "Small Penis," p. 569.

5. Patricia K. Donahoe, David M. Powell, and ry M. Lee, "Clinical Management of Intersex Ab- malities," *Current Problems in Surgery* 28 (1991): -79, p. 540.

6. Diamond and Sigmundson, "Sex Reassign- nt," pp. 300–301.

7. Cheryl Chase, personal communication.

8. Quoted in Justine M. Schober, "Long-Term tcomes for Intersex," *Pediatric Surgery and Urology: ng Term Outcomes*, ed. Pierre D. E. Mouriquand iladelphia: William B. Saunders, forthcoming). ark D. Stringer, Pierre D. E. Mouriquand, Keith T. lham, Edward R. Howard. *Pediatric Surgery and ology: Long Term Outcomes*. Philadelphia: William Saunders, 1998.]

29. H. M. Malin, personal communication, January 1997, to Justine M. Schober, quoted in Schober, ong-Term Outcome."

30. Brendan P. Minogue and Robert Taraszewski, he Whole Truth and Nothing But the Truth?" se study], *Hastings Center Report* 18, no. 5 (1988): -35.

31. Anita Natarajan, "Medical Ethics and Truth lling in the Case of Androgen Insensitivity Syn- ome," *Canadian Medical Association Journal* 154 96): 568–70. (For responses to Natarajan's recom- endations by AIS women and a partner of an AIS man, see *Canadian Medical Association Journal* 154 96]: 1829–33.)

32. Anonymous, "Be Open and Honest with Sufferers," *British Medical Journal* 308 (1994): 1041–42.

33. Martha Coventry, "Finding the Words," *Chrysalis: The Journal of Transgressive Gender Identities* 2 (1997): 27–30.

34. Sherri A. Groveman, "Letter to the Editor," *Canadian Medical Association Journal* 154 (1996): 1829, 1832.

35. B. Diane Kemp, "Letter to the Editor," *Canadian Medical Association Journal* 154 (1996): 1829.

36. Sherman Elias and George J. Annas, "The Whole Truth and Nothing But the Truth?" [case study], *Hastings Center Report* 18, no. 5 (1988): 35–36, p. 35.

37. Groveman, "Letter to the Editor," p. 1829.

38. Newman, Randolph, and Anderson, "Surgical Management," p. 651.

39. "Is Early Vaginal Reconstruction Wrong for Some Intersex Girls?" *Urology Times* (February 1997): 10–12.

40. Intersexuals are understandably tired of hearing that "long-term follow-up data is needed" while the surgeries continue to occur. On this, see especially the guest commentary by David Sandberg, "A Call for Clinical Research," *Hermaphrodites with Attitude* (fall/winter 1995–1996): 8–9, and the many responses of intersexuals in the same issue.

41. George J. Annas, "Siamese Twins: Killing One to Save the Other," *Hastings Center Report* 17, no. 2 (1987): 27–29.

42. See, for example, M. Morgan Holmes, "Medical Politics and Cultural Imperatives: Intersex Identities beyond Pathology and Erasure" (M.A. thesis, York University, 1994); Chase, "Hermaphrodites with Attitude"; Geoffrey Cowley, "Gender Limbo," *Newsweek*, May 19, 1997, pp. 64–66; Natalie Angier, "New Debate Over Surgery on Genitals," *New York Times*, May 13, 1997; "Special Issue: Intersexuality," *Chrysalis: The Journal of Transgressive Gender Identities* 2 (1997). Intersexual autobiographies are also from peer support groups, including the Intersex Society of North America. For information about support groups, see the special issue of *Chrysalis*, vol. 2, 1997.

43. Suzanne J. Kessler, "Meanings of Genital Variability," *Chrysalis: The Journal of Transgressive Gender Identities* 2 (1997): 33–37.

44. Omnibus Consolidated Appropriations Bill, H.R. 3610, PL. 104–208.

45. Milton Diamond and Keith Sigmundson, "M agement of Intersexuality: Guidelines for Dealing Persons with Ambiguous Genitalia," *Archives of P atric and Adolescent Medicine* 151 (1997): 1046–50.

CHAPTER 16

The Discovery of Hyperkinesis: Notes on the Medicalization of Deviant Behavior[1]

PETER CONRAD

INTRODUCTION

THE INCREASING MEDICALIZATION of eviant behavior and the medical institution's role as an agent of social ontrol has gained considerable notice (Freidson 1970; Pitts 1968; Kitterie 971; Zola 1972). By medicalization we mean defining behavior as a medal problem or illness and mandating or licensing the medical profession provide some type of treatment for it. Examples include alcoholism, rug addiction and treating violence as a genetic or brain disorder. This edefinition is not a new function of the medical institution: psychiatry and ublic health have always been concerned with social behavior and have traditionally functioned as agents of social control (Foucault 1965; Szasz 1970; Rosen 1972). Increasingly sophisticated medical technology has extended the potential of this type of social control, especially in terms of psychotechnology (Chorover 1973). This approach includes a variety of medical and quasi-medical treatments or procedures: psychosurgery, psychotropic medications, genetic engineering, Antibuse, and methadone. This paper describes how certain forms of behavior in children have become defined as a medical problem and how medicine has become a major agent for their social control since the discovery of hyperkinesis. By discovery we mean both origin of the diagnosis and treatment for this disorder; and discovery of children who exhibit this behavior. The first section analyzes the discovery of hyperkinesis and why it suddenly became popular in the 1960s. The second section will discuss the medicalization of deviant behavior and its ramifications.

THE MEDICAL DIAGNOSIS OF HYPERKINESIS

Hyperkinesis is a relatively recent phenomenon as a medical diagnostic category. Only in the past two decades has it been available as a recognized diagnostic category and only in the last decade has it received widespread notice and medical popularity. However, the roots of the diagnosis and treatment of this clinical entity are found earlier. Hyperkinesis is also known as Minimal Brain Dysfunction, Hyperactive Syndrome, Hyperkinetic Disorder of Childhood, and by several other diagnostic categories. Although the symptoms and the presumed etiology vary, in general the behaviors are quite similar and greatly overlap.[2] Typical symptom patterns for diagnosing the disorder include: extreme excess of motor activity (hyperactivity); very short attention span (the child flits from activity to activity); restlessness; fidgetiness; often wildly oscillating mood swings (he's fine one day, a terror the next); clumsi aggressive-like behavior; impulsivity; in sc he can not sit still, cannot comply with rules low frustration level; frequently there ma sleeping problems and acquisition of speech be delayed (Stewart et al. 1966; Stewart ı Wender 1971). Most of the symptoms for the order are deviant behaviors.[3] It is six time prevalent among boys as among girls. We us term hyperkinesis to represent all the diagn categories of this disorder.

THE DISCOVERY OF HYPERKINESIS

It is useful to divide the analysis into what m be called *clinical factors* directly related to th agnosis and treatment of hyperkinesis and s *factors* that set the context for the emergen the new diagnostic category.

CLINICAL FACTORS

Bradley (1937) observed that amphetamine d had a spectacular effect in altering the beh of school children who exhibited behavior d ders or learning disabilities. Fifteen of the t children he treated actually became more dued in their behavior. Bradley termed the e of this medication paradoxical, since he expe that amphetamines would stimulate childre they stimulated adults. After the medication discontinued the children's behavior return premedication level.

A scattering of reports in the medical liter on the utility of stimulant medications for "c hood behavior disorders" appeared in the two decades. The next significant contribu was the work of Strauss and his associates (St and Lehtinen 1947) who found certain beh (including hyperkinesis behaviors) in po cephaletic children suffering from what called minimal brain injury (damage). This irst time these behaviors were attributed to new organic distinction of minimal brain age.

his disorder still remained unnamed or else it called a variety of names (usually just "child-l behavior disorder"). It did not appear as a ific diagnostic category until Laufer et al. 7) described it as the "hyperkinetic impulse rder" in 1957. Upon finding "the salient char-ristics of the behavior pattern ... are strik-y similar to those with clear cut organic cau-n" these researchers described a disorder no clear-cut history or evidence for organic-Laufer et al. 1957).

1966 a task force sponsored by the U.S. Pub-Health Service and the National Association Crippled Children and Adults attempted to fy the ambiguity and confusion in terminol-and symptomology in diagnosing children's avior and learning disorders. From over three en diagnoses, they agreed on the term "mini-brain dysfunction" as an overriding diagnosis would include hyperkinesis and other disor-(Clements 1966). Since this time M.B.D. been the primary formal diagnosis or label. e middle 1950s a new drug, Ritalin, was syn-ized, that has many qualities of ampheta-es without some of their more undesirable effects. In 1961 this drug was approved by the A. for use with children. Since this time e has been much research published on the of Ritalin in the treatment of childhood be-or disorders. This medication became the tment of choice" for treating children with rkinesis.

nce the early sixties, more research appeared he etiology, diagnosis and treatment of hy-inesis (cf. DeLong 1972; Grinspoon and er 1973; Cole 1975)—as much as three-quar-concerned with drug treatment of the disor-There had been increasing publicity of the rder in the mass media as well. The *Reader's le to Periodical Literature* had no articles on hyperkinesis before 1967, one each in 1968 and 1969 and a total of forty for 1970 through 1974 (a mean of eight per year).

Now hyperkinesis has become the most common child psychiatric problem (Gross and Wilson 1974: 142); special pediatric clinics have been established to treat hyperkinetic children, and substantial federal funds have been invested in etiological and treatment research. Outside the medical profession, teachers have developed a working clinical knowledge of hyperkinesis' symptoms and treatment (cf. Robin and Bosco 1973); articles appear regularly in mass circulation magazines and newspapers so that parents often come to clinics with knowledge of this diagnosis. Hyperkinesis is no longer the relatively esoteric diagnostic category it may have been twenty years ago, it is now a well-known clinical disorder.

SOCIAL FACTORS

The social factors affecting the discovery of hyperkinesis can be divided into two areas: (1) The Pharmaceutical Revolution; (2) Government Action.

(1) The Pharmaceutical Revolution. Since the 1930s the pharmaceutical industry has been synthesizing and manufacturing a large number of psychoactive drugs, contributing to a virtual revolution in drug making and drug taking in America (Silverman and Lee 1974).

Psychoactive drugs are agents that effect the central nervous system. Benzedrine, Ritalin, and Dexedrine are all synthesized psychoactive stimulants which were indicated for narcolepsy, appetite control (as "diet pills"), mild depression, fatigue, and more recently hyperkinetic children. Until the early sixties there was little or no promotion and advertisement of any of these medications for use with childhood disorders.[4] Then two major pharmaceutical firms (Smith, Kline and French, manufacturer of Dexedrine, and

CIBA, manufacturer of Ritalin) began to advertise in medical journals and through direct mailing and efforts of the "detail men." Most of this advertising of the pharmaceutical treatment of hyperkinesis was directed to the medical sphere; but some of the promotion was targeted for the educational sector also (Hentoff 1972). This promotion was significant in disseminating information concerning the diagnosis and treatment of this newly discovered disorder.[5] Since 1955 the use of psychoactive medications (especially phenothiazines) for the treatment of persons who are mentally ill, along with the concurrent dramatic decline in inpatient populations, has made psychopharmacology an integral part of treatment for mental disorders. It has also undoubtedly increased the confidence in the medical profession for the pharmaceutical approach to mental and behavioral problems.

(2) Government Action. Since the publication of the U.S.P.H.S. report on M.B.D. there have been at least two significant governmental reports on treating school children with stimulant medications for behavior disorders. Both of these came as a response to the national publicity created by the *Washington Post* report (1970) that probably five to ten percent of the 62,000 grammar school children in Omaha, Nebraska, were being treated with "behavior modification drugs to improve deportment and increase learning potential" (quoted in Grinspoon and Singer 1973). Although the figures were later found to be a little exaggerated, it nevertheless spurred a Congressional investigation (U.S. Government Printing Office 1970) and a conference sponsored by the Office of Child Development (1971) on the use of stimulant drugs in the treatment of behaviorally disturbed school children.

The Congressional Subcommittee on Privacy chaired by Congressman Cornelius E. Gallagher held hearings on the issue of prescribing drugs for hyperactive school children. In general, the committee showed great concern over the facility in which the medication was prescribed; more specifically that some children at least wer ceiving drugs from general practitioners w primary diagnosis was based on teachers' and ents' reports that the child was doing poorl school. There was also a concern with the sence of follow-up studies on the long term fects of treatment.

The H.E.W. committee was a rather ha convened group of professionals (a majority w M.D.s) many of whom already had com ments to drug treatment for children's beha problems. They recommended that only M. make the diagnosis and prescribe treatment, the pharmaceutical companies promote the tr ment of the disorder only through medical ch nels, that parents should not be coerced to acc any particular treatment and that long term low up research should be done. This re served as blue ribbon approval for treating hy kinesis with psychoactive medications.

DISCUSSION

We will focus discussion on three issues: H children's deviant behavior became concept ized as a medical problem; why this occur when it did; and what are some of the impli tions of the medicalization of deviant behav

How does deviant behavior become concep alized as a medical problem? We assume t before the discovery of hyperkinesis this type deviance was seen as disruptive, disobedient, bellious, anti-social or deviant behavior. Perh the label "emotionally disturbed" was someti used, when it was in vogue in the early sixties, a the child was usually managed in the context the family or the school or in extreme cases, t child guidance clinic. How then did this cons lation of deviant behaviors become a medical d order?

The treatment was available long before t disorder treated was clearly conceptualized. was twenty years after Bradley's discovery of t "paradoxical effect" of stimulants on certain c t children that Laufer named the disorder described its characteristic symptoms. Only he late fifties were both the diagnostic label the pharmaceutical treatment available. The rmaceutical revolution in mental health and increased interest in child psychiatry pro-ed a favorable background for the dissemina- of knowledge about this new disorder. The er probably made the medical profession more ly to consider behavior problems in children within their clinical jurisdiction.

There were agents outside the medical profes- itself that were significant in "promoting" erkinesis as a disorder within the medical nework. These agents might be conceptual-d in Becker's terms as "moral entrepreneurs," se who crusade for creation and enforcement he rules (Becker 1963).[6] In this case the moral repreneurs were the pharmaceutical compa-s and the Association for Children with Learn- Disabilities.

The pharmaceutical companies spent consid-ble time and money promoting stimulant dications for this new disorder. From the mid- 1960s on, medical journals and the free row away" magazines contained elaborate ad-tising for Ritalin and Dexedrine. These ads ex-ined the utility of treating hyperkinesis and ged the physician to diagnose and treat hyper-etic children. The ads run from one to six ges. For example, a two page ad in 1971 stated:

> M.B.D.... MEDICAL MYTH OR DIAGNOSABLE DISEASE ENTITY What medical practitioner has not, at one time or another, been called upon to examine an impulsive, excitable hyperkinetic child? A child with difficulty in concentrating. Easily frustrated. Unusually aggressive. A classroom rebel. In the absence of any organic pathology, the conduct of such children was, until a few short years ago, usually dismissed as spunkiness, or evidence of youthful vitality. But it is now evident that in many of these children the hyperkinetic syndrome exists as a distinct medical entity. This syndrome is readily diagnosed through patient histories, neurologic signs, and psychometric testing—has been classified by an expert panel convened by the United States Department of Health, Education, and Welfare (H.E.W.) as Minimal Brain Dysfunction, M.B.D.

The pharmaceutical firms also supplied sophisticated packets of "diagnostic and treatment" information on hyperkinesis to physicians, paid for professional conferences on the subject, and supported research in the identification and treatment of the disorder. Clearly these corporations had a vested interest in the labeling and treatment of hyperkinesis; CIBA had $13 million profit from Ritalin alone in 1971, which was 15 percent of the total gross profits (Charles 1971; Hentoff 1972).

The other moral entrepreneur, less powerful than the pharmaceutical companies, but nevertheless influential, is the Association for Children with Learning Disabilities. Although their focus is not specifically on hyperkinetic children, they do include it in their conception of Learning Disabilities along with aphasia, reading problems like dyslexia and perceptual motor problems. Founded in the early 1950s by parents and professionals, it has functioned much as the National Association for Mental Health does for mental illness: promoting conferences, sponsoring legislation, providing social support. One of the main functions has been to disseminate information concerning this relatively new area in education, Learning Disabilities. While the organization does have a more educational than medical perspective, most of the literature indicates that for hyperkinesis members have adopted the medical model and the medical approach to the problem. They have sensitized teachers and schools to the conception of hyperkinesis as a medical problem.

The medical model of hyperactive behavior has become very well accepted in our society.

Physicians find treatment relatively simple and the results sometimes spectacular. Hyperkinesis minimizes parents' guilt by emphasizing "it's not their fault, it's an organic problem" and allows for nonpunitive management or control of deviance. Medication often makes a child less disruptive in the classroom and sometimes aids a child in learning. Children often like their "magic pills," which make their behavior more socially acceptable, and they probably benefit from a reduced stigma also. There are, however, some other, perhaps more subtle ramifications of the medicalization of deviant behavior.

THE MEDICALIZATION OF DEVIANT BEHAVIOR

Pitts has commented that "medicalization is one of the most effective means of social control and that it is destined to become the main mode of *formal* social control" (1968: 391). Kitterie (1971) has termed it "the coming of the therapeutic state."

Medicalization of mental illness dates at least from the seventeenth century (Foucault 1965; Szasz 1970). Even slaves who ran away were once considered to be suffering from the disease *drapetomania* (Chorover 1973). In recent years alcoholism, violence, and drug addiction as well as hyperactive behavior in children have all become defined as medical problems, both in etiology or explanation of the behavior and the means of social control or treatment.

There are many reasons why this medicalization has occurred. Much scientific research, especially in pharmacology and genetics, has become technologically more sophisticated, and found more subtle correlates with human behavior. Sometimes these findings (as in the case of XYY chromosomes and violence) become etiological explanations for deviance. Pharmacological technology that makes new discoveries affecting behavior (e.g., Antibuse, methadone and stimulants) is used as treatment for deviance part this application is encouraged by the pres of the medical profession and its attachmen science. As Freidson notes, the medical pro sion has first claim to jurisdiction over anyth that deals with the functioning of the body especially anything that can be labeled ill (1970: 251). Advances in genetics, pharmacol and "psychosurgery" also may advance m cine's jurisdiction over deviant behavior.

Second, the application of pharmacolog technology is related to the humanitarian tr in the conception and control of deviant beh ior. Alcoholism is no longer sin or even m weakness, it is now a disease. Alcoholics are longer arrested in many places for "public dru enness," they are now somehow "treated," eve it is only to be dried out. Hyperactive child are now considered to have an illness rather th to be disruptive, disobedient, overactive prob children. They are not as likely to be the "b boy" of the classroom; they are children wit medical disorder. Clearly there are some real manitarian benefits to be gained by such a m ical conceptualization of deviant behav There is less condemnation of the deviants (th have an illness, it is not their fault) and perh less social stigma. In some cases, even the m ical treatment itself is more humanitarian soc control than the criminal justice system.

There is, however, another side to the m icalization of deviant behavior. The four aspe of this side of the issue include (1) the problem expert control; (2) medical social control; (3) t individualization of social problems; and (4) t "depoliticization" of deviant behavior.

1. *The problem of expert control.* The medi profession is a profession of experts; they have monopoly on anything that can be conceptu ized as illness. Because of the way the medic profession is organized and the mandate it h from society, decisions related to medical dia noses and treatment are virtually controlled medical professionals.

ome conditions that enter the medical do-n are not *ipso facto* medical problems, espe-ly deviant behavior, whether alcoholism, eractivity or drug addiction. By defining a blem as medical it is removed from the public m where there can be discussion by ordinary ple and put on a plane where only medical ple can discuss it. As Reynolds states,

'he increasing acceptance, especially among he more educated segments of our populace, of echnical solutions—solutions administered by isinterested politically and morally neutral ex-erts—results in the withdrawal of more and nore areas of human experience from the realm of public discussion. For when drunkenness, ju-enile delinquency, sub par performance and ex-reme political beliefs are seen as symptoms of an nderlying illness or biological defect the merits nd drawbacks of such behavior or beliefs need ot be evaluated (1973: 220–21).

The public may have their own conceptions of viant behavior but that of the experts is usually minant.

2. *Medical social control.* Defining deviant be-vior as a medical problem allows certain things be done that could not otherwise be consid-d; for example, the body may be cut open or choactive medications may be given. This atment can be a form of social control.

In regard to drug treatment Lennard and Asso-tes point out: "Psychoactive drugs, especially ose legally prescribed, tend to restrain individ-ls from behavior and experience that are not nplementary to the requirements of the dom-ant value system" (1971: 57). These forms of edical social control presume a prior definition deviance as a medical problem. Psychosurgery an individual prone to violent outbursts re-ires a diagnosis that there was something wrong th his brain or nervous system. Similarly, pre-ribing drugs to restless, overactive and disrup-e school children requires a diagnosis of hy-rkinesis. These forms of social control, what Chorover (1973) has called "psychotechnology," are very powerful and often very efficient means of controlling deviance. These relatively new and increasingly popular forms of social control could not be utilized without the medicalization of deviant behavior. As is suggested from the discovery of hyperkinesis, if a mechanism of medical social control seems useful, then the deviant behavior it modifies will develop a medical label or diagnosis. No overt malevolence on the part of the medical profession is implied: rather it is part of a complex process, of which the medical profession is only a part. The larger process might be called the individualization of social problems.

3. *The individualization of social problems.* The medicalization of deviant behavior is part of a larger phenomenon that is prevalent in our society, the individualization of social problems. We tend to look for causes and solutions to complex social problems in the individual rather than in the social system. This view resembles Ryan's (1971) notion of "blaming the victim"; seeing the causes of the problem in individuals rather than in the society where they live. We then seek to change the "victim" rather than the society. The medical perspective of diagnosing an illness in an individual lends itself to the individualization of social problems. Rather than seeing certain deviant behaviors as symptomatic of problems in the social system, the medical perspective focuses on the individual diagnosing and treating the illness, generally ignoring the social situation. Hyperkinesis serves as a good example. Both the school and the parents are concerned with the child's behavior; the child is very difficult at home and disruptive in school. No punishments or rewards seem consistently to work in modifying the behavior; and both parents and school are at their wits' end. A medical evaluation is suggested. The diagnoses of hyperkinetic behavior lead to prescribing stimulant medications. The child's behavior seems to become more socially acceptable, reducing problems in school and at home. But there is an alternate perspective. By

focusing on the symptoms and defining them as hyperkinesis we ignore the possibility that behavior is not an illness but an adaptation to a social situation. It diverts our attention from the family or school and from seriously entertaining the idea that the "problem" could be in the structure of the social system. And by giving medications we are essentially supporting the existing systems and do not allow this behavior to be a factor of change in the system.

4. *The depoliticization of deviant behavior.* Depoliticization of deviant behavior is a result of both the process of medicalization and individualization of social problems. To our Western world, probably one of the clearest examples of such a depoliticization of deviant behavior occurred when political dissenters in the Soviet Union were declared mentally ill and confined in mental hospitals (cf. Conrad 1972). This strategy served to neutralize the meaning of political protest and dissent, rendering it the ravings of mad persons.

The medicalization of deviant behavior depoliticizes deviance in the same manner. By defining the overactive, restless and disruptive child as hyperkinetic we ignore the meaning of behavior in the context of the social system. If we focused our analysis on the school system we might see the child's behavior as symptomatic of some "disorder" in the school or classroom situation, rather than symptomatic of an individual neurological disorder.

CONCLUSION

I have discussed the social ramifications of the medicalization of deviant behavior, using hyperkinesis as the example. A number of consequences of this medicalization have been outlined, including the depoliticization of deviant behavior, decision-making power of experts, and the role of medicine as an agent of social control. In the last analysis medical social control may be the central issue, as in this role medicine becomes a *de facto* agent of the *status quo.* ' medical profession may not have entirely sou this role, but its members have been, in gene disturbingly unconcerned and unquestionin their acceptance of it. With the increasing n ical knowledge and technology it is likely more deviant behavior will be medicalized medicine's social control function will expa

NOTES

1. This paper is a revised version of a paper prese at the meetings of the Society for the Study of So Problems in San Francisco, August 1975. It was tially supported by a National Science Foundation sertation grant (SOC 74 22043). I would like to th Drs. Martin Kozloff, James E. Teele, John McKi and the anonymous referees for comments on ea drafts of this paper.

2. The U.S.P.H.S. report (Clements 1966) inclu 38 terms that were used to describe or distinguish conditions that it labeled Minimal Brain Dysfuncti Although the literature attempts to different M.B.D., hyperkinesis, hyperactive syndrome, and eral other diagnostic labels, it is our belief that in p tice they are almost interchangeable.

3. For a fuller discussion of the construction of diagnosis of hyperkinesis, see Conrad (1976), especi chapter 6.

4. The American Medical Association's change policy in accepting more pharmaceutical advertis in the late fifties may have been important. Proba the F.D.A. approval of the use of Ritalin for childre 1961 was more significant. Until 1970 Ritalin was vertised for treatment of "functional behavior pr lems in children." Since then, because of an F.D order, it has only been promoted for treatment M.B.D.

5. The drug industry spends fully 25 percent of budget on promotion and advertising. See Colema al. (1966) for the role of the detail men and how phy cians rely upon them for information.

6. Freidson also notes the medical professional r as moral entrepreneur in this process also: "The p

on does treat the illnesses laymen take to it, but it seeks to discover illness of which the laymen may even be aware. One of the greatest ambitions of the sician is to discover and describe a "new" disease or drome..." (1970: 252).

REFERENCES

Becker, Howard S. 1963. *The Outsiders*. New York: e Press.

Bradley, Charles. 1937. "The Behavior of Children eiving Benzedrine." *American Journal of Psychiatry* March): 577–85.

Charles, Alan. 1971. "The Case of Ritalin." *New Re-lic* 23 (October): 17–19.

Chorover, Stephen L. 1973 "Big Brother and Psy-technology." *Psychology Today* (October): 43–54.

Clements, Samuel D. 1966. *Task Force I: Minimal in Dysfunction in Children*. National Institute of urological Diseases and Blindness, monograph no. Washington, D.C.: U.S. Department of Health, Ed-tion, and Welfare.

Cole, Sherwood. 1975. "Hyperactive Children: The e of Stimulant Drugs Evaluated." *American Journal Orthopsychiatry* 45 (January): 28–37.

Coleman, James, Elihu Katz, and Herbert Menzel. 6. *Medical Innovation*. Indianapolis: Bobbs-Merrill.

Conrad, Peter. 1972. "Ideological Deviance: An alysis of the Soviet Use of Mental Hospitals for Po-cal Dissenters." Unpublished manuscript.

——. 1976. "Identifying Hyperactive Children: A idy in the Medicalization of Deviant Behavior." .D. dissertation, Boston University.

DeLong, Arthur R. 1972. "What Have We Learned m Psychoactive Drugs Research with Hyperac-es?" *American Journal of Diseases in Children* 123 ebruary): 177–80.

Foucault, Michel. 1965. *Madness and Civilization*. ew York: Pantheon.

Friedson, Eliot. 1970. *Profession of Medicine: A udy of the Sociology of Applied Knowledge*. New rk: Dodd Mead.

Grinspoon, Lester, and Susan Singer. 1973. "Am-etamines in the Treatment of Hyperactive Children." *Harvard Educational Review* 43 (November): 515–55.

Gross, Mortimer B., and William E. Wilson. 1974. *Minimal Brain Dysfunction*. New York: Brunner Mazel.

Hentoff, Nat. 1972. "Drug Pushing in the Schools: The Professionals." *Village Voice* 22 (May): 21–23.

Kitterie, Nicholas. 1971. *The Right to Be Different*. Baltimore: Johns Hopkins University Press.

Laufer, M. W., E. Denhoff, and G. Solomons. 1957. "Hyperkinetic Impulse Disorder in Children's Behavior Problems." *Psychosomatic Medicine* 19 (January): 38–49.

Lennard, Henry L., and Associates. 1971. *Mystification and Drug Misuse*. New York: Harper & Row.

Office of Child Development. 1971. *Report of the Conference on the Use of Stimulant Drugs in Treatment of Behaviorally Disturbed Children*. Washington, D.C.: Office of Child Development, Department of Health, Education and Welfare, January 11–12.

Pitts, Jesse. 1968. "Social Control: The Concept." Pp. 381 96 in David Sills (ed.), *International Encyclopedia of the Social Sciences*, Volume 14. New York: Macmillan.

Reynolds, Janice M. 1973. "The Medical Institution." Pp. 198–324 in Larry T. Reynolds and James M. Henslin (eds.), *American Society: A Critical Analysis*. New York: David McKay.

Robin, Stanley S., and James J. Bosco. 1973. "Ritalin for School Children: The Teachers Perspective." *Journal of School Health* 47 (December): 624–28.

Rosen, George. 1972. "The Evolution of Social Medicine." Pp. 30–60 in Howard E. Freeman, Sol Levine, and Leo Reeder (eds.), *Handbook of Medical Sociology*. Englewood Cliffs, N.J.: Prentice Hall.

Ryan, William. 1970. *Blaming the Victim*. New York: Vintage.

Silverman, Milton, and Philip R. Lee. 1974. *Pills, Profits and Politics*. Berkeley: University of California Press.

Stewart, Mark A. 1970. "Hyperactive Children." *Scientific American* 222 (April): 794–98.

Stewart, Mark A., A. Ferris, N. P. Pitts, and A. G. Craig. 1966. "The Hyperactive Child Syndrome."

American Journal of Orthopsychiatry 36 (October): 861–67.

Strauss, A. A., and L. E. Lehtinen. 1947. *Psychopathology and Education of the Brain Injured Child,* Vol. 1. New York: Grune and Stratton.

Szasz, Thomas. 1970. "Justice in the Therapeutic State." *Comprehensive Psychiatry* 11 (5): 433–44.

U.S. Government Printing Office. 1970. "Federal Involvement in the Use of Behavior Modification Drugs on Grammar School Children of the Rig Privacy Inquiry: Hearing before a Subcommittee o Committee on Government Operations." Wash ton, D.C.: 91st Congress, 2nd session (September

Wender, Paul. 1971. *Minimal Brain Dysfunctio Children.* New York: John Wiley and Sons.

Zola, Irving. 1972. "Medicine as an Institution o cial Control." *Sociological Review* 20 (Noveml 487–504.

CHAPTER 17

Suffering and the Social Construction of Illness: The Delegitimation of Illness Experience in Chronic Fatigue Syndrome

NORMA C. WARE

THIS ARTICLE BUILDS ON retrospective ccounts of illness experience in chronic fatigue syndrome to address ne suffering engendered by the socially constituted nature of illness.[1] s specific focus is the suffering associated with delegitimation, defined ere as the experience of having one's perceptions and definitions of illness systematically disconfirmed (Kleinman 1992).[2]

To organize and frame the discussion, I draw upon the concept of illness reality. In applying this construct to the analysis of cultural categories of illness, Good and Good have defined an "illness reality" as "a 'syndrome' of typical experiences, a set of words, experiences, and feelings which typically 'run together' for members of a given society, a set of experiences associated through networks of meaning and social interaction" (1982: 148; see also Good 1977:27). My intent is to depict a set of words, experiences, and feelings that "run together" for individuals suffering from chronic fatigue syndrome.[3]

BACKGROUND

Chronic fatigue syndrome is a debilitating condition of unknown etiology that came to the attention of the medical community and the general public in the mid-1980s. Its symptoms center on the experience of severe, persistent, and unexplained fatigue, but they also include a diffuse constellation of other complaints, such as muscle and joint pain, headache, sore throat, fever, weakness, dizziness, concentration difficulties, and memory loss (Centers for Disease Control 1990; Holmes et al. 1988). A significant number of chronic fatigue syndrome patients also suffer from depression before or after the onset of illness (Hickie et al. 1990; Kruesi, Dale, and Straus 1989).

Early etiological research on this illness focused on the Epstein-Barr virus as the probable cause of the symptoms (Jones et al. 1985; Straus et al. 1985). This initial explanation was abandoned when subsequent studies failed to replicate the association between elevated antibodies to Epstein-Barr virus and the syndrome (Swartz 1988).

The origin of chronic fatigue syndrome is presently a subject of lively debate among medical researchers. Some scientists continue to search for a viral cause; retroviruses (DeFreitas et al. 1991), enteroviruses (Gow et al. 1991), and pes-viruses other than Epstein-Barr have rece been posited as potential etiological agents. (ers emphasize the role of immune dysfunctio the disorder (Lloyd et al. 1989). Sleep abnor ities (McCluskey 1992) and disturbances of hypothalamic-pituitary-adrenal axis (as a f common pathway) (Demitrack et al. 1991) h also been put forward as explanations. Ano line of inquiry centers on the relationshi chronic fatigue syndrome to psychiatric ill (David 1991). Etiological models integrating logical and psychological perspectives are beginning to appear (Kendell 1991; Koma 1991).

The configuration of symptoms curre known as chronic fatigue syndrome closely sembles the clinical profile of neurasthenia historically minded observers are beginning point out (Abbey and Garfinkel 1991; Greenb 1990; Wessely 1990). Neurasthenia enjoyed c siderable popularity as a diagnosis in late 1 and early 20th-century U.S. medicine, whe provided clinicians and patients with a spectable physical explanation for compla that might otherwise have been interpreted indications of hypochondriasis, malingering, outright insanity (Sicherman 1977). As a dise construct, it was gradually dismantled and s sumed under various affective and anxiety dis ders as psychiatric nosology became more phisticated and the usefulness of so broad a unwieldy a category was increasingly called i question.

Other medically unexplained, fatigue-relat illnesses have also gained temporary prominen in U.S. medical history, only to come to simi ends. Exhaustion accompanied by dizziness, p pitations, and other symptoms in Civil War v erans coalesced into Da Costa's or "effort" sy drome in the 1870s (Da Costa 1871). Da Cost syndrome flowered as a medical diagnosis for se eral decades, then was redefined and dismissed a form of neurosis in the 1940s. Chronic bruc

, a form of persistent fatigue attributed ini- y to the effects of bacterial infection (Evans 7), was later shown to be related to "psycho- cal vulnerability" (Imboden, Canter, and ff 1961). It subsequently disappeared.

n the 1960s and 1970s, chronic fatigue of un- wn etiology was often attributed to hypo- emia. Today, diffuse somatic syndromes in ch fatigue plays a salient role may be sified as chronic fatigue syndrome or, alter- ively, as fibromyalgia (if pain *is* predominant), didiasis hypersensitivity syndrome, or "total rgy syndrome" (Stewart 1987; Straus 1991). us the configuration of symptoms currently t known as chronic fatigue syndrome is not v, but rather has been constructed and recon- icted in popular and professional discourse r time.

Epidemiological research on fatigue is fraught h difficulties of design and measurement rufferman 1991; Lewis and Wessely 1992). ly a few attempts to assess the prevalence of ronic fatigue *syndrome* have been made to date. liminary estimates from this work suggest that es fulfilling all criteria for the CDC definition y be rare in clinical as well as community pop- tions (Gunn, Connell, and Randal 1992; Price l. 1991; Komaroff, personal communication).[4]

In contrast, complaints of disabling fatigue in- e and outside doctors' offices are widespread. cent data from the National Ambulatory Care rvey indicate that fatigue accounts for approx- ately 6 million internal medicine visits each ar (Nelson and McLemore 1988).[5] Studies of e frequency of severe or extraordinary fatigue in neral practice estimate its prevalence at 10 to % (e.g., Buchwald et al. 1987; Kroenke et al. 38). Community surveys suggest that the preva- nce of excessive fatigue in nonclinical popula- ns may reach similar levels (e.g., Chen 1986; ox et al. 1987; see Lewis and Wessely 1992 for a view).

Others have also applied the concept of dele- timation to the anthropological study of suffering but in somewhat different ways. Kleinman (1992), for example, in an examination of the experience and meaning of, chronic pain, uses the term to refer to the loss of a "legitimate" world, that is, a world consisting of those ways of being that are culturally valued and defined as normative. Pain is construed, for the purposes of this particular analysis, as an effort to resist or transform the lost life-world, to "re-legitimate" one's existence.

Whereas Kleinman is concerned with the delegitimation of experience, Das (1991) focuses more on the social order. She seeks both to expose the social origins of suffering and to demonstrate how suffering as experience may be transformed through social discourse into an authorization, a legitimation, of existing structures of power. We may think of Das's work, therefore, as directed more toward the social production than the social construction of suffering.

THE RESEARCH

Fifty individuals were interviewed as part of the research reported here. Interviewees were referred by Anthony Komaroff, Director of the Division of General Medicine and Primary Care, Brigham and Women's Hospital, Boston, from the approximately 350 chronically fatigued patients he is currently following. These patients sought help for a debilitating fatigue that significantly interfered with their work or home responsibilities; approximately 80% meet the U.S. (Holmes et al. 1988), the British (Sharpe et al. 1991), or the Australian (Lloyd et al. 1990) operational case definition of chronic fatigue syndrome. The study sample is similar in age, sex, and educational background to the larger group but tended to have fewer objective laboratory test abnormalities.

The interviews were conducted over a period of approximately 18 months, beginning in the winter of 1989 and ending in the summer of 1990. Each interview sought the elicitation of data on life history and illness experience using a systematic series of open-ended questions. Interviews were tape-recorded and transcribed.

Eighty percent of those interviewed were women; 92% were white. Their ages ranged from 23 to 66 years, with a mean age of 39. Early anecdotal accounts of chronic fatigue syndrome reported it to be an illness of the educated and professional classes—a so-called yuppie disease (*Time Magazine* 1987). Almost half (48%) of this group of subjects, however, had left school before completing a bachelor's degree; 22% had a high school education or less. Furthermore, the occupations of the 43 participants who reported having at some point been members of the labor force were almost equally divided between trades, clerical occupations, or direct service delivery (27, or 56%) and professional or managerial activity (e.g., consulting, teaching, administration).

Length of illness in the group at the time of data collection ranged from 1.5 to 25 years. Fifty percent of the interviewees had been ill for five years or more at the time the interviews took place. The mean length of illness for the sample was 5.7 years.

DEFINING CHRONIC FATIGUE SYNDROME AS "NOT REAL": THE EXPERIENCE OF DELEGITIMATION

Two types of delegitimizing encounters appeared regularly in interviewees' reports of their experience with chronic fatigue syndrome. The first stems from the apparent insignificance of the symptoms. Because everyone from time to time endures aches and pains, sore throat, feelings of depression, and fatigue, such complaints can be construed as minor, if discomfiting, consequences of everyday living rather than as indications of serious illness. Perceptions of the trivialization of symptoms by others converge fo
ferers in the thematic phrase: "You're tired? W
all tired! So what!"

> What you get [when you talk to people abou
> illness] is, "Well jeez, a lot of people are t
> What the hell is that? I'm tired, and I go to w
> A lot of people are in pain." Maybe they say, "
> tsk, have another cup of tea."
>
> If you have cancer, you can tell your fri
> you have cancer and your friends underst
> You cannot tell your friends you are tired. W
> are they going to say? "I'm tired too!" Several
> ple have said that to me "I'm tired too!"
>
> People think, "Oh, you've got a sore throat,
> you're tired. So? I've had sore throats and
> been nauseous. So?"

The second, and more damaging, delegitin
ing experience for chronic fatigue patients is
bodied in physicians' definition of the illnes
psychosomatic—"all in your head." Interview
report being given two different rationales for
definition. The first is that no observable evide
of disease in the form of clinical signs or labora
findings can be found. The second is the fact
the illness has yet to be fully accepted as a di
nostic entity in the standard professional nosolo

Study participants repeatedly complained
being disbelieved or not taken seriously beca
they "don't look sick." They are neither thin a
pale nor obviously disabled. They may funct
relatively normally, at least for a time, in work a
social settings. Convinced that the severity of
subjective experience of the illness is belied
outward appearance, they react with intense fr
tration to being told that they "look great!"

> And that's part of this illness. That everybody w
> always say to you, "Well, you *look* great!" Well,
> tan and all that. What do you want?
>
> The thing I hear from everybody is, "Gee, y
> look much too good to be sick!" I hear that all
> time because I'm not emaciated and I'm not st

> ering, and of course when people see me, they ee me on my good days, when I can get out of the partment. They don't see me on my bad days hen I can't get out of bed!
>
> Unless you're in a wheelchair or in bed, people on't really believe that you're sick. They just ind of look at you and say, "Well, you don't *look* ick! You don't act sick!" It's just obvious that eople don't believe you or think that it's serious.
>
> Because I'm not in agony or carrying a broken eg, there's always that little doubt, "Well, how ad really *is* it?" I tell you—it's bad. It's bad. I'm ure if I had a rash, or was vomiting, or my arm ropped off, it would be lots easier for people to e nice to me. I *look* healthy as a horse! You hould see me in the summer when I've been siting around and I have a tan. People look at me nd say, "God, you look wonderful!" And I have o say, "I feel awful!"

Part of the etiological controversy that esently surrounds chronic fatigue syndrome ms from the fact that the illness has yet to be rebly associated with any identifiable organic thology. Laboratory tests undertaken for diagstic purposes therefore prove consistently unisfying. Chronic fatigue patients have typically dergone extensive testing ordered by physins. When the results of every test come back gative, the conclusion is that there is nothing ysically wrong.

For chronic fatigue syndrome sufferers, the k of recognition of the illness has meant that ysicians could not definitively diagnose their ndition. Many experienced this as betrayal by e medical profession and responded by consultg another (sometimes many other) doctors in arch of an explanation for their distress. When is effort failed, they turned to alternative health re providers or fell back on various illness manement strategies of their own devising.

Thus, the absence of observable evidence of thology, together with the ambiguous status of the illness in professional medicine, precluded the possibility of a physical diagnosis for many chronic fatigue syndrome sufferers. And if an illness is not physical, it must, it follows, be mental. The cause of the symptoms was therefore often hypothesized to be depression, stress, or some other form of psychological disturbance.

> That's been my experience [with doctors] over and over again. They really try. They really listen. And then they try a whole bunch of things that they think might turn something up, and when everything fails, they just think you're nuts. And then they get sort of angry.
>
> They [doctors] would say things like, "You can't be experiencing what you are experiencing. You need to see a psychologist. You're not as sick as you think you are."
>
> I was going to a neurologist, and he could find nothing wrong with me. "Well, there's nothing wrong on your X-ray but why don't you try taking this, because a lot of women"—he used the word "women"—"have a lot of trouble with depression that could cause other symptoms." I was really sensitive at that stage about being told I was depressed when things had never been better. And I still have problems with that, because I still don't feel like I'm depressed.[6]

Forty-five (90%) of those interviewed reported delegitimizing experiences of the sort described above. Those who did not indicated that their symptoms had been accepted by others as real, either on the basis of observable evidence (e.g., swollen glands) or because they had heard of chronic fatigue syndrome and considered it a physical illness.

What, then, is the illness reality that emerges from these two forms of delegitimation? The trivialization of symptoms serves to characterize the sufferer as not sick. To classify complaints as part of normal life in effect disqualifies them as symptoms. The implications of the psychosomatic label are slightly different. In popular conceptions, a psychosomatic illness is an illness that exists, but as a product of the mind. Psychosomatically ill people are sick, they exhibit symptoms that, while "mental" in origin, are nonetheless located in the body. They are not, however, embodied in the sense of manifesting themselves either as physical sensation or observable bodily dysfunction. Part of the popular cultural meaning of psychosomatic illness is that its symptoms are defined as "imagined." Thus chronic fatigue sufferers repeatedly find themselves judged to be either not sick or suffering from an imaginary illness. In either case, their complaints and their experience are discounted as being "not real."

SUFFERING AND DELEGITIMATION

The experience of being repeatedly disconfirmed in their definition of reality led many to self-doubt. Those who had had such experiences described in frustrated tones how at one point or another they felt compelled to accept the possibility that what they were feeling might, after all, be "all in their heads" and that that might mean they were "crazy."

> I was beginning to think I was crazy! I couldn't believe I could be this fatigued for this long.... I've been fatigued because of the schedule I was keeping, but it didn't keep me from doing anything. No matter how tired I was, I could still go another 10 hours. I thought I was imagining it. I thought, "Maybe I'm really depressed and that's what's causing it."
>
> I thought I was crazy. I thought I was a hypochondriac. There were things I didn't want to tell the doctor because I thought he would think I was a fruitcake!
>
> I remember standing in front of the mirror, and I looked wretched. People told me I looked like I was going to die! And yet the doctor said it was just a viral illness and that it would go away. And I'd look in the mirror and think, "Are crazy? Maybe there's nothing wrong with Maybe it's all in your head."

In fearing that their illness might, after al psychosomatic, self-doubters confront the p bility of psychological disorder and the stign entails. The suffering of self-doubt thus lies in prospect of adding the burden of a stigmati identity to that of living with a chronic illness is severely debilitating, basically untreatable, of questionable authenticity in the eyes of oth

The ambiguous nature of chronic fatigue drome causes some to retreat into secrecy. Ra than expose themselves to the pain of being believed, those who opt for secrecy actively tr hide the fact that they are sick. In casual con sations, they deliberately omit any referenc their condition. If asked how they are, they variably reply brightly, "Fine!" They make g efforts to "pass" as healthy by struggling to h onto jobs, to lead seemingly normal social li or simply to continue to perform the rout functions of daily living. For these individu dissembling, as difficult and demanding as it seems preferable to the risk of being disc firmed in their experience of their illness.[7]

In explaining their reasons for choosing crecy, study participants cited the awkwardn and embarrassment of trying to explain to so one that they have an illness whose symptoms ill-defined, that has no "real" name or kno cause, and that (at least at the time) most peo have never heard of. The lack of shared kno edge of the illness and of meaningful terms which to describe it made it difficult to arg convincingly for chronic fatigue syndrome a disease. As more than one person put it, it wou be easier in more ways to have some serious b immediately recognizable disease like canc

> Cancer would be better, I shouldn't say that, b cause I don't think it would be better. But would be easier to share with somebody. I thin could tell somebody I had cancer, that I was de

ıg with cancer, I can't tell people about this, ecause, first of all, I don't know what to call it. don't know how to describe it. Chronic fatigue yndrome? People have never heard of such a ıing! It doesn't mean anything to them! It oesn't sound real.

'hose who choose secrecy, however, not only y the burden of keeping the secret, they also rive themselves of the catharsis of talking ut what is most on their minds and of receiving nfort in discovering there are others who care l may provide help when needed. Ironically, y also preclude the possibility of being affirmed heir experience of their illness. The suffering secrecy thus lies in the alienation it entails. \s we have seen, the lack of recognition of onic fatigue syndrome meant that many pa- ıts found themselves consulting physician r physician in the search for a diagnosis— en over months or even years. The failure of dical professionals to name their condition left ients feeling not only betrayed but also with no ans of coping. Without a diagnosis, there was treatment—no way of fighting the illness. Not owing whether what they had was life threat- ing or what course it would take made life de- ions and planning for the future impossible. e sense of paralysis that ensued was conveyed ecially clearly by one individual, who also ntrasted the experience of chronic fatigue syn- ome to that of having cancer.

It would be easier in many ways if someone was to say to me, "OK. We've found out what's wrong with you. You've got a tumor the size of a grape-fruit and you've got two years to live." OK. Now I know. That's what it is. I can get my affairs in order and sell my long-term bonds. OK. This is it. We pay off the car. We take a trip to Bermuda. I don't have to wonder what it is that I'm going to do with the rest of my life.

Of the various forms of suffering that experi- ıces of delegitimation can engender, none was as devastating for this group as the humiliation that resulted from having their subjective perceptions and sensations of illness either trivialized or dismissed as psychosomatic. Other authors have written of the potential for shame in the medical encounter when illness is experienced by the sick person as a deficit or when the vulnerability of the patient is overlooked by the physician (Kleinman 1988; Lazare 1987). The shame of chronic fatigue sufferers, however, stems not from the fact of having an illness but from being told that they do not. Their shame is the shame of being wrong about the nature of reality.

CONTESTING THE DEFINITION

Part of depicting the social process through which illness realities are constructed is to show how they are contested. To contest is to challenge and attempt to reconstitute a given definition of a situation by advocating an alternative interpretation.

Most efforts by study participants to dispute the definition of their illness were directed toward the designation of chronic fatigue syndrome as psychosomatic. The challenge to this definition took two principal forms. One was to argue that the illness is after all physical; the other was to present evidence that one is not psychologically impaired.

One way of making the case for the physical nature of chronic fatigue syndrome was to redefine psychosomatic as somatopsychic. In this approach, attention is directed away from the presumed psychological origins of the bodily complaints toward a possible organic explanation of psychiatric symptoms. If the cause of the illness can be assumed to be depression or some other psychological disorder, it can also be claimed that psychological disorders have biological roots.

I maintain that the psychological component is based strictly on neurological problems. I realize that a big part of it was a depressive episode. But it was a neurological problem. There's some brain dysfunction there.

I don't think it's psychological at all. I don't like having this illness, and sometimes I'm not as bubbly as I'd like to be, because it's hard to take. And sometimes I tend to be short-tempered. But I don't think that the psychological—no, not the psychological—the cognitive things I'm experiencing, or physiological things that I'm experiencing, come from a psychological origin. I think it's physiological.

The presence of "observable evidence" was invoked to support a second line of reasoning in which the definition of chronic fatigue syndrome as a psychosomatic illness was contested. In struggling to convince themselves, as well as others, of the organic nature of their distress, patients would point to the presence of physical signs of pathology.

Every so often I ask myself, "Could I have this? Or is it psychological?" And then I feel these massive glands sticking out and I realize [I wouldn't] have a fever and swollen glands and aches like I have [if I were depressed]. The thing that makes me sure I have chronic fatigue syndrome is the pain and the swollen glands and the fever, the definite physical symptoms I don't believe would be psychosomatic.

[I knew I was really sick] because I had actual physical symptoms, even though nothing showed up on the tests . . . like sore throat, headache, nausea, temperatures that showed up on a thermometer. One test showed that there was some kind of actual weakness in the muscles. It showed up on this little graph. That was great.

The case for defining chronic fatigue syndrome as a physical illness could also be made by analogy. Likening the condition to a well-known and unquestionably biological ailment clearly implies that it should be considered biological as well. Opportunities for drawing such analogies arose when patients were called upon to explain their condition.

I say, "Well, it's kind of like mono. You've h of mono. The Epstein-Barr virus? Well, it kir recurs in people. It appears at certain times makes me lazy and gives me a fever." I say, going through different research studies, they've changed the name, and they're not re sure, but there's definitely something there cause there's some kind of 'titer' that's high stuff."

If arguing for a physical definition of chrc fatigue syndrome is one way of rejecting a chosomatic label, another is to find ways of pr ing that one is not, in fact, "crazy." Most often involved challenging the idea that depress causes this illness. Many such challenges be by invoking personal experiences of previous pressive episodes, the point being to distingu depression from the experience of chronic tigue syndrome. Depression, according to one terpretation, could be traced to some identifia event or situation in the world, whereas malaise in chronic fatigue syndrome was f floating, unattached, seeming to "come ou nowhere." The difference between loss of in est in activities in depression and fatigue chronic fatigue syndrome was another frequer cited distinction. Individuals who had been pressed spoke of having lost interest in thin contrasting this with the feeling of having the terest but not the energy to be active since onset of chronic fatigue syndrome. "This is depression but exhaustion, and they are not same thing," is the message these claims are tended to convey.

To insist that depression is not the cause chronic fatigue syndrome is not to deny that i a part of it. Depressed feelings after illness on were acknowledged by a large proportion of t study sample. Those who had known depressi since becoming ill with chronic fatigue sy drome interpreted these feelings in one of t ways. Either they were intrinsic to the syndror itself—a symptom, like muscle aches, joint pai or fever—or they resulted from the experience onic fatigue syndrome, the predictable outne of months or years of being seriously ill. : are not depressed, we're sick! And if we *are* ressed, it's *because* we're sick!" is the essence he argument against depression as the cause hronic fatigue syndrome.

SUMMARY AND CONCLUSION

aim here has been to focus attention on exiences of delegitimation as socially constied, nonbodily suffering in illness. The reality structed for sufferers of chronic fatigue synme through delegitimizing experiences is t their illness is not "real" at all but rather a fabition based either on the needless exaggeran of everyday complaints (in which case they malingerers) or on the perception of imagiy symptoms (in which case they are "crazy"). either case, the self-doubt and the threat of gma, the secrecy and the social isolation that ults, the psychological paralysis induced by : ambiguities of the illness, and the shame of ing wrong about "really" being sick all conoute to the psychic suffering of the chronic faue victim. In spite, or perhaps because, of this fering, patients felt called upon to challenge s version of reality either by making the case it chronic fatigue syndrome *is* a real (i.e., physl) illness or by presenting evidence to prove it they were not psychologically disturbed.

A well-developed critique of biomedical thinkg and practice now exists in medical anthrology. The historically rooted and culturally nstituted nature, of mind-body and other dusms, biological reductionism, and scientific raonality has been repeatedly pointed out, along th the epistemological and clinical shortcomgs of a natural science model of illness and ealing (e.g., Lock and Gordon 1988; Good 93).

Assaults on biomedicine have also been ounted from within the profession itself. Biopsychosocial" theories of etiology, calls for "holistic" approaches to care, and curriculum innovations emphasizing the social, psychological, and moral dimensions of suffering and the emotional needs of patients represent attempts to reform medicine "from the inside."

Yet it is the standard biomedical paradigm that accounts for the delegitimatizing experiences encountered by chronic fatigue syndrome sufferers. The definition of "medically invisible" bodily complaints as psychogenic and therefore imaginary is a direct reflection of scientific materialism, which accords primacy to substance, equates the real with the physically observable, and discounts or bypasses altogether the subjective experience of the patient. Thus, not surprisingly, delegitimation in chronic fatigue testifies to the intractability of the biomedical model. As long as biomedicine remains efficacious, politically entrenched, and consistent with core values and concepts in Western cultural tradition, we may expect this to continue to be the case (Gordon 1988).

Kirmayer (1988) has pointed to the moral implications of a diagnosis of psychosomatic illness and interpreted them in terms of the symbolic meanings attached to mind-body dualism in Western metaphysics, e.g., agency and accident, reason and emotion, control and chaos, accountability and blamelessness. In the case of "real" physical disease, medicine contrives through conceptual and practical means to distance the self from the body, thereby exempting the individual from personal responsibility for illness. In the case of psychological disorder, however, defining a problem as "mental" or "emotional" means linking it to the values associated with mind in Western metaphysics—hence the notion that psychiatric illness represents a failure of intentionality and volition, a lapse of rational self-control that must ultimately be recognized to be "one's own fault." Despite the fact that psychosomatic medicine was originally conceivable as an antidote to biological reductionism, an attempt to bring mind and body together in biomedicine in more or less equal union, in reality psychosomatic diagnoses have come to be classed with psychiatric disorders, reproducing dualistic thinking and sharing the stigmatized status of mental illness as a disability we "bring on ourselves." In making explicit the similarities between qualities of "mind" and the construction of the person in Western tradition, Kirmayer also argues for biomedicine as a sociomoral phenomenon that will resist change in the absence of a restructuring of categories and definitions at the level of culture.

An appreciation of the cultural underpinnings of delegitimizing experiences in chronic fatigue syndrome also opens the door to understanding their personal meaning. What is at issue in the struggle over the proper definition of reality in chronic fatigue—physical or psychosomatic condition, real or unreal illness—is whether patients will be accorded the status of sane persons who are genuinely sick. If so, much of their psychic, if not their physical, suffering will be alleviated. If not, they must continue to deal with the implications of having a "not real" disorder.

The delegitimizing experiences reported by sufferers of chronic fatigue syndrome are strikingly similar to those encountered by chronic pain patients. As in the case of chronic fatigue, individuals who live with chronic pain routinely find their complaints of subjective distress discounted by medical professionals who, in the absence of an identifiable biological explanation, define the problem as psychosomatic and the pain itself as imaginary (Hilbert 1984; Kleinman 1988). Indeed, the same distinction between real (physical) and unreal (psychological) disorder that is crucial to the experience of chronic fatigue syndrome appears no less central in chronic pain, where patients also struggle to deflect stigmatization by defining their condition as organic (Jackson 1990, 1992).

The elaboration of suffering as an analytical category for understanding the lived, felt quality of human events requires that various forms of suffering be identified and articulated. This article experiments with delegitimation as a way of representing one particular form of nonbc suffering in illness. As defined here, for exam delegitimation is likely to apply best to condit classified in popular or professional consci ness as psychosomatic. Reconfigured, howeve might also prove useful for understanding exp ence in other types of psychological disorder c illnesses that are unquestionably physical highly stigmatized. For this reason, and beca it seems to reflect experience more directly, w less built-in interpretation, than some other c gories of potential relevance to the study of fering, delegitimation merits further explora by those interested in carrying out experien near analysis in medical anthropology.

ACKNOWLEDGMENTS

The research on which this article is based was ried out in collaboration with Arthur Kleinman, M and Anthony Komaroff, M.D. Data collection completed while the author was an NIMH-sponso Postdoctoral Research Fellow in Medical Ant pology at Harvard Medical School (grant 5T32MH18006). A grant from the Robert Wood Jo son Foundation (No. 13984) provided additional fur The advice and support of Professor Kleinman in veloping the work are particularly appreciated. Tha are extended also to Mary Jo DelVecchio Good, J Jackson, Alan Harwood, and several anonymous M reviewers for their helpful comments on earlier dra as well as to those who gave interviews in the stu

NOTES

1. The definition of suffering within as well as o side of illness is a complicated matter and not cen to the aims of this discussion. For present purposes rather loose definition of suffering as "the subjective perience of enduring pain from which there is no i mediately visible escape" will suffice.

2. In adopting the term "delegitimation" to refer these kinds of experiences, I do not mean to imply t chronic fatigue syndrome has been accorded "leg mate" status by the medical profession. "Delegitin

" is used here to represent sufferers' perceptions interpretations of their experiences and implies assumption of legitimacy on their part. The par-y constructed status of chronic fatigue syndrome as sease category in the medical lexicon is a separate e that is also discussed.

. The illness reality construct has been applied in arch on clinical encounters between doctors and ents to characterize the process through which rted symptoms are made meaningful by mapping n onto existing cultural models of illness and ling. See Atkinson 1977; Gaines 1979; Kleinman ɔ.

. This may, of course, point to inadequacies in the inition when applied to epidemiological research ufferman 1991).

. In fact, a review of NAMCS statistics through the os and early 1980s reveals a marked drop in the nber of physician visits reportedly prompted by fa-ıe. Interestingly, this may reflect a change in the inition of the construct rather than an actual de-ase. It seems that in 1977 narrower coding criteria for gue were implemented in tabulating the data, re-ting in an immediate 17% drop in incidence (Barof-and Legro 1991).

6. The tendency in professional medicine to dis-ınt the complaints of women means that gender st also be examined as part of an analysis of illness erience in chronic fatigue syndrome. The politics gender in chronic fatigue syndrome is the focus of e of several additional articles planned as part of this earch.

7. Concealment of disability as a strategy for avoid-g delegitimation is discussed in the context of ronic pain by Hilbert (1984).

REFERENCES

Abbey, Susan E., and Paul E. Garfinkel. 1991. Jeurasthenia and Chronic Fatigue Syndrome: The ıle of Culture in the Making of a Diagnosis." *Ameri-n Journal of Psychiatry* 148 (12): 1638–46.

Atkinson, P. 1977. "The Reproduction of Medical ıowledge." In *Health Care and Health Knowledge.* Dingwall et al., eds. London: Croom Helm.

Barofsky, Ivan, and Marcia West Legro. 1991. "Definition and Measurement of Fatigue." *Reviews of Infectious Diseases* 13 (Suppl. 1): S94–S108.

Buchwald, D., et al. 1987. "Frequency of 'Chronic Epstein-Barr Virus Infection' in a General Medical Practice." *Journal of the American Medical Association* 257:2303–07.

Centers for Disease Control. 1990. *Chronic Fatigue Syndrome: An Information Pamphlet.* NIH Publication No. 90-484. Washington, D.C.: National Institute of Allergy and Infectious Diseases.

Chen, M. 1986. "The Epidemiology of Self-Perceived Fatigue among Adults." *Preventive Medicine* 15: 74–81.

Cox, B., et al. 1987. *The Health and Lifestyle Survey.* London: Health Promotion Research Trust.

Da Costa, J. M. 1871. "On Irritable Heart: A Clinical Study of a Form of Functional Cardiac Disorder and Its Consequence." *American Journal of Medical Science* 121:17–52.

Das, Veena. 1991. "Moral Orientations to Suffering: Legitimation, Power and Healing." Manuscript in files of author, Department of Sociology, School of Economics, University of Delhi, Delhi, India.

David, A. S. 1991. "Postviral Fatigue Syndrome and Psychiatry." *British Medical Bulletin* 47(4): 966–88.

De Freites, S., et al. 1991. "Retroviral Sequences Related to Human T-Lymphotrophic Virus Type II in Patients with Chronic Fatigue Immune Dysfunction Syndrome." *Proceedings of the National Academy of Sciences USA* 88 (7): 2922–26.

Demitrack, M. A., et al. 1991. "Evidence for Impaired Activation of the Hypothalamic-Pituitary-Adrenal Axis in Patients with Chronic Fatigue Syndrome." *Journal of Clinical Endocrinology and Metabolism* 73 (6): 1224–34.

Evans, A. 1947. "Brucellosis in the United States." *American Journal of Public Health* 37: 139–51.

Gaines, Atwood. 1979. "Definitions and Diagnoses: Cultural Implications of Psychiatric Help-Seeking and Psychiatrists' Definition of the Situation in Psychiatric Emergencies." *Culture, Medicine and Psychiatry* 3: 381–418.

Good, Byron J. 1977. "The Heart of What's the Matter: The Semantics of Illness in Iran." *Culture, Medicine and Psychiatry* 1 (1): 125–58.

——. 1993. *Medicine, Rationality and Experience.* Cambridge: Cambridge University Press.

Good, Byron I., and Mary Jo DelVecchio Good. 1982. "Toward a Meaning-Centered Analysis of Popular Illness Categories: 'Fright Illness' and 'Heart Distress' in Iran." In *Cultural Conceptions of Mental Health and Therapy.* A. J. Marsala and G. M. White, eds. Dordrecht: D. Reidel.

Gordon, Deborah R. 1988. "Tenacious Assumptions in Western Medicine." In *Biomedicine Examined.* Margaret Lock and Deborah R. Gordon, eds. Dordrecht: Kluwer.

Gow, J. W., et al. 1991. "Enteroviral RNA Sequences Detected by Polymerase Chain Reaction in Muscle of Patients with Postviral Fatigue Syndrome." *British Medical Journal* 302 (6778): 692–96.

Greenberg, Donna. 1990. "Neurasthenia in the 1980's: Chronic Mononucleosis Syndrome, Chronic Fatigue Syndrome, and Anxiety and Depressive Disorders." *Psychosomatics* 31 (2): 129–37.

Grufferman, Seymour. 1991. "Issues and Problems in the Conduct of Epidemiologic Research on Chronic Fatigue Syndrome." *Reviews of Infectious Diseases* 13 (Suppl. l): S60–S67.

Gunn, W. J., D. Connell, and B. Randal. 1992. "Epidemiology of CFS: The Centers for Disease Control Study." Paper presented at the CIBA Foundation Symposium on Chronic Fatigue Syndrome (No. 173), London, May 11–14.

Hickie, Ian, et al. 1990. "The Psychiatric Status of Patients with Chronic Fatigue Syndrome." *British Journal of Psychiatry* 156: 534–40.

Hilbert, R. A. 1984. "The Acultural Dimensions of Chronic Pain: Flawed Reality Construction and the Problem of Meaning." *Social Problems* 31 (4): 365–78.

Holmes, Gary P., et al. 1988. "Chronic Fatigue Syndrome: A Working Case Definition." *Annals of Internal Medicine* 108: 387–89.

Imboden, J. C., A. Canter, and L. E. Cluff. 1961. "Convalescence from Influenza: A Study of the Psychological and Clinical Determinants." *Archives of Internal Medicine* 108: 393–99.

Jackson, Jean E. 1990. "The Stigma of Severe Chronic Pain." Manuscript, Department of Anthropology, Massachusetts Institute of Technology, C bridge, Mass.

——. 1992. "After a While No One Believes Real and Unreal Pain." In *Pain as Human Experie An Anthropological Perspective.* Mary Jo DelVecc Good et al. eds. Berkeley: University of Califc Press.

Jones, James F., et al. 1985. "Evidence for Ac Epstein-Barr Virus Infection in Patients with Pe tent Unexplained Illnesses: Elevated Anti-Early A gen Antibodies." *Annals of Internal Medicine* 1–7.

Kendell, R. E. 1991. "Chronic Fatigue, Viruses, Depression." *Lancet* 337: 160–61.

Kirmayer, Laurence J. 1988. "Mind and Bod Metaphors: Hidden Values in Biomedicine." In *medicine Examined.* Margaret Lock and Deboral Gordon, eds. Dordrecht: Kluwer.

Kleinman, Arthur. 1980. *Patients and Healers in Context of Culture.* Berkeley: University of Califo Press.

——. 1988. *The Illness Narratives: Suffering, H ing and the Human Condition.* New York: Basic Bo

——. 1992. "Pain and Resistance: The Dele mation and Relegitimation of Local Worlds." In *P as Human Experience: An Anthropological Perspect* Mary Jo DelVecchio Good et al., eds. Berkeley: U versity of California Press.

Komaroff, Anthony L. 1991. Remarks delivered the Workshop on the Definition and Medical O come Assessment of Chronic Fatigue Syndrome in search, National Institutes of Health, Bethesda, M March 18–19.

Kroenke, K., et al. 1988. "Chronic Fatigue in mary Care: Prevalence, Patient Characteristics, a Outcome." *Journal of the American Medical Assoc tion* 260:929–34.

Kruesi, Markus J. P., Janet Dale, and Stephen Straus. 1989. "Psychiatric Diagnoses in Patients W Have Chronic Fatigue Syndrome." *Journal of Clini Psychiatry* 50 (2): 53–56.

Lazare, Aaron. 1987. "Shame and Humiliation the Medical Encounter." *Archives of Internal Medic* 147: 1653–58.

ewis, G., and S. Wessely. 1992. "The Epidemiology atigue: More Questions than Answers." *Journal of demiology and Community Health* 46 (2): 92–97.

loyd, Andrew R., et al. 1989. "Immunological Ab-nalities in the Chronic Fatigue Syndrome." *Med-Journal of Australia* 151: 122–24.

——. 1990. "Prevalence of Chronic Disease Syn-ne in an Australian Population." *Medical Journal of tralia* 153: 522–28.

ock, Margaret, and Deborah R. Gordon, eds. 1988. *medicine Examined.* Dordrecht: Kluwer.

AcCluskey, D. R. 1992. "Pharmacological Ap-aches to Therapy of Chronic Fatigue Syndrome." er presented at the CIBA Foundation Symposium Chronic Fatigue Syndrome, London, May 11–14.

Nelson, C., and T. McLemore. 1988. *The National bulatory Medical Care Survey, Vital and Health tistics.* Series 13, no. 93. Hyattsville, Md.: National nter for Health Statistics, U.S. Department of alth and Human Services.

Price, Rumi K., et al. 1991. "Estimating the Preva-ce of Chronic Fatigue Syndrome (CFS) and Asso-ted Symptoms in the Community." *Public Health ports* 107 (5): 514–22.

Sharpe, M. C., et al. 1991. "A Report-Chronic Fatigue Syndrome: Guidelines for Research." *Journal of the Royal Society of Medicine* 84: 118–21.

Sicherman, Barbara. 1977. "The Uses of a Diagnosis: Doctors, Patients and Neurasthenia." *Journal of the History of Medicine and Allied Sciences* 32: 33–54.

Stewart, Donna E. 1987. "Environmental Hypersensitivity Disorder, Total Allergy and Twentieth Century Disease: A Critical Review." *Canadian Family Physician* 33: 405–10.

Straus, Stephen E. 1991. "History of Chronic Fatigue Syndrome." *Reviews of Infectious Diseases* 13 (Suppl. 1): S2–S7.

Straus, Stephen E., et al. 1985. "Persisting Illness and Fatigue in Adults with Evidence of Epstein-Barr Virus Infection." *Annals of Internal Medicine* 102: 7–16.

Swartz, Morton N. 1988. "The Chronic Fatigue Syndrome: One Entity or Many?" *New England Journal of Medicine* 319: 1726–28.

Time Magazine. 1987. "Stealthy Epidemic of Exhaustion: Doctors Are Perplexed by the Mysterious 'Yuppie Disease.'" June 29: 52.

Wessely, Simon. 1990. "Old Wine in New Bottles: Neurasthenia and 'ME.'" *Psychological Medicine* 20: 35–53.

CHAPTER 18

The Premenstrual Syndrome: A Brief History

JOHN T. E. RICHARDSON

PREMENSTRUAL SYMPTOMS AND PREMENSTRUAL SYNDROME

MOST MENSTRUATING WOMEN regula experience a variety of physical, psychological and behavioural chang during the time between ovulation and menstruation. One of the earli accounts of these changes was given by Horney ([1], translated as [2]) 1931 in a paper which was entitled "Die prämenstruellen Verstimmunge (Premenstrual Tensions):

> It is remarkable that so little attention has been paid to the fact that disturbanc occur not only during menstruation but even more frequently, though less o trusively, in the days before the onset of menstrual flow. These disturbances a generally known; they consist of varying degrees of tension, ranging from a fee ing that everything is too much, a sense of listlessness or of being slowed dow

nd intensities of feelings of self-depreciation to ıe point of pronounced feelings of oppression nd of being severely depressed. All these feelings re frequently intermingled with feelings of irriability or anxiousness [2, p. 99].

s Horney's account implies, there had previly been little recognition of these symptoms popular culture. Janiger, Riffenburgh and sh [3] reported the findings of a fairly exten- survey of historical and anthropological rces. They commented that, while there were ny examples of cultural myths, taboos and sustitions associated with menstruation, they found no reports relating to premenstrual ıptoms. Moreover, although there are isolated erences to these symptoms in historical writs, it is also only in modern times that clinicians e identified them as a characteristic feature the premenstrual phase. For instance, Hipcratic physicians described a pathological conion of uterine gaseous distension, where the umulation of black bile in the uterus was nifested in headache, vertigo, melancholia, ck urine and vaginal discharge [4, p. 59]. In 16th century, da Monte speculated on the reionship between menstruation and certain ascts of depression [5], while in the 19th century ichard [6] referred to "dysmenorrhoeal affecns":

> Some females at the period of the catemenia undergo a considerable degree of nervous excitement: morbid dispositions of mind are displayed by them at these times, a wayward and capricious temper, excitability in the feelings, moroseness in disposition, a proneness to quarrel with their dearest relatives, and sometimes a dejection of mind approaching to melancholia [6, p. 207].

With the benefit of contemporary research, ese examples may be taken to illustrate two reects in which accounts of paramenstrual sympms before the present century were fundamenlly inadequate: first, they failed to distinguish clearly between symptoms associated with the late luteal phase of the cycle and symptoms associated with menstruation (or "catamenia") itself; and, second, the conditions they described were supposed to be pathological states affecting only a small minority of women [7].

Although precisely contemporaneous with Horney's description, a paper by Frank [8] is usually credited as giving the first modern clinical account of premenstrual symptoms. Frank also used the term "premenstrual tension" to emphasize the cyclical emotional disturbances that were associated with the second half of the menstrual cycle. However, in 1953 Greene and Dalton [9] argued that emotional tension was only one of many components of this condition, and they proposed that instead it should be referred to as "premenstrual syndrome." That year another commentator suggested that the syndrome was composed of

> marked general tension and irritability, together with one or more of the following symptoms: anxiety, depression, bloated abdominal feelings, swelling of subcutaneous tissues, nausea, fatigue, painful swelling of the breasts, headaches, dizziness, and palpitations [10, p. 1014].

In Western countries, at least, many physicians nowadays assume that there is a specific clinical condition of premenstrual syndrome (or "PMS") which has emotional, somatic and behavioural components. Brush and Goudsmit [11] concluded that there was

> a useful consensus of opinion ... supporting the following as having significantly high incidence: irritability (sometimes extreme), depression, anxiety, breast swelling and pain, headaches, abdominal bloating, poor concentration, poor coordination, food cravings, lethargy, weight gain and change in libido [11, p. 5].

What needs to be emphasized at this point, however, is that this condition has only a "brief history," to quote the title of my paper. The idea that there are certain characteristic symptoms that are associated with the premenstrual phase of the menstrual cycle has been acknowledged by physicians and in the general culture for little more than 60 years, while the idea that these symptoms define a clinical "syndrome" is only 40 years old at the time of writing.

AETIOLOGY OF PREMENSTRUAL SYNDROME

In trying to understand the underlying cause of PMS, a natural place to start is the study of women's hormones. After all, PMS is supposed to be a feature of the menstrual cycle, and the menstrual cycle is driven by hormonal mechanisms. In his original paper on premenstrual tension, Frank [8] speculated that it was produced by an excessive accumulation of "the female sex hormone" (that is, oestrogen) because of renal dysfunction. He argued that it should be treated either by medication to encourage the excretion of oestrogen or by radiological treatment of the ovaries to attenuate its production. However, Abraham [12] pointed out that this explanation was wholly inadequate, as renal dysfunction would result in an elevated concentration of oestrogen which had been rendered biologically inactive by the liver.

Greene and Dalton [9] proposed that PMS was produced by water retention, and that the latter was due to abnormal elevation of the ratio between the circulating levels of oestrogen and progesterone. They argued that it could be treated by the injection or implantation of progesterone or else by the oral ingestion of synthetic progestogens. Smith [13] pointed out that a fundamental difficulty with this idea is that the first half of the cycle is characterized by large amounts of circulating oestrogen and very little progesterone in all women and yet is found to be relatively free of any mood disorders.

Subsequently, a variety of other theories w proposed that also implicated some imbala between the ovarian hormones in the aetio of premenstrual symptoms. However, resea studies have failed to find any specific relat ships between the concentrations of these h mones and either mood or behaviour. M specifically, as one reviewer recently c mented, "no consistent or identifiable patt has been established that can different women with PMS from control subjects" [14 50]. Certainly, major endocrinological ab malities are not characteristic of women w PMS.

Other theories have implicated a variety extra-ovarian factors, such as a deficiency of p doxine (vitamin B6), high levels of monoam oxidase activity, high levels of prolactin, o withdrawal reaction to beta-endorphin. H ever, none of these models has given rise t form of treatment for PMS that has proved to consistently effective in appropriately control clinical trials [14, 15]. In fact, excessive supp mentation with vitamin B6 produces nonspec peripheral axonal degeneration, leading to p gressive sensory ataxia without any apprecia influence upon premenstrual symptoms [16,

In her own original account, Horney [1] cribed premenstrual symptoms to the repress wish for a child and to frustrated libidinal ener which she claimed was directly released by normal physiological processes of preparation pregnancy. Deutsch [18] similarly claimed th they originated in fantasies relating to pregnan and childbirth engendered by the first menst ation. Subsequently, a number of other auth have sought to implicate psychological factors the aetiology of premenstrual symptoms. O common idea is that PMS is linked to a neuro predisposition, but any observed association he may be due to the fact that similar items tend be used in personality tests and in questionnai on premenstrual symptoms.

Iore recent research has suggested an associ-n with episodes of psychiatric illness, and es-ially with depression and other affective dis-ers [19]. As Goudsmit observed, "A common clusion is that in most women, the appear-e and/or reporting of premenstrual symptoms ie result of some personality flaw which is re-d to prevailing unresolved conflicts or con-rent psychosocial and cultural influences" , p. 21]. However, Goudsmit also pointed out t most of the evidence for a psychogenic basis purely correlational in nature, so that psy-logical factors might be a consequence of suf-ng from premenstrual symptoms rather than ir underlying cause.

Moreover, much of this research is based on study of psychiatric patients and other untyp-l samples of subjects, from whom it is clearly alid to generalize to the population of women general. In fact, Horney [1] had originally sug-ted that premenstrual symptoms were seldom nnected with psychological disturbances, and e recent study confirmed that in most cases n severe premenstrual symptomatology oc-rs in the absence of other psychopathology [21].

More convincing evidence for psychosocial tors in the aetiology of premenstrual symp-ns is the fact that evaluations of different forms treatment for such symptoms are typically alified by a very high placebo effect [22]. As e author summarized the position, "uncon-lled studies virtually always show positive sults, no matter what the treatment, whereas equately controlled double-blind studies fre-ently show negative findings" [13, p. 45]. In-ed, in one study reported by Magos, Brincat d Studd [23], 94% of the control subjects re-rted an overall improvement in their premen-ual symptoms as the result of an inactive acebo, and 84% considered it to be more effec-e than other forms of treatment that they had ed. Given results of this sort, it is perhaps not rprising that in a survey of general practitioners over 80% claimed to be successful in treating pre-menstrual symptoms [24].

Although premenstrual symptoms are experi-enced by women in all of the cultures that have been studied to date, the frequency and the sever-ity of particular symptoms vary amongst different cultural groups [3, 25]. For example, an interna-tional study conducted by the World Health Or-ganization [26] found that the incidence of mood changes such as irritability, lethargy and depres-sion varied between 23% amongst Sundanese women in Indonesia and 73% amongst Muslim women in Yugoslavia. Moreover, like other re-productive phenomena such as menarche, lacta-tion, menopause and menstruation itself [27–30], the cultural meaning of premenstrual symptoms appears to vary between different societies. In some cultures, such as those of Bahrain and southern Italy, both somatic and emotional symptoms are a common feature of women's ex-perience, yet many women have no concept of a "premenstrual syndrome" [25]. Johnson went so far as to claim that PMS was a Western culture-specific disorder. As he pointed out:

> This particular taxon appears only recently in in-dustrial cultures: it has only been formalized dur-ing the past two decades. PMS involves bizarre behavior which is recognized, defined, and treated as a specific syndrome only by bio-med-ical healers in Western, industrial cultures [31, p. 347].
>
> PMS can be seen as internally related to our culture, and can be *best* understood as a social and cultural phenomenon, even though there may be psychological or psychiatric determi-nants and consequences. It is not suggested here that premenstrual symptoms do not exist, but rather than the phenomenon of premenstrual syndrome is best studied as a social, rather than individual, reality [31, p. 350].

Some authors have argued that socially mediated expectations and beliefs may determine the incidence of premenstrual symptoms. Parlee suggested that these beliefs "may provide a set of cognitive categories for the subject to use in labeling what would under other circumstances be experienced as non-specific states of arousal" [32, p. 248]. Fradkin and Firestone [33] used a journal article, a videotape and group discussion to tell a group of women that "premenstrual tension was due not to biology but to negative societal myths." Subsequently, these women reported fewer premenstrual symptoms and less premenstrual mood disturbance.

A study reported by Ruble [34] is often cited as a demonstration of the role of learned associations and psychosocial influences upon a woman's description of her current state. Ruble encouraged different subjects to believe that they were either premenstrual or intermenstrual. When asked to describe the moods and symptoms which they had experienced over the previous day or two, the former subjects reported a significantly higher degree of severe physical symptoms, such as headaches, fatigue and swelling. Nevertheless, Goudsmit [20] pointed out that there were in fact no significant differences between the two groups in Ruble's study in terms of their reports of irritability, anxiety and depression, or of changes in their concentration or behaviour.

It is in fact well established that cyclical symptoms may persist in women who have undergone simple hysterectomy, although obviously in such cases there is no menstrual flow to act as an overt marker of this cycle. Bäckström, Boyle and Baird came to the conclusion that "neither the presence of the uterus nor the occurrence of menstruation are necessary for the manifestation of the premenstrual tension syndrome" [35, p. 350]. This implies that PMS should not strictly be regarded as a *premenstrual* syndrome and on the face of it supports a psychosocial explanation of PMS rather than a biological one.

However, Osborn [36] came to exactly the opposite conclusion. The argument here is that socially mediated expectations should be effec only as long as menstruation was experien but that hormonal factors would continue to erate in the absence of menstruation as lon ovulation continued to occur. There is in one report in the literature of persistent cyc symptoms after hysterectomy combined with removal of both ovaries [37]. This finding never to my knowledge been replicated, bu Osborn's argument this would imply a cere basis for PMS rather than an ovarian one.

Nevertheless, it is beyond question tha Western societies there are quite determin culturally shared attitudes and beliefs about influence of the menstrual cycle upon wom experience and behaviour. These attitudes beliefs are held by both women and men, they are known to be acquired by both g and boys before the onset of puberty [38]. In f the expectations of premenarcheal girls tend parallel the symptom reports and attitudes older women [39]. Hence, the actual experie *of* menstruation seems to have little effect u girls' attitudes *towards* menstruation.

There is also evidence of a general tende on the part of both men and women to ascr negative moods experienced by women arou the time of menstruation to the biological p cess of menstruation itself, but to ascribe p cisely the same moods experienced by women other times of the menstrual cycle to external f tors. Koeske and Koeske [40] found that this at butional pattern was stronger in the case women than in the case of men and was not served in the case of positive moods.

Campos and Thurow [41] investigated bo the incidence of particular moods and wome attributions of their own mental states at differe times in the menstrual cycle. They found that ritability and tension occurred more often arou the time of menstruation, while depression a happiness did not. Independent of this, howev the likelihood that irritability, tension, or depr sion would be ascribed to the process of menstr n was greater around the time of menstrua- than at other times of the cycle. Similar find- were obtained in a subsequent study by nnan [42].

Vhat I would therefore conclude is that at sent the aetiology of premenstrual symptoms yet unknown. They are experienced as being narily psychological in nature, they vary ely in their incidence across different cultural ups, and they respond to inactive placebos as ctively as to active preparations. The balance vidence suggests that women's experience of menstrual symptoms probably has more to do h cultural or psychological factors than with logical ones; that is, it represents "a recreation acit cultural knowledge about the effect of the roductive system on women's behaviour" [43, 50]. Of course, the same may well be true of er reproductive health experiences such as t flushes and other menopausal symptoms –47], and like these premenstrual symptoms y tend to be related to how different cultures menstruation and to the general role of men in society.

A PREMENSTRUAL SYNDROME?

further point that needs to be made is that in king about "PMS" the very use of the term ndrome" has certain connotations about ich at least some researchers are exceeding eptical. As Sampson pointed out, "The term ndrome' typically refers to a group of symp- ms that occur together and characterize a med- l or 'abnormal' condition" [48, p. 38]. Many of ese arguments have recently been rehearsed in hapter by Ussher [49], and I shall simply sum- arize them very briefly.

The first issue has to do with the empirical sis for using the word "syndrome." There is in ct a tremendous range of possible symptoms at women report and no agreement over any ore" set of symptoms that would support a diagnosis of PMS. I investigated this issue myself in a study published previously by administering a checklist of 44 symptoms to a large number of women university students [50]. They were patently not a random sample of the general population, but the general distribution of their symptoms reports was very similar to that found in previous studies using more representative samples.

A factor analysis of their responses produced six factors which could be readily interpreted as indices of cognitive impairment, emotionality, faintness, social impairment, behavioural impairment and fluid retention, respectively. These factors were all positively, though weakly, correlated with one another, and a higher-order analysis indicated the existence of a single underlying second-order factor on which they were all significantly loaded. This suggests that the "premenstrual syndrome" is not a simple set of regularly co-occurring symptoms, but a "monarchial hierarchy" in which a number of distinct symptom clusters are tied together by a single overarching second-order factor.

It is in fact becoming increasingly accepted that "PMS" is at best a loose heterogeneous grouping of symptoms rather than a single diagnostic entity. This in turn would motivate the exploration of alternative forms of treatment for this condition. However, one recent review estimated that as many as 327 different treatments for PMS had been proposed [51], and most of these lack any coherent rationale or research basis.

The second issue is that talking about PMS as a "syndrome" implies the existence of a clinical condition that is statistically abnormal. In fact, estimates of the prevalence of PMS have varied between 5% and 95% of all menstruating women. According to at least some studies therefore, a majority of women suffer from this alleged "syndrome." As Tonks remarked, "The incidence figures are so high as to make this condition statistically normal" [52, p. 405]. Conversely, some would argue that it was the woman who did not have premenstrual symptoms who was statistically abnormal, and that the concept of "PMS" actually served to reinforce stereotypes of femininity.

A third issue is that the notion of a "syndrome" implies a condition that can be diagnosed consistently both across different assessors and across different occasions. A distinctive feature of PMS is that it is diagnosed solely from self-reports [22]. Indeed, women typically present with a self-diagnosis of PMS that is based upon retrospective reports of premenstrual changes in mood and behaviour. Although it has been argued that such retrospective reports are both reliable and accurate [53], and although they can provide the basis for a provisional clinical diagnosis [54, p. 369; 55, p. 718], in recent years clinical practice (particularly in the United States) has demanded that they be confirmed by prospective daily self-reports from two successive cycles [56]. Nevertheless, there is poor agreement between different procedures for evaluating changes in prospective reports within a single menstrual cycle and poor consistency between the reports obtained from successive menstrual cycles [57].

The final point is that the notion of a "syndrome" also implies the existence of a pathological condition that demands and indeed legitimates intervention and treatment by medical authorities. In the United Kingdom, this view of PMS seems to have been largely accepted by default. However, in the United States there has been much more discussion and debate. The Work Group set up to revise the third edition of the American Psychiatric Association's *Diagnostic and Statistical Manual of Mental Disorders* did recognize that it was necessary "to narrow the boundaries of the syndrome to those that would define a disorder" [58, p. 271]. Despite opposition from, among others, the American Psychological Association, the resulting concept of "late luteal phase dysphoric disorder" (LLPDD) was listed as an example under "Unspecified Mental Disorders" in the text of DSM-III-R and included in an appendix as a "proposed diagnostic cate[gory] needing later study" to "facilitate further syst[em]atic clinical study and research" [54, pp. xxv, 3

Critics of this decision argued that it gave [for]mal recognition to a highly controversial d[iag]nostic category and that it created consider[able] potential for misuse against women on the pa[rt of] clinicians, employers and insurance compan[ies]. In fact, Horney had herself commented that [pre]menstrual symptoms "frequently occur in ot[her]wise healthy women and usually do not [give] the impression of a pathological process" [2 100]. At the same time, it has transpired that fe[wer] than half of all women who are referred or w[ho] present with PMS for clinical assessment sat[isfy] the DSM-III-R criteria for LLPDD [19, A subsequent Work Group that was set up to [re]vise DSM-III-R did not consider that the [evi]dence justified the inclusion of this conditio[n as] an accepted diagnostic entity, but they nevert[he]less sought to acknowledge the occurrence of [se]vere dysphoria in the premenstrual phase [59 249]. Consequently, renamed "premenstrual d[ys]phoric disorder," this condition was include[d in] an appendix to DSM-IV to encourage furt[her] study and also listed as a "depressive disorder [not] otherwise specified" within the main text [55, 350, 715].

PMS AS A LEGAL DEFENCE

Under English law, it is possible for a person [ac]cused of homicide to submit a plea of "dim[in]ished responsibility": in other words, that at t[he] time of the killing, they were suffering from me[n]tal abnormalities such as would substantially i[m]pair their responsibility for their actions. If s[uc]cessful, this defense entitles the accused to [be] found guilty not of murder but of the less[er] charge of manslaughter. In three different cas[es] medical evidence of severe PMS has been a[c]cepted as providing an adequate basis for a plea [of] manslaughter with diminished responsibili[ty] reover. in each of these cases, the medical ev- nce was also taken into account by way of mit- ion in determining sentencing [60–62].

n 1982, a defence based on PMS was em- yed in the United States in a case where the endant was charged with the assault of her ghter. A motion for dismissal was denied, but h the charges and the defence were subse- ntly withdrawn when the defendent agreed to ad guilty to the lesser charge of harassment, she was discharged on the condition that she lerwent psychological assessment and coun- ing. A defence based on PMS was also re- ted in a case heard before the U.S. Bankruptcy urt in 1983 that concerned medical costs in- red as the result of an assault by stabbing. nedek [63] and Katz and Taub [61] discussed h these cases and concluded that a defence to minal charges based on PMS would be un- ely to succeed in the United States, given the agreement within the medical community as its status as a diagnostic entity. Nevertheless, a fence based on PMS has been employed in a mber of state civil cases with mixed success. wis [64] discussed these and the previous cases d concluded that it would in principle be pos- le for a PMS defence to succeed, given appro- ate legal arguments and evidence. However, acknowledged that this could be seen as rein- cing a social stereotype that women were the tims of hormonal fluctuations and thus un- itable for positions of responsibility. The oader implications for both criminal justice d civil rights of citing PMS as a legal defence d indeed been discussed previously by De- ney, Lupton and Toth [65].

CONCLUSIONS

sum up, then, the concept of PMS has a ghly contentious status whether as a diagnostic tegory for practitioners or as an entity for psy- ological research. First, the concept is related the experience of women within contempo- rary Western cultures. Second, the aetiology of this condition is unclear, but it seems to depend upon social, cultural and psychological factors as much as upon biological ones. Third, the relevant symptoms do not appear to possess the empirical integrity to talk about a "syndrome." Fourth, the relevant symptoms may be normal rather than abnormal from a statistical point of view. Fifth, both clinicians and feminists have questioned whether the relevant symptoms amount to a pathological condition that warrants and legitimates medical intervention and treatment. The position has been well summarized by Golub:

> According to Webster's *New Collegiate Dictionary*, a syndrome is "a group of signs and symptoms that occur together and characterize a particular abnormality." Using this definition, premenstrual syndrome does not exist. To date no abnormality has been found, though many have been postulated. At best, PMS can be characterized as a group of psychological and somatic symptoms that are limited to the week preceding menstruation and are relieved by the onset of menses [66, p. 181].

ACKNOWLEDGMENTS

The author is grateful to two anonymous reviewers for their comments on an earlier version of this paper.

REFERENCES

1. Horney K. "Die prämenstruellen Verstimmungen." *Z. Psychoanal. Pädag.* 5, 161, 1931.

2. Horney K. "Premenstrual Tension." In *Feminine Psychology* (Edited and translated by Kelman H.), p. 99. Routledge and Kegan Paul, London, 1967.

3. Janiger O., Riffenburgh R., and Kersh R. "Cross Cultural Study of Premenstrual Symptoms." *Psychosomatics* 13, 226, 1972.

4. Ricci J. V. *The Genealogy of Gynaecology*. Blakiston, Philadelphia, 1950.

5. Bonuzzi L. "The Contribution to Psychiatry by Padua University." *Br. J. Psychiat.* 128, 223, 1976.

6. Prichard J. C. *Treatise on Insanity and Other Disorders Affecting the Mind.* Sherwood, Gilbert and Piper, London, 1835.

7. Richardson J. T. E. "The Menstrual Cycle, Cognition, and Paramenstrual Symptomatology." In *Cognition and the Menstrual Cycle* (Edited by Richardson J. T. E.), p. 1. Springer, Berlin, 1992.

8. Frank R. T. "The Hormonal Causes of Premenstrual Tension." *Archs. Neurol. Psychiat. Chicago* 26, 1053, 1931.

9. Greene R. and Dalton K. "The Premenstrual Syndrome." *Br. Med. J.* 1, 1007, 1953.

10. Rees L. "The Premenstrual Tension Syndrome and Its Treatment." *Br. Med. J.* 1, 1014, 1953.

11. Brush M. G. and Goudsmit E. M. "General and Social Considerations in Research on Menstrual Cycle Disorders with Particular Reference to PMS." In *Functional Disorders of the Menstrual Cycle* (Edited by Brush M. G. and Goudsmit E. M.), p. 1. Chichester: Wiley, 1988.

12. Abraham G. "The Premenstrual Tension Syndromes." In *Contemporary Obstetric and Gynecologic Nursing* (Edited by McNall L. K.), p. 170. C. V. Mosby, St. Louis, 1980.

13. Smith S. L. "Mood and the Menstrual Cycle." In *Topics in Psychoendocrinology* (Edited by Sacher E. J.), p. 19. Grune and Stratton, New York, 1975.

14. Parry B. L. "Biological Correlates of Premenstrual Complaints." In *Premenstrual Dysphorias* (Edited by Gold J. H. and Severino S. K.), p. 47. American Psychiatric Press, Washington, D.C., 1994.

15. Rivera-Tovar A., Rhodes R., Pearlstein T. B., and Frank E. In *Premenstrual Dysphorias,* (Edited by Gold J. H. and Severino S. K.), p. 99. American Psychiatric Press, Washington, D.C., 1994.

16. Schaumberg H., Kaplan J., Windebank A., Vick N., Rasmus S., Pleasure D., and Brown M. J. "Sensory Neuropathy from Pyridoxine Abuse: A New Megavitamin Syndrome." *New Engl. J. Med.* 309, 445, 1983.

17. Berger A. and Schaumberg H. H. "More on Neuropathy from Pyridoxine Abuse." *New Engl. J. Med.* 311, 986, 1984.

18. Deutsch H. *The Psychology of Women: A Psy analytic Interpretation.* Vol. 1. Grune and Stra New York, 1944.

19. Endicott J. "Differential Diagnoses and Co bidity." In *Premenstrual Dysphorias* (Edited by C J. H. and Severino S. K.), p. 3. American Psychi Press, Washington, D.C., 1994.

20. Goudsmit E. M. "Psychological Aspects of menstrual Symptoms." *J. Psychosom. Obstet. Gyn* 2, 20, 1983.

21. Haskett R. F., Steiner M., Osmun J. N., and roll B. J. "Severe Premenstrual Tension: Delineatic the Syndrome." *Biol. Psychiat.* 15, 121, 1980.

22. Parlee M. B. "Commentary on the Literature view." In *Premenstrual Dysphorias* (Edited by C J. H. and Severino S. K.), p. 149. American Psychia Press, Washington, D.C., 1994.

23. Magos A. L., Brincat M., and Studd J. W "Treatment of the Premenstrual Syndrome by Sub taneous Oestradiol Implants and Cyclical C Norethisterone: Placebo Controlled Study." *Br. M J.* 292, 1629, 1986.

24. Alexander D. A., Taylor R. J., and Fordyce I "Attitudes of General Practitioners Towards Prem strual Symptoms and Those Who Suffer from The *J. R. Coll. Gen. Practnrs* 36, 10, 1986.

25. Dan A. J. and Monagle L. "Sociocult Influences on Women's Experiences of Perimenstr Symptoms." In *Premenstrual Dysphorias* (Edited Gold J. H. and Severino S. K.), p. 201. American I chiatric Press, Washington, D.C., 1994.

26. World Health Organization. "A Cross-Cultu Study of Menstruation: Implications for Contracept Development and Use." *Stud. Family Plan.* 12, 3, 19

27. Ford C. S. *A Comparative Study of Human production.* Yale University Publications in Anthrop ogy, No. 32. Human Relations Area Files Press, N Haven, Conn., 1964.

28. Frayser S. G. *Varieties of Sexual Experience: Anthropological Perspective on Human Sexual* Human Relations Area Files Press, New Have Conn., 1985.

29. Furth C. and Shu-yueh C. "Chinese Medici and the Anthropology of Menstruation in Contem rary Taiwan." *Med. Anthrop. Q.* 6, 27, 1992.

ɔ. Harrell B. B. "Lactation and Menstruation in ▪tural Perspective." *Am. Anthrop.* 83, 796, 1981.

▪1. Johnson T. M. "Premenstrual Syndrome as a ▪tern Culture-Specific Disorder." *Culture Med. Psy-▪t.* 11, 337, 1987.

2. Parlee M. B. "Positive Changes in Moods and Ac-▪tion Levels during the Menstrual Cycle in Experi-ıtally Naive Subjects." In *The Menstrual Cycle.* Vol. *Synthesis of Interdisciplinary Research* (Edited by ▪ A. J., Graham E. A., and Beecher C. P.), p. 247. ▪inger, Berlin, 1980.

;3. Fradkin B. and Firestone P. "Premenstrual Ten-ı, Expectancy, and Mother-Child Relations." *J. ▪av. Med.* 9, 245, 1986.

▪34. Ruble D. N. "Premenstrual Symptoms: A Re-ɪrpretation." *Science, N. Y.* 197, 291, 1977.

▪35. Backstrom C. T., Boyle H., and Baird D. T. "Per-▪ence of Symptoms of Premenstrual Tension in Hys-ɜctomized Women." *Br. J. Obstet. Gynaec.* 88, 530, ›1.

36. Osborn M. "Physical and Psychological Deter-▪nants of Premenstrual Tension: Research Issues and 'roposed Methodology." *J. Psychosom. Res.* 25, 363, ı.

37. Gray L. A. "The Use of Progesterone in Nervous ısion States." *5th. Med. J., Nashville* 34, 1004, 1941.

38. Clarke A. E. and Ruble D. N. "Young Adoles-▪nts' Beliefs Concerning Menstruation." *Child Dev.* 231, 1978.

39. Brooks-Gunn J. and Ruble D. N. "The Devel-ment of Menstrual-Related Beliefs and Behaviors ring Early Adolescence." *Child Dev.* 53, 1567, ▪2.

40. Koeske R. K. and Koeske G. F. "An Attributional ▪proach to Moods and the Menstrual Cycle." *J. Pers. ▪c. Psychol.* 31, 473, 1975.

41. Campos F. and Thurow C. "Attributions of ▪oods and Symptoms to the Menstrual Cycle." *Pers. ▪c. Psychol. Bull.* 4, 272, 1978.

42. Brennan B. M. "The Effect of Menstrual Cycle ▪ase and Instructional Set on Self-Report of Current ▪d Retrospective States." *Diss. Abstr. Int.* 41, 1479B, ▪80.

43. Rodin M. "The Social Construction of Premen-▪rual Syndrome." *Soc. Sci. Med.* 35, 49, 1992.

44. George T. "Menopause: Some Interpretations of the Results of a Study among a Non-Western Group." *Maturitas* 10, 109, 1988.

45. Kaufert P. A. and Gilbert P. "Women, Menopause, and Medicalization." *Cult. Med. Psychiat.* 10, 7, 1986.

46. Lock M. "Ambiguities of Aging: Japanese Experience and Perceptions of Menopause." *Cult. Med. Psychiat.* 10, 23, 1986.

47. Lock M. *Encounters with Aging: Mythologies of Menopause in Japan and North America.* University of California Press, Berkeley, 1993.

48. Sampson G. A. "Definition of Premenstrual Syndrome and Related Conditions." In *Functional Disorders of the Menstrual Cycle* (Edited by Brush M. G. and Goudsmit E. M.), p. 37. Wiley, Chichester, 1980.

49. Ussher J. M. "The Demise of Dissent and the Rise of Cognition in Menstrual-Cycle Research." In *Cognition and the Menstrual Cycle* (Edited by Richardson J. T. E.), p. 132. Springer, Berlin, 1992.

50. Richardson J. T. E. "Student Learning and the Menstrual Cycle: Premenstrual Symptoms and Approaches to Studying." *Educ. Psychol.* 9, 215, 1989.

51. Blumenthal S. J. and Nadelson C. C. "Mood Changes Associated with Reproductive Life Events: An Overview of Research and Treatment Strategies." *J. Clin. Psychiat.* 49, 466, 1988.

52. Tonks C. M. "Premenstrual Tension." In *Contemporary Psychiatry (Br. J. Psychiat,* special publication no. 9), edited by T. Silverstone and B. Barraclough, p. 399. British Medical Association, London, 1975.

53. Richardson J. T. E. "Questionnaire Studies of Paramenstrual Symptoms." *Psychol. Women Q.* 14, 15, 1990.

54. American Psychiatric Association. *Diagnostic and Statistical Manual of Mental Disorders,* 3rd ed., rev. American Psychiatric Association, Washington, D.C., 1987.

55. American Psychiatric Association. *Diagnostic and Statistical Manual of Mental Disorders,* 4th ed. American Psychiatric Press, Washington, D.C., 1994.

56. Parry B. L., Rosenthal N. E., and Wehr T. A. "Research Techniques Used to Study Premenstrual Syndrome." In *Premenstrual Syndrome: Current Findings*

and Future Directions (Edited by Osofsky H. J. and Blumenthal S. J.), p. 87. American Psychiatric Press, Washington, D.C., 1985.

57. Schnurr P. P., Hurt S. W., and Stout A. L. "Consequences of Methodological Decisions in the Diagnosis of Late Luteal Phase Dysphoric Disorder." In *Premenstrual Dysphorias* (Edited by Gold J. H. and Severino S. K.), p. 19. Washington, D.C.: American Psychiatric Press, 1994.

58. Spitzer R. L. and Williams J. B. W. "The Revision of DSM-III: Process and Changes." In *International Classification in Psychiatry: Unity, and Diversity* (Edited by Mezzich J. E. and van Cranach M.), p. 263. Cambridge University Press, Cambridge, 1988.

59. Gold J. H. and Severino S. K., eds. *Premenstrual Dysphorias: Myths and Realities*, p. 249. American Psychiatric Press, Washington, D.C., 1994.

60. Allen H. "At the Mercy of Her Hormones: menstrual Tension and the Law." *m/f* 9, 19, 1984.

61. Katz A. and Taub J. "Medico-Legal Aspects o Premenstrual Syndrome." In *Hormones and Beh* (Edited by Dennerstein L. and Fraser I.), p. 213. cerpta Medica, Amsterdam, 1986.

62. Laws S. "The Sexual Politics of Pre-Mens Tension." *Women's Stud. Int. Forum* 6, 19, 1983.

63. Benedek E. P. "Premenstrual Syndrome: A V from the Bench." *J. Clin. Psychiat.* 49, 498, 1964.

64. Lewis J. W. "Premenstrual Syndrome as a C inal Defense." *Archs Sexual Behav.* 19, 425, 1990.

65. Delaney J., Lupton M. J., and Toth E. *The Cu A Cultural History of Menstruation*. New York: Dut 1976.

66. Golub S. *Periods: From Menarche to M opause*. Sage, Newbury Park, Calif., 1992.

CHAPTER 19

The Politics of Menopause: The "Discovery" of a Deficiency Disease

FRANCES B. McCREA

IN THE 1960S THE MEDICAL profession ı the United States hailed the contraceptive pill as the "great liberator" of omen, and estrogens in general as the fountain of youth and beauty. rominent gynecologists "discovered" that menopause was a "deficiency isease," but promised women that estrogen replacement therapy would t them avoid menopause completely and keep them "feminine forever." et within a few years, U.S. feminists in the vanguard of an organized omen's health movement defined the health care system, including strogen treatment, as a serious social problem. The male-dominated ıedical profession was accused of reflecting and perpetuating the social ideology of women as sex objects and reproductive organs. Treating women with dangerous drugs was defined as exploitation and an insidious form of social control.

These issues raised several questions: How did such diametrically opposed definitions evolve? How, under what conditions, and by whom does a certain behavior become defined as deviant or sick? In what context does a putative condition become defined as a social problem?

I believe that definitions of health and illness are socially constructed and that these definitions are inherently political. "Deviant behaviors that were once defined as immoral, sinful or criminal," according to Conrad and Schneider (1980: 1), "have now been given new medical meanings" which are profoundly political in nature" and have "real political consequences." Indeed "in many cases these medical treatments have become a new form of social control."

I interpret the definition of menopause from this framework. During the 19th century, Victorian physicians viewed menopause as a sign of sin and decay; with the advent of Freudian psychology in the early 20th century, it was viewed as a neurosis; and as synthetic estrogens became readily available in the 1960s, physicians treated menopause as a deficiency disease (McCrea 1981). Perhaps more important than these differences, however, are four themes which pervade the medical definitions of menopause. These are: (1) women's potential and function are biologically destined; (2) women's worth is determined by fecundity and attractiveness; (3) rejection of the feminine role will bring physical and emotional havoc; (4) aging women are useless and repulsive.

In this paper I first analyze the rise of the disease definition of menopause and show that this definition reflects and helps create the prevailing ageism and sexism of our times. Then I show how the disease definition has been challenged from inside the medical community. Finally I examine how feminists outside the medical c munity have also challenged the disease mo claiming that menopause is normal and r tively unproblematic.

MENOPAUSE AS DISEASE

The roots of the disease definition of menopa can be traced back to the synthesis of estrog The earliest interest in these hormones grew of efforts to find a cure for male impotence (B ton 1944; Page 1977). In 1889, Charles Édou Brown-Sequard, a French physiologist, repo to the Societé de Biologie in Paris that he exp enced renewed vigor and rejuvenation after jecting himself with extracts from animal te cles. Four years later another French scien Regis de Bordeaux, used an ovarian extract in tion to treat a female patient for menopausal " sanity." And in 1896 a German physician, T odore Landau, used desiccated ovaries to tr menopausal symptoms at the Landau Clinic Berlin. In the late 1920s, Edgar Allen and Edw Doisey isolated and crystallized theelin (la known as estrone) from the urine of pregn women. In 1932 Samual Geist and Frank Sp man described in the *American Journal of C stetrics and Gynecology* their efforts to tr menopausal women with theelin. Such tre ments, however, were expensive and suppl of the drug limited, since it was derived fro human sources. These problems were solved 1936 when Russell Marker and Thomas O wood developed a synthetic form of estrog known as diethylstilbesteral (DES). This che and potent hormone substance could be ma readily available to a large number of wom and paved the way for the development of t contraceptive pill. The last step in the develo ment of hormone therapy occurred in 1943 wh James Goodall developed an estrogen extra from the urine of pregnant mares. Termed co jugated equine estrogen and manufactured rst under the brand name Premarin, it was y about half as potent as synthetic estrogen, it created fewer unpleasant side effects.

By the early 1960s exogenous estrogen (that is, ogen originating outside the human body) widely available in the United States, and inexpensive and easy to administer. It was d to treat various conditions of aging. But if es- gens were to become the cure, what was to be disease?

> Medicine] is active in seeking out illness.... One of the greatest ambitions of the physician is o discover and describe a "new" disease or syn- drome and to be immortalized by having his name used to identify the disease. Medicine, then, is oriented to seeking out and finding ill- ness, which is to say that it seeks to create social meanings of illness where that meaning or inter- pretation was lacking before. And insofar as ill- ness is defined as something bad—to be eradi- cated or contained—medicine plays the role of what Becker called the "moral entrepreneur" (Freidson 1970: 252).

The moral entrepreneur who, during the 60s, led the crusade to redefine menopause as disease was the prominent Brooklyn gynecolo- t Robert A. Wilson. As founder and head of the ilson Foundation, established in New York in 63 to promote estrogens and supported by $1.3 illion in grants from the pharmaceutical indus- (Mintz and Cohn 1977). Wilson's writings re crucial to the acceptance of menopause as "deficiency disease" and the large-scale routine ministration of Estrogen Replacement Ther- y (ERT). He claimed that menopause was a rmone deficiency disease similar to diabetes d thyroid dysfunction. In an article published the *Journal of the American Medical Associa- on*, Wilson (1962) claimed that estrogen pre- nted breast and genital cancer and other prob- ms of aging. Even though his methodology was eak,[1] this article launched a campaign to promote estrogens for the prevention of menopause and age-related diseases.

A year later, writing with his wife Thelma in the *Journal of the American Geriatrics Society*, Wilson and Wilson (1963) advocated that women be given estrogens from "puberty to grave." Crucial to the popular acceptance of the disease model of menopause was Robert Wilson's widely read book *Feminine Forever* (1966a) which claimed that menopause is a malfunction threatening the "feminine essence." In an article summarizing his book, Wilson described menopausal women as "living decay" (1966b: 70) but said ERT could save them from being "condemned to witness the death of their womanhood" (1966b: 66). He further proclaimed that menopause and aging could be allayed with ERT and listed 26 physiological and psychological symptoms that the "youth pill" could avert—including hot flashes, osteoporosis (thinning of bone mass), vaginal atrophy (thinning of vaginal walls), sagging and shrinking breasts, wrinkles, absent-mindedness, irritability, frigidity, depression, alcoholism, and even suicide.

Wilson also was aware of the physician's potential and even mandate for social control. The first paragraph of a chapter titled "Menopause—The Loss of Womanhood and Good Health" states:

> ... I would like to launch into the subject of menopause by discussing its effect on men. Menopause covers such a wide range of physical and emotional symptoms that the implications are by no means confined to the woman. Her husband, her family, and her entire relationship to the outside world are affected almost as strongly as her own body. Only in this broader context can the problem of the menopause—as well as the benefits of hormonal cure—be properly appreciated (1966a: 92).

Wilson gives an example of how he helped a distressed husband who came to him for help with the following complaint:

> She is driving me nuts. She won't fix meals. She lets me get no sleep. She picks on me all the time. She makes up lies about me. She hits the bottle all day. And we used to be happily married (1966a: 93).

This man's wife, Wilson says, responded well to "intensive" estrogen treatment and in no time resumed her wifely duties (1966a: 94). In another chapter Wilson conjures up visions of Ira Levin's (1972) novel *The Stepford Wives:*

> In a family situation, estrogen makes women adaptable, even-tempered, and generally easy to live with. Consequently, a woman's estrogen carries significancy beyond her own well-being. It also contributes toward the happiness of her family and all those with whom she is in daily contact. Even frigidity in women has been shown to be related to estrogen deficiency. The estrogen-rich woman, as a rule, is capable of far more generous and satisfying sexual response than women whose femininity suffers from inadequate chemical support (Wilson 1966: 64).

From Wilson's own words it is obvious that the disease label is not neutral. This label, like any disease label, decreases the status and the autonomy of the patient while increasing the status and power of the physician. When seen as part of a political process, knowledge and skill are claimed by a group to advance its interests. True or false the knowledge, disinterested or interested the motive, claims of knowledge function as ideologies ... insofar as claims to knowledge and skill are essential elements in a political process ... it is highly unlikely that they can remain neutrally descriptive (Freidson 1971: 30).

By individualizing the problems of menopause, the physician turns attention away from any social structural interpretation of women's conditions. The locus of the solution then becomes the doctor-patient interaction in which the physician is active, instrumental, and authoritative while the patient is passive and dependent. The inherent authority of physicians is institutionalized in ways that minimize relia[nce] on explanation and persuasion. This clin[ical] mentality is "intrinsically imperialistic, claim[ing] more for the profession's knowledge and s[kill] and a broader jurisdiction than in fact can [be] justified by demonstrable effectiveness" (Fr[eid]son 1971: 31). Such imperialism is independen[t of] the particular motivation of the physician. [Not] only could it function as "crude self-interest," [but] also as "a natural outcome of the deep com[mit]ment to the value of his work developed by [the] thoroughly socialized professional" (1971: 31).

A number of prominent U.S. physicians s[up]ported Wilson's claims. Robert Greenb[latt] (1974), former president of the American G[eri]atrics Society, claimed that about 75 perc[ent] of menopausal women are acutely estrog[en] deficient and advocated ERT for them, eve[n if] they were without symptoms. Another crusa[der] for ERT, Helen Jern, a gynecologist at the N[ew] York Infirmary, wrote a book of case studies p[ro]claiming the miraculous recoveries made by [el]derly women placed on ERT:

> I know the remarkably beneficial effect of est[ro]gen as energizer, tranquilizer and anti-dep[res]sant. I know that it stimulates and maintains me[n]tal capacity, memory, and concentration, resto[res] zest for living, and gives a youthful appe[ar]ance.... Hormone therapy, once begun, sho[uld] be continued throughout a woman's lifetime. I[t is] my firm belief that many female inmates of nu[rs]ing homes and mental institutions could be [re]stored to full physical and mental health throu[gh] adequate hormone therapy (Jern 1973: 1560).

David Reuben proclaimed in his best-selli[ng] book *Everything You Wanted to Know about Se[x]*:

> As estrogen is shut off, a woman comes as close [as] she can to being a man. Increased facial ha[ir,] deepened voice, obesity, and decline of brea[sts] and female genitalia all contribute to a masc[u]line appearance. Not really a man but no long[er]

functional woman, these individuals live in a ·orld of intersex. Having outlived their ovaries, ıey have outlived their usefulness as human be- ıgs (Reuben 1969: 287).

Βut women need not despair. Reuben (1969:) proclaimed that with estrogen replacements men can "turn back the clock," and adequate ounts of estrogens throughout their lives will tect them against breast and uterine cancer. Throughout the late 1960s and early 1970s, lson's book was excerpted widely in traditional men's journals, and over 300 articles promot- estrogens appeared in popular magazines hnson 1977). During the same period an ag- ssive advertising campaign, capitalizing on disease label, was launched by the U.S. phar- ceutical industry. ERT products were widely ertised in medical literature and promotional terial as amelioratives for a variety of psycho- ical, as well as somatic, problems. One adver- ment depicted a seated woman clutching an line ticket, with her impatient husband stand- behind her glancing at his watch. The copy d:

> Bon Voyage? Suddenly she'd rather not go. She's waited thirty years for this trip. Now she doesn't have the "bounce." She has headaches, hot flashes, and she feels tired and nervous all the time. And for no reason she cries (Seaman and Seaman 1977: 281).

Another advertisement promoted ERT "for e menopausal problems that bother him the ost" (Seaman and Seaman, 1977: 281). Yet an- her advertisement stated: "Any tranquilizer ight calm her down ... but at her age, estrogen ay be what she really needs" (Seaman and Sea- an 1977: 281). Such advertisements paid off: be- een 1963 and 1973 dollar sales in the United ates for estrogen replacements quadrupled J.S. Bureau of the Census 1975). As one Har- rd researcher stated, "few medical interven- ons have had as widespread application as exogenous estrogen treatment in post-menopausal women" (Weinstein 1980). By 1975, with prescriptions at an all-time high of 26.7 million (Wolfe 1979) estrogens had become the fifth most frequently prescribed drug in the United States (Hoover et al. 1976). A 1975 survey in the Seattle-Tacoma area of Washington State revealed that 51 percent of all post-menopausal women had used estrogens for at least three months, with a median duration of over 10 years (Weiss et al. 1976).

Indeed, 1975 was a watershed year for estrogen therapy: sales were at an all-time high and physicians routinely used estrogens to treat a wide variety of purported menopausal symptoms. Yet within a few years this trend changed as estrogen therapy came under attack from inside and outside the medical community.

MEDICAL CONTROVERSY

Researchers had suspected an association between estrogens and cancer since the 1890s (Johnson 1977). Experimental animal studies, conducted in the 1930s and 1940s, claimed that estrogenic and progestinic substances were carcinogenic (Cook and Dodds 1933; Gardner 1944; Perry and Ginzton 1937). Novak and Yui (1936) warned that estrogen therapy might cause a pathological buildup of endometrial tissue.

Most investigators trace the roots of the ERT controversy back to 1947. In that year Dr. Saul Gusberg, then a young cancer researcher at the Memorial Sloane-Kettering Hospital and Columbia University in New York City, made a histologic link between hyperplasia (proliferation of the cells) and adenocarcinoma in the female endometrium (lining of the uterus). After a significant increase in endometrial cancer among estrogen users, Gusberg (1947: 910) wrote:

> Another human experiment has been set up in recent years by the widespread administration of estrogens to post-menopausal women. The rela-

> tively low cost of stilbestrol [synthetic estrogen] and the ease of administration have made its general use promiscuous.

Why was more attention not paid to these early warnings? In addition to the low cost and ease of administering estrogens mentioned by Gusberg, most scientists judged these early cancer studies to be scientifically unsound: those based on animal studies were dismissed as not applicable to humans. Perhaps most importantly, physicians found estrogens to be remarkably effective in alleviating vasomotor disturbances (hot flashes) and vaginal atrophy (Page 1977: 54). In his book *The Ageless Woman*, Sherwin Kaufman (1967: 61) described menopausal symptoms as the result of hormone deficiency, and lamented:

> Many women are obviously in need of estrogen replacements but are so afraid of "hormones" that it requires a good deal of explanation to persuade them that estrogen does not cause cancer and may, on the contrary, make them feel much better.

Kaufman regretted that some of his colleagues also share this unwarranted fear of cancer:

> Some doctors prescribe estrogens reluctantly.... Historically, and too often hysterically, estrogens have been endowed with malignant potentialities. Paradoxically, it has been pointed out that even conservative physicians may not hesitate to give sedatives or tranquilizers, yet they stop at the suggestion of estrogen replacement therapy. This is baffling to a good many doctors (1967: 67).

Kaufman confessed that "Years ago, I used to discontinue such treatment [ERT] after a few months," but "today I am in no rush to stop" (1967: 64).

The ERT controversy erupted in 1975 when two epidemiological studies, by research teams from Washington University (Smith et al. 1975) and the Kaiser-Permanente Medical Center in Los Angeles (Ziel and Finkle 1975) found a link between post-menopausal estrogen therapy endometrial cancer. The two studies, accor to Ziel[2] were written independently of each o and published side by side in the prestig *New England Journal of Medicine*. By 1980, r more studies, all done in the United States, c cluded that women on ERT were four to 20 ti more likely to develop endometrial cancer t non-users (Ziel 1980). Moreover, the risk of c cer purportedly increased with the duration dose of estrogens. Indeed, according to Gusb (1980: 729), endometrial cancer has "superse cervical cancer as the most common malign tumor of the female reproductive tract."

At a 1979 Consensus Development Con ence on Estrogen Use and Post-Menopau Women sponsored by the National Institute Aging, researchers unanimously concluded t ERT substantially increases the risk of endor trial cancer.[3] The final report of the conferer concluded that ERT is only effective in the tre ment of hot flashes and vaginal atrophy, and used at all, should be administered on a cycli basis (three weeks of estrogen, one week off), lowest dose for the shortest possible time.[4] A candidate for post-menopausal estrogen, the port recommended, "should be given as mu information as possible about both the bene and risks and then, with her physician, reach individualized decision regarding whether to ceive estrogens" (Gastel et al. 1979: 2).

Not only has the treatment of menopau come under criticism, the disease label has a been challenged by medical researchers. Sa Gusberg who first warned of the ERT-canc link, called the deficiency disease label menopause "nonsense," adding "People are b ginning to be more sensible about this, and re ize that not a great trauma has happened to t average woman going through the menopaus (quoted in Reitz 1977: 198). Research present at the Consensus Development Conference 1979 claimed that although ovarian productio of estrogen declines after the menopause, old nen need less estrogen. Moreover, production he hormone by the adrenal glands partially npensates diminished ovarian production for st women (Ziel and Finkle 1976). Further-re, only 10 to 20 percent experience severe or apacitating symptoms, and even those are erally temporary and decline over time (Gas-et al. 1979; McKinley and Jeffreys 1974).

esearchers have also criticized the disease del on ideological grounds. Ziel and Finkle 76: 737), two well-known cancer researchers, ued that the disease model was based on a tra-onal view of women's role:

> Because they desire the preservation of cosmetic youth and the unflagging libido of the patients, physicians have championed estrogen replacement therapy in the hope of attaining a maximal quality of life for their patients.

The female patient, in turn, "is readily de-led by her wish to preserve her figure and her ysician's implication that estrogen promises rnal youth" (1976: 739).

Despite a strong consensus in the research mmunity that ERT increases the risk of cancer, cticing physicians continued to prescribe the ig. As one San Francisco gynecologist stated er the 1975 cancer studies were published:

> I think of the menopause as a deficiency disease like diabetes. Most women develop some symptoms whether they are aware of them or not, so I prescribe estrogens for virtually all menopausal women for an indefinite period (quoted in Brody, 1975: 55).

Even though U.S. prescriptions for ERT have adily declined since the 1975 cancer studies, me 16 million were written in 1978 (Wolfe, 79). Indeed, a 1978 Detroit-area survey showed at two-thirds of all women who saw their physi-ans about menopausal complaints received trogens and 50 percent received tranquilizers Dosey and Dosey, 1980). In fact, a 1978 drug alysis by the U.S. Food and Drug Administration (FDA) concluded that menopausal estrogens, even after a major decline, were still "grossly overused" (Burke et al., 1978). My analysis[5] of 1979 estrogen replacement prescriptions revealed that 31 percent were still written for such vague diagnostic categories as "symptoms of senility," "special conditions without sickness," and "mental problems"—in violation of FDA specifications.[6]

Other measures of physicians' endorsement of ERT are authoritative references which describe menopause as a morbid condition for which estrogen therapy is indicated. For example, *The Merck Manual* (Berkow, 1980), a book of diagnosis and therapy widely used by physicians, lists menopause under "Ovarian Dysfunction." Modell's (1980) *Drugs of Choice* lists it under "Diseases of the Endocrine system." Both sources advocate estrogens for treatment. *Drugs of Choice* states that "objective studies" evaluating the risks and benefits are "not currently available" (1980: 540). Likewise, *Current Medical Diagnosis and Treatment* (Krupp and Chatton, 1980: 731) lists menopause under "Endocrine Disorders" and notes that "estrogen therapy has been recommended for life" but "the advisability of this practice remains unsettled." *Current Therapy* (Kantor, 1980: 839) lists as benefits of ERT "improvement of disposition and unreasonable outburst of temper" and "avoidance of the shrinking and sagging of breasts." Attention is called to recent cancer claims, but "when doses are small and administration is in interrupted courses, any potential risk is indeed small and perhaps theoretic." But a patient who has been frightened by "magazine articles" or "Food and Drug Administration bulletins" may "psychologically block the benefits" of ERT (Kantor, 1980: 839).

U.S. physicians have viewed the use of ERT as a political issue, and their endorsement of the therapy as an exercise of professional control. Editorials in the *Journal of the American Medical Association* have been critical of outside interference in the doctor-patient relationship. A 1979 editorial criticized the FDA Commissioner for mandating a "biased" warning: "In doing so he has officially expressed his distrust of the medical profession" (Landau, 1979: 47). A 1980 editorial castigated the FDA for creating unnecessary "public anxiety." Contradicting almost all the then-current U.S. research, the editorial concluded that "Estrogens already rank among the safest of all pharmaceuticals" (Meier and Landau, 1980: 1658).

MENOPAUSE AS NORMAL

In the late 1960s and early 1970s, U.S. feminists began to challenge medical authority by questioning the legitimacy of the disease model of menopause. They argued that menopause is not a disease or sickness but a natural process of aging, through which most women pass with minimum difficulty.[7] The medical problems that do arise can be effectively treated or even prevented by adequate nutrition and exercise combined with vitamin supplements. According to feminists, the menstrual and menopausal myths are a form of social control. If women are perceived as physically and emotionally handicapped by menstruation and menopause, they cannot and may not compete with men. The health care system legitimates sexism, under the guise of science, by depicting women's physical and mental capabilities as dependent on their reproductive organs.

Schur (1980: 6) calls these struggles over collective definitions "stigma" contests, wherein subordinate groups reject their deviant label. Although economic, legal, and political power are often involved in stigma contests, "what is essentially at stake in such situations is the power of moral standing or acceptability." Thus, stigma contests are always partly symbolic, since prestige and status are important issues (Gusfield, 1966; 1967). Stigmatized individuals must rectify a "spoiled identity" (Goffman, 1963) through collective efforts. In the United States, feminists have tried to neutralize stigma by claiming menopause is a normal experience of nor women.

On these ideological grounds, feminists h opposed the routine use of ERT. For example article, published in *Ms.* in 1972, before str medical evidence against ERT was uncove maintained that menopause was not a traum experience for most women. Because me pause freed women from the risk of pregnanc was viewed as a sexually liberating event. E seen as an attempt to keep women "feminine ever," was thus viewed as a male exploitation, egating women to the status of sex obj (Solomon, 1972). Four years later, offering a fe inist interpretation of the menstrual and me pausal taboo, Delaney et al. (1976: 184) stated t "the main fault of Feminine Forever lies no the medicine but in the moralizing."

After medical evidence became available strengthen the ideological arguments, femi criticism became widespread. In *Women and Crisis in Sex Hormones* (Seaman and Seam 1977), the ERT controversy received a 70-pa analysis titled "Promise Her Anything But G Her... Cancer." These authors warned agai the increasing medicalization of normal fem functions:

> Pregnancy or non-pregnancy are hardly diseas and neither is menopause. The latter is a norn developmental state wherein reproductive pacity is down; the temporary hot flashes so women experience may be compared to t high-to-low voice register changes adolesce boys evidence when their reproductive capac is gearing up. We no longer castrate young b to preserve their male sopranos, nor should treat hot flashes with a cancer-and-choleste pill (1977: xi).

In a collection of feminist critiques, Grossm and Bart (1979: 167), two social scientists, make similar claim in a chapter titled "Taking M Out of Menopause":

. [the] actions of the medical and pharmaceuti-al groups dramatize the sexism and general in-umanity of the male-dominated, profit-oriented J.S. medical system. A "deficiency disease" was nvented to serve a drug that could "cure" it, de-pite the suspicion that the drug caused cancer in vomen. That the suspicion has been voiced for so nany years before anyone would investigate it is et another example of how unimportant the vell-being of women is to men who control re-earch and drug companies who fund much of it.

e 1981 edition of *The Ms. Guide to a Woman's alth* warns women that "Estrogen replace-nt therapy (ERT) is a dangerously overused atment. Avoid it if at all possible" (Cooke and vorkin, 1981: 310). The chapter on menopause eatedly states that the change of life is not a ease but a normal process. Similarly, *The New oman's Guide to Health and Medicine* states he truth is that menopause is a positive or at st neutral experience for many women" (Der-shire, 1980: 269). Several other U.S. feminist blications, such as *Majority Report* (Lieber-n, 1977) and *Off Our Backs* (Moira, 1977) have en strong stances against ERT. *Mother Jones* ndemned ERT in an article titled "Feminine aight to the Grave" (Wolf, 1978).

Though most of the criticism has been voiced younger feminists, some older women have posed ERT. Reitz (1977: 181) referred to ERT "The No. 1 Middle-Age Con" and proclaimed:

> I accept that I'm a healthy woman whose body is changing. No matter how many articles and books I read that tell me I'm suffering from a deficiency disease, I say I don't believe it. I have never felt more in control of my life than I do now and I feel neither deficient nor diseased. I think that people who are promoting this idea—that something is wrong with me because I am 50 – have something to gain or are irresponsible or stupid.

Collins (1977: 3) in an article in *Prime Time*, a ublication devoted to ageist issues, stated:

> Even today the literature . . . defines menopause as a deficiency disease. Of course that may sell estrogen, and we'll stay out of the controversy over whether that's a good thing or not. But it certainly echoes once more the male prejudice against menopausal and post-menopausal women.

Health-related associations and consumer groups have also joined feminists in their opposition to ERT. *Consumer Reports* (1976), the official publication of Consumers Union, published a lengthy article warning women of the risks; Citizens Health, Ralph Nader's organization, opposes (and regularly testifies against) ERT (Wolfe, 1979). Smaller groups such as Coalition for Medical Rights of Women (Brown, 1978) and National Action Forum for Older Women (1979) have all warned women of the risks of ERT and advocated alternate treatment (diet, exercise, and vitamin supplements) for menopause. Menopause workshops and self-help groups have sprung up across the United States (Page, 1977).

After the 1975 cancer studies several feminist and consumer groups, including the National Health Network and Consumers Union, began to pressure the FDA to warn consumers dangers of ERT. On July 22, 1977, after two years of public hearings, the FDA issued a ruling that a "patient package insert" (PPI), warning of the risk of cancer and other dangers, be included with every estrogen and progesterine prescription. On October 5, 1977, in an effort to block this regulation, the Pharmaceutical Manufacturing Association—together with the College of Obstetricians and Gynecologists, the National Association of Chain Drug Stores, the American Society of Internal Medicine, and various state and county medical societies—responded by filing a civil suit in the Wilmington, Delaware, Federal District Court against the FDA. The plaintiffs charged that the FDA lacked statutory authority to require the patient package insert warning, and that such a requirement was an unconstitutional interference with the practice of medicine. They also asserted that such a regulation is "arbitrary, capricious (and) an abuse of discretion" (*Pharmaceutical Manufacturers Association v. Food and Drug Administration*, 1980).

To represent the interests of women patients, the National Women's Health Network, Consumers Union, Consumers Federation of America, and Women's Equity Action League filed as interveners in the lawsuit in support of the FDA. Three years later, in 1980, Federal District Judge Walter K. Stapleton upheld the FDA decision, giving estrogen replacements the distinction of being one of only four classes[8] of drugs which require such patient package inserts in the United States (*Pharmaceutical Manufacturers Association v. Food and Drug Administration*, 1980). Regulation, however, does not mean compliance, and the feminist victory appears more symbolic than instrumental. A 1979 FDA survey of 271 drug stores in 20 U.S. cities revealed that only 39 percent of all ERT prescriptions were accompanied by the required insert (Morris et al., 1980). Moreover, under the administration of President Ronald Reagan, the FDA has suspended all proposed PPI regulations and is reconsidering existing ones (National Women's Health Network, 1981).[9]

CONCLUSION

In this article I have characterized the medical-feminist struggle over the collective definition of menopause as a stigma contest. Feminists have attempted to show that menopause is not an event that limits women's psychological or physical capacities, but a natural part of aging. Physicians have tried to explain the problems of middle-aged women through a medical model. In so viewing the life course, including menopause, physicians have tended to see problems experienced during menopause as either "all in the head" or the result of a deficiency disease, to be treated with tranquilizers or hormones.

The aging woman has a particularly vulner
status in our society. She is no longer the obje
adoration and romanticism that youthful wor
frequently are. Menopause usually comes
time when children leave home, and husba
frequently seek younger sexual partners. Phys
changes taking place in her body might be c
pounded, and negatively interpreted, by the
of status and primary social role. Clearly, s
women are vulnerable to the promise of a "you
pill which purports to allay the aging process.
to blame all the problems that aging women
perience on menopause is a classic case of bl
ing the victim. The medical model individ
izes the problem, and deflects responsibility fr
the social structure which assigns aging wor
to a maligned and precarious status.

The vulnerable status of women makes fer
ground for medical imperialism. A health c
system, based on fee-for-service, is conducive
defining more and more life events as illnesse
disease definition of menopause has served
interests of both the medical profession and
pharmaceutical industry. Until these structu
arrangements change, the hormone deficier
definition of menopause, or some equivalent
it, is likely to prevail.

Feminists, particularly those in the wome
health movement (Ruzek 1979) have exposed
sexism in women's health care. Publicatic
such as *Our Bodies, Ourselves* (Boston Wome
Health Collective 1976) offered a new definiti
of women's role in health care. No longer pass
consumers of male-dominated medicine, wom
asserted the right to control their own bodi
Feminists in the health movement have begun
demystify menopause and have made it a top
for discussion. By making their stigma cont
part of a broad-based social movement, femini
have been able to define women's health care
a social problem (Mauss 1975).

Yet in their efforts to fight off the stigma
menopause, some feminists have inadverten

tributed to ageism. Most criticisms have been -ed by younger feminists who have not gone ough menopause. Their main focus has been the medicalization of childbirth and menstru-n, and they have extrapolated their analysis menopause without adequate appreciation of problems of aging women. By emphasizing natural and unproblematic nature of meno-se, they have overlooked the minority of men who do need medical attention. Such men might feel shame or guilt for suffering ough what others claim is normal or unprob-iatic (Posner 1979).

Moreover, most feminist studies of menopause e ignored structural factors, restricting their lyses to ideological and social psychological ies. Most feminists in the health movement women's oppression rooted in arguments of logical inferiority. Feminists have tried to set-the nature-nurture debate by showing that ferences in socialization, not biology, account women's inferior status. In their attempt to rthrow the dictum "biology is destiny," femi-ts have argued that menstruation, childbirth, d menopause are natural events and, in most ses, do not warrant medical intervention. They arge that myths surrounding these events func-n as social control. In so doing, feminists have empted to substitute a new ideology (biology is elevant) for an old one (biology is destiny).

The women's health movement, largely iddle-class, has approached the problems of omen's health care from a point most visible to e middle-class consumer: the private office the gynecologist or psychiatrist. Focusing on ctor-patient interaction, they have advocated lf-help outside the established health care sys-m. Admirable though these actions are, they e not sufficient to change the collective status women. Nor will the call by radical feminists r self-help, alternative health care accomplish is goal; it only takes the struggle to the margins the established order (Fee 1975).

Neither ideological nor social-psychological analyses challenge the private health care system or the economic and social infrastructure which support it. What is needed are studies which elucidate the structural affinities between the economics of health care and the status of women. Such scholarship might point the way toward more meaningful change.

NOTES

The author thanks Gerald Markle for his collaboration in the research; John Gilmore, Daryl Kelley, Ronald Kramer, Ellen Page-Robin, Ronald Troyer, and the anonymous Social Problems reviewers for their criticisms of earlier drafts; and Agnes McColley for typing the manuscript.

1. For example, Wilson (1962) stated that 86 of the 304 women had undergone a total hysterectomy either before or during treatment without giving a reason for the hysterectomy (Johnson 1977)

2. Harry Ziel, February 1, 1983; personal communication.

3. Other U.S. studies claimed that ERT increased the risk of breast cancer, atherosclerosis, myocardial infarction, pulmonary emboli, thrombophlebitis, gall bladder disease, and diabetes (Gastel, Coroni-Huntley, and Brody 1979).

4. In Great Britain researchers are skeptical of the cancer link. They claim that sequential therapy (the addition of progestin for the last five to 13 days of a 20-to-30-day course of estrogen) would eliminate the potential risk of cancer. U.S. researchers claim that sequential treatment may not prevent endometrial cancer (Ziel 1980: 451) and the dangers associated with progestins have not been fully evaluated (Gastel, Coroni-Huntley, and Brody 1979). British researchers also promote ERT for the prevention of osteoporosis and, at this time, the established cancer risk outweighs the potential benefit of the treatment. For a discussion of the cancer and osteoporosis debates, see McCrea and Markle (1984).

5. The data for this analysis are proprietary, and were obtained from the IMS National Disease and Therapeutics Index, IMS America, Ltd., Ambler, Pennsylvania. IMS collects these data from a representative panel of 1,500 physicians who, four times a year, report case history information on private patients seen over a 48-hour period. For each prescription written, physicians report their diagnosis.

6. The FDA has found menopausal estrogens "effective" only for the treatment of vasomotor symptoms and atrophic vaginitis, and "probably" effective for "estrogen deficiency-induced osteoporosis, and only when used in conjunction with other important therapeutic measures such as diet, calcium, physiotherapy, and good general health-promoting measures." Furthermore, the FDA states that estrogens are not effective for nervous symptoms or depression "and should not be used to treat such conditions" (*Physicians Desk Reference* 1982: 641).

7. Although the majority of U.S. feminists, particularly those in the women's health movement, have defined menopause as unproblematic, there are notable exceptions. For example, Posner (1979: 189) charges that feminists "... have been led into the ideological trap of denying their own hormones." Lock (1982) argues that physicians ought to pay more attention to physiology, and not dismiss women's medical complaints as psychological. British feminists also want more medical services made available in the treatment of menstruation and menopause (McCrea and Markle 1984; Sayers 1982).

8. The other three are oral contraceptives, progestational drug products, and isoproterenol inhalation preparations used by asthmatics.

9. This was confirmed by the FDA official in charge of the PPI program, Louis Morris, May 11, 1983: personal communication.

REFERENCES

Berkow, Robert. 1980. *The Merck Manual of Diagnosis and Therapy*. 13th edition. Rahway, N.J.: Merck.

Boston Women's Health Book Collective. 1976. *Our Bodies, Ourselves*. New York: Simon and Schuster.

Brody, Jane. 1975. "Physicians' Views Uncha on Use of Estrogen Therapy." *New York Times,* cember 5: 55.

Brown, Sheryl. 1978. "The Second Forty Years." *ond Opinion* 1: 1–10.

Burke, Laurie, Dianne Crosby, and Chang 1978. "Estrogen Prescribing in Menopause." Paper sented at the annual meeting of the American Pu Health Association, Washington, D.C., Novemb 1977. Updated June 23, 1978.

Buxton, C.L. 1944. "Medical Therapy during Menopause." *Journal of Endocrinology* 12: 591–96.

Collins, Marjorie. 1977. "We Are Witness to Age in the Medical Profession." *Prime Time* 5: 3–5.

Conrad, Peter, and Joseph W. Schneider. 1980. *viance and Medicalization: From Badness to Sickn* St. Louis: Mosby.

Consumer Reports. 1976. "Estrogen Therapy: Dangerous Road to Shangri La." *Consumer Report* 642–45.

Cook, J. W., and E. C. Dodds. 1933. "Sex Hormo on Cancer-Producing Compounds." *Nature* 131:

Cooke, Cynthia, and Susan Dworkin. 1981. *The Guide to a Woman's Health*. New York: Berkeley P lishing.

Delaney, Janice, Mary Lupton, and Emilly T 1976. *The Curse*. New York: E. P. Dutton.

Derbyshire, Caroline. 1980. *The New Wom Guide to Health and Medicine*. New York: Apple Century Croft.

Dosey, Mary, and Michael Dosey. 1980. "The C macteric Women." *Patient Counseling and Health ucation* 2 (first quarter): 14–21.

Fee, Elizabeth. 1975. "Women and Health Care Comparison of Theories." *International Journal Health Services* 5: 397–415.

Freidson, Eliot. 1970. *Profession of Medicine*. N York: Harper and Row.

———. 1971. *The Professions and Their Prospec* Beverly Hills, Calif.: Sage.

Gardner, W. U. 1944. "Tumors in Experimental A imals Receiving Steroid Hormones." *Surgery* 16: 8.

Gastel, Barbara, Joan Coroni-Huntley, and Jac Brody. 1979. "Estrogen Use and Post-Menopau nen: A Basis for Informed Decisions." Summary nclusion, National Institute on Aging Consensus elopment Conference. Bethesda, Maryland, September 13–14.

Geist, Samuel H., and Frank Spielman. 1932. "Therautic Value of Theelin in Menopause." *American nal of Obstetrics and Gynecology* 23: 710.

Goffman, Erving. 1963. *Stigma.* Englewood Cliffs, .: Prentice Hall.

Greenblatt, Robert. 1974. *The Menopausal Syn-ne.* New York: Medcom Press.

Grossman, Marilyn, and Pauline Bart. 1979. "Tak-Men out of Menopause." Pp. 163–84 in Ruth Hubd, Mary Sue Henifin, and Barbara Fried, eds., *men Looking at Biology Looking at Women.* Boston: K. Hall.

Gusberg, Saul. 1947. "Precursors of Corpus Carcina Estrogens and Adenomatous Hyperplasia." *erican Journal of Obstetrics and Gynecology* 54: ;–26.

———. 1980. "Current Concepts in Cancer." *New gland Journal of Medicine* 302: 729–31.

Gusfield, Joseph. 1966. *Symbolic Crusade.* Urbana: iversity of Illinois Press.

———. 1967. "Moral Passage: The Symbolic Process Public Designations of Deviance." *Social Problems* 175–88.

Hoover, Robert, Laman Gray, Philip Cole, and an Mac Mahon. 1976. "Menopausal Estrogens and east Cancer." *New England Journal of Medicine* 295: 1–05.

Jern, Helen. 1973. *Hormone Therapy of the enopause and Aging.* Springfield, Ill.: Charles C. omas Publishers.

Johnson, Anita. 1977. "The Risks of Sex Hormones Drugs." *Women and Health* 1: 8–11.

Kantor, Herman. 1980. "Menopause." Pp. 838–40 in oward F. Conn, ed., *Current Therapy.* Philadelphia: . B. Saunders.

Kaufman, Shirwin. 1967. *The Ageless Woman.* Enewood Cliffs, N.J.: Prentice Hall.

Krupp, Marcus, and Milton Chatton. 1980. *Current edical Diagnosis and Treatment.* Los Altos, Calif.: nge Medical Publications.

Landau, Richard. 1979. "What You Should Know about Estrogens." *Journal of the American Medical Association* 241: 47–51.

Levin, Ira. 1972. *The Stepford Wives.* New York: Random House.

Lieberman, Sharon. 1977. "But You Will Make Such a Feminine Corpse..." *Majority Report* 6 (February 19–March 4): 3.

Lock, Margaret. 1982. "Models and Practice in Medicine: Menopause as Syndrome or Life Transition?" *Culture, Medicine and Psychiatry* 6: 261–80.

McCrea, Frances. 1981. "The Medicalization of Normalcy? Changing Definitions of Menopause." Paper presented at the International Interdisciplinary Congress on Women, Haifa, Israel, December 28–January 1, 1982.

McCrea, Frances, and Gerald Markle. 1984. "The Estrogen Replacement Controversy in the USA and UK: Different Answers to the Same Questions." *Social Studies of Science* 14, no. 1 (February): 1–26.

McKinley, Sonja M., and Margot Jeffreys. 1974. "The Menopausal Syndrome." *British Journal of Preventive and Social Medicine* 28: 108–15.

Mauss, Armand. 1975. *Social Problems as Social Movements.* Philadelphia: J. B. Lippincott.

Meier, Paul, and Richard Landau. 1980. "Estrogen Replacement Therapy." *Journal of the American Medical Association* 243: 1658.

Mintz, Morton, and Victor Cohn. 1977. "Hawking the Estrogen Fix." *Progressive* 41: 24–25.

Modell, Walter. 1980. *Drugs of Choice, 1980–1981.* St. Louis: Mosby.

Moira, Fran. 1977. "Estrogens Forever: Marketing Youth and Death." *Off Our Backs* (March): 12.

Morris, Louis, Ann Meyers, Paul Gibbs, and Chang Lao. 1980. "Estrogen PPIs: A Survey." *American Pharmacy* 20 (June): 318–22.

National Action Forum for Older Women. 1979. "Forum." *Newsletter of the National Action Forum for Older Women* 2 (2): 8.

National Women's Health Network. 1981. "Network Fights to Save PPI Program." *National Women's Health Network Newsletter* 6 (6): 1–2.

Novak, Emil, and Enmei Yui. 1936. "Relation of

Endometrial Hyperplasia to Adenocarcinoma of the Uterus." *American Journal of Obstetrics and Gynecology* 321: 596–674.

Page, Jane. 1977. *The Other Awkward Age: Menopause.* Berkeley, Calif.: Ten Speed Press.

Perry, I. H., and L. L. Ginzton. 1937. "The Development of Tumors in Female Mice Treated with 1: 2: 5: 6 Dibenzanthracone and Theelin." *American Journal of Cancer* 29: 680.

Physicians' Desk Reference. 1982. *Physicians' Desk Reference,* 36th ed. Oradell, N.J.: Medical Economics.

Posner, Judith. 1979. "It's All in Your Head: Feminist and Medical Models of Menopause (Strange Bedfellows)." *Sex Roles* 5: 179–90.

Reitz, Rosetta. 1977. *Menopause: A Positive Approach.* Radnor, Penn.: Chilton.

Reuben, David. 1969. *Everything You Always Wanted to Know about Sex But Were Afraid to Ask.* New York: David McKay.

Ruzek, Sheryl Burt. 1979. *The Women's Health Movement.* New York: Praeger.

Sayers, Janet. 1982. *Biological Politics.* London: Tavistock.

Schur, Edwin. 1980. *The Politics of Deviance.* Englewood Cliffs, N.J.: Prentice Hall.

Seaman, Barbara, and Gideon Seaman. 1977. *Women and the Crisis in Sex Hormones.* New York: Rawson Association Publishers.

Smith, Donald D., Prentice Ross, J. Thompson Donovan, and Walter L. Herrmann. 1975. "Association of Exogenous Estrogen and Endometrial Carcinoma." *New England Journal of Medicine* 293: 1164–67.

Solomon, Jean. 1972. "Menopause: A Rite of Passage." *Ms.* (December) 1: 16–18.

U.S. Bureau of the Census. 1975. *Pharmaceutical Preparations, Except Biologicals.* Current Industrial Reports, Series Ma-28G(73)-1. Washington, D.C.: U.S. Government Printing Office.

Weinstein, Milton. 1980. "Estrogen Use in Post-Menopausal Women—Costs, Risks and Benefits." *New England Journal of Medicine* 303: 308-16.

Weiss, Noel S., Daniel Szekely, and Donal Austin. 1976. "Increasing Incidence of Endome Cancer in the United States." *New England Journ Medicine* 294: 1259–62.

Wilson, Robert. 1962. "Roles of Estrogen and P esterine in Breast and Genital Cancer." *Journal o American Medical Association* 182: 327–31.

———. 1966a. *Feminine Forever.* New York: Evans.

———. 1966b. "A Key to Staying Young." *Look* (uary): 68–73.

Wilson, Robert, and Thelma Wilson. 1963. " Fate of Nontreated Post-Menopausal Woman: A for the Maintenance of Adequate Estrogen from berty to the Grave." *Journal of the American Geria Society* 11: 347–61.

Wolfe, Sidney. 1978. "Feminine Straight to Grave." *Mother Jones* (May): 18–20.

———. 1979. *Women in Science and Technol Equal Opportunity Act,* 1979. Testimony before Committee on Labor and Human Resources, S committee on Health and Scientific Research. 9 Congress, 1st session. Washington, D.C.: U.S. Gove ment Printing Office.

Ziel, Harry K. 1980. "The Negative Side of Lo Term Postmenopausal Estrogen Therapy." Pp. 450 in Louis Lasagna, ed., *Controversies in Therapeut* Philadelphia: W. B. Saunders.

Ziel, Harry K., and William D. Finkle. 1975. " creased Risks of Endometrial Carcinoma among Us of Conjugated Estrogens." *New England Journal Medicine* 293: 1167–70.

———. 1976. "Association of Estrone with the I velopment of Endometrial Carcinoma." *Americ Journal of Obstetrics and Gynecology* 134: 735–40.

CASE CITED

Pharmaceutical Manufacturers Association v. Fo and Drug Administration, 484 F. Supp. 1179, 1980.

CHAPTER 20

Aging, Culture, and the Framing of Alzheimer Disease

MARTHA HOLSTEIN

ALZHEIMER DISEASE (AD) has assumed most mythic proportions in American society. This disease affects over ur million people and has stimulated the expenditure of substantial pub- c and private resources in the search for the key to its complex and prob- ly multiple etiologies, its threat to fundamental sources of human iden- ty, and its affect on others in addition to the patient. In spite of these penditures, AD is a refractory disorder that is unlikely to be "cured" any me in the near future. Instead, scientific investigators now have a more odest goal—to delay the onset of symptoms by five years. Sociologists, an- ropologists, psychologists, and others are interested in how this disorder r disorders) is perceived, how different perceptions shape responses to the patient, and how psychological factors contribute to symptom formation.

This vast research enterprise and the enormous public consciousness about AD's devastation are surprisingly recent. Senile Dementia of the Alzheimer type (SDAT) or Dementia of the Alzheimer Type (DAT), terms commonly employed to distinguish an Alzheimer-type dementia from other dementias, became firmly established as a disease category approximately twenty years ago. Before the mid-70's, most physicians considered AD, a disease that affected individuals in their forties and fifties and occasionally even younger, to be quite rare. Older people with symptoms and brain pathologies comparable to those of younger patients were diagnosed with senile dementia, senility, senile psychoses, or organic brain syndrome. This mixture of diagnostic labels revealed how poorly developed the science (or art) of differential diagnosis was with respect to mental conditions that affect older people. It also reflected the customary view that mental decline in old age is common and essentially untreatable.

Today, neither senility as a diagnostic label nor the idea that mental decline may be an inevitable feature of growing old is acceptable. The dominant discourse about AD holds that dementia of the Alzheimer type (DAT) is a disease without age boundaries that is qualitatively and quantitatively different from "normal" aging except that age represents the single most important risk factor for its onset. It seeks, in Gubrium's (1986) words, "unity in diversity." The causes of AD are located deep within our DNA.

These transitions in the concept of AD graphically illustrate how negotiation processes establish that certain physical and/or mental conditions deserve the disease label—a decision that often cannot be singularly explained by scientific discovery. For example, while most physicians in the United States accepted AD as a diagnostic label by 1920, the relatively few recognized cases of AD lacked definitive neuropathological signs and commonly accepted behavioral sympto The familiar plaques and tangles appeare other diseases and conditions; postmortem r ropathologic examination could rarely sepa younger from older patients, although the br of younger patients seemed to be more seve diseased. While this lack of specificity necessa limited the definitiveness of conclusions ab the exact nature of AD, it did not preclude in tigators from deciding that AD was *not* senile mentia (SD). The few dissenting voices (New 1948; Neumann and Cohn 1953)—includ that of Dr. Alzheimer in a 1911 paper—had no dience for many years.

Thus, Drs. Fuller, Southard, and their c temporaries adopted the diagnostic label "/ heimer disease," tentatively proposed by famed nosologist Emil Kraepelin to differenti it from the familiar condition known as se dementia. SD was too encumbered to m the needs of the time. Its very name announ that it was a condition of old age. Conventio conceptions about disease and health were ba on age norms. The belief that mental decl in old age is an expected part of an overall patt of decline meant that what was clearly "abn mal" at 50 might be quite "normal" at 70. Th physicians were uncertain if SD was a disease "normal," though perhaps extreme, physiolo cal aging.

Assumptions, beliefs, and uncertainties abc involutionary processes and the accompanyi mental and physical changes were captured nosology and created a relatively closed conce tual account. This system left little room younger patients like Frau Auguste D., Dr. A heimer's patient, whose age and condition ini ated the flurry of attention. Rarely requiri articulation, these views were embedded in me ical history, education, and popular attitud They filtered perceptions and influenced ev the most careful work. Given the state of resear on aging at the time, these assumptions faced fe challenges.

ı contrast, the new diagnostic label "Alzhei- · disease" was unhampered by medical and lay ᴡs about mental illness, senility, senile de- ntia, and cultural meanings of old age; as h, it presented a chance for scientific investi- on and perhaps remediation. Physicians logi- y determined that AD, which could only be ved as pathological, was a presenile disease re- d to, but different from, SD. This solution did compel physicians to resolve their perplexi- about normalcy and pathology in old age, but d allow them to retain assumptions about dis- e classification and time-honored etiologic ws about SD. Thus, despite admitted uncer- ıty, medical opinion in the United States in o almost universally supported a dual under- nding of SD and AD. In this view, AD was a e disorder affecting individuals in the prese- ım; its etiological link to processes associated h early or atypical involution was assumed hout being explained.

In the remainder of this chapter, I focus on how tors internal and external to science influenced conceptualization of AD as different from SD much of this century. In particular, I consider w shifting medical and cultural perceptions of age and ways of classifying mental disease pported this distinction and later its reversal. ese factors are important because they helped nstitute the conceptual world of investigators, ıich, in turn, filtered their experiences. Con- ptual worlds are critical; they bring some ob- rvations, interpretive possibilities, and options to focus while obscuring others. They establish rizons of possibility. How any issue is framed is, erefore, always a choice; it can be framed oth- wise. "Evidence conforms to conceptions just often as conceptions conform to evidence ... alogously to social structures, every age has its vn dominant conceptions as well as remnants of st ones and rudiments of those in the future" 'leck 1985 [1935], 28).

The conceptual framework of physicians who ıdied postmortem neuropathology in the early twentieth century helps explain why their original uncertainty evolved into a firm belief system that separated SD from AD for over fifty years. Today, other conceptual frameworks shape thinking and conclusions about DAT, and newer and different frameworks hover on the horizon. These too are negotiated positions that dovetail with prevailing professional views about aging and old age, other critical social and professional forces, and changing scientific discoveries.

THE CONCEPTUAL WORLD: CULTURE, AGING, AND DEMENTIA

Writers have been writing about old age for as long as there have been written words. As historian Carole Haber pointed out, "No scheme ever omitted old age as a separate and distinct segment of the life cycle " (1983, 49). American notions about old age have varied. By the late nineteenth century, however, old age had become associated with an almost unrelenting pattern of decay in which the line between the normal and the pathological was quite indistinct. Contemporary historians of old age and aging disagree about why Americans held such negative views of aging in the late nineteenth and early twentieth centuries, but the result was widely shared cultural biases against the elderly. Studies such as one by George Miller Beard (1881) portrayed old age (which, incidentally, started roughly at the age of 45) as the "inevitable casualty in the great 'race of life'" (Cole 1991,164); inventiveness and creativity dissipated. In a similar vein, William Krause (1900), an upstate New York neurologist, asserted that senility, decline, and decay were synonymous to the medical mind:

> The sturdy frame, once the personification of grace and strength now resembles the mighty oak of the forest, slowly decaying at the center until, only the bark remaining, it topples over from its own sheer weight.... The brow, the wrinkled

> face, the stooped frame and shuffling gait all are omens of that dissolution that comes without pain, without disease. The nerve currents from the spent storage centers become gradually weaker until the flash of the final spark and the circuit is broken. (648)

In his valedictory address at the Johns Hopkins University School of Medicine in February 1905, no less a figure than the renowned physician William Osler argued that men over the age of 40 were comparatively useless and those over 60 absolutely useless (Cole 1991, 170–71). To some practitioners, old age was often depicted as a medical problem in toto. Thus, one physician advised older people: "Go into medical training, as it were, for the remainder of the battle of life, like a pugilist for the coming fight, for there will soon come to him the need for all the reserve power of his system, hemotogenic, neuronogenic thyrogenic, peptogenic, metabolic, phagocytic, etc. The doctor, as the dock to the ocean voyaging ships, should be often sought for needed repair in order that further voyaging may be safer" (Hughes 1909, 67).

Using the words *senile dementia* and *senility* interchangeably to describe mental deterioration in old age, physicians rarely distinguished between simple forgetfulness and its more malignant form. I. J. Nascher, a physician known as the "father" of modern geriatrics, for example, described a 76-year-old woman's behavioral changes as her hearing, memory, and reasoning power became impaired as a "garrulous dement." An aged merchant, once a dominant personality, became a "pliant non-entity" (Nascher 1911, 48–59). He made these observations despite his general view that old age itself was not a pathological condition but rather a distinct physiological stage of life (Achenbaum 1995). A decade later, famed psychiatrists Smith Ely Jelliffe and William Alanson White (1923) described a "normal" old age in terms of certain inevitabilities—memory loss, inability to recognize others, marked egotism, occasional irritability, and interference. Alfred Scott Warthin (1929) marked that central nervous system involu meant:

> loss of memory, failing powers of observation tention and concentration, slowness of all n tal reactions, lessened ability to initiate id increasing errors of judgment, loss of effecti irritability, retrograde amnesia, pseudo-remi cence, automatism, aphasia, psychical fati and weakness, daytime sleeping and noctu insomnia, melancholia, changes and perversi in personal habits, illusions and delusions, lo orientation, and ultimately the fully develo stage of "second childhood" and senile dem tia. (106)

Theoretical support for a decline-and-loss p adigm flowed easily from the application of laws of conservation of energy and entropy (th modynamics) to organic phenomena (Rab bach 1990): if the body behaved like a machi then like a machine, it would wear down. cording to a popular metaphor, each body ha limited fund of vitality. Once depleted, the b had few reserves; these losses led to the physi and mental transformations associated with age (Haber 1983).

These descriptions indicate why "normal was such a slippery concept, why it had sign cance far beyond the medical encounter, a why age norms were so influential in shapi thinking. Ideas about normalcy helped form cial expectations and social responses to old a In most instances, American physicians adopt the position taken some years earlier by the gr experimental physiologist Claude Bernard that is the line between the normal and path logical was one of degree. Imagine, howev where this line would be drawn if the literatu repeatedly described old age in Nascher's Warthin's terms. Physicians also tended to gen alize from their patients' characteristics to the e tire population. Finding mutual support amo their peers and the period's medical literatu they formed impressions about the mental a sical changes that might accompany old age. 1ost older people they encountered had re- ed lung capacity, for example, or displayed iificant memory loss, they would assume that se conditions were normal. Notions about mality constituted a shared understanding ɔng most physicians and older people and ir families; as such, they did not demand any ernal verification. Whether old age itself was hological may have been unclear; it seemed ently obvious, however, that it was riddled h medically adverse conditions for which pal- ion rather than cure was the highest hope.

This tendency to think of "normal" aging in es- tially negative terms continued well beyond d-twentieth century (Ferraro 1959; Eros 1959; ies and Kaplan 1956; Palmer, Braceland, and stings 1943). No sharp lines, no mini-mental tus exams, no differential diagnosis divided ɔrmal" senility from senile dementia. Where draw that line "must often be an arbitrary one" othschild 1956, 308). Noted British neurologist acdonald Critchely (1939) shared the uncer- nty of his American colleagues. He com- ented that the "frontiers between healthy and normal old age—between senescence and se- ity—[are] so ill-defined as to be scarcely rec- nizable." Often it "becomes merely a matter of rsonal opinion whether a particular symptom physical sign is to be regarded as normal or thological" (Critchely 1939, 488).

Normal or pathological? A disease or part of e aging process? These oppositional and irre- lvable categories provided the conceptual unterpoint for thinking about AD. If AD could understood as being different from SD—that as a clearly pathological condition affecting ople under 65 that may or may not be related processes of aging—then it could be detached om all the uncertainty that surrounded demen- a and aging. It did not demand resolution of hat seemed so unclear. In a psychiatric world ominated by the search for the organic under- nnings of mental disease, this new condition ould also serve the professional needs of psychiatrists. AD was a disorder in which signs and symptoms could be linked to neuropathology. As such, it met the prevailing requirement for defining a condition as a disease—that is, it was organically based and located in identifiable and ever smaller components of the body (for a detailed description of this argument, see Holstein 1996).

As research on aging took shape in the middle third of the twentieth century, this inherited frame of reference limited the problems that research on aging would address. For example, while physicians did not treat SD lightly, it was not central to an emerging research agenda. In the popular culture, advice books that instructed people in the maintenance of good health (Haber 1983) had little to say about SD. Popularly, the notion that senility was "just old age" apparently prevailed and contributed to a general therapeutic and research nihilism. In these circumstances, American physicians had little incentive (and even fewer resources) to conduct research on the mental conditions that affected older patients. While biologists like Elie Metchnikoff dreamed of a time when "normal" or "physiological" aging would replace what he saw as "utterly pathological" (Achenbaum 1995), old age and its diseases remained among "the most obscure subjects in the field of biology" (Rothschild and Kasanin 1936, 318). Something would have to change before questions about old age became sufficiently compelling for investigators to break free from the conceptual limits imposed by traditional views of aging.

NOSOLOGY AND ETIOLOGY

These views provided the underpinnings for nosologic categories for mental and other diseases. Age was an important framework for thinking about disease. I. J. Nascher, for example, had adapted the familiar stages of life metaphor when he suggested that age was a convenient and visible marker of many of life's events, including specific physiological norms. Age also served as an important basis for classifying mental illness and so helped shape what investigators selected for notice (Beach 1987; Bick 1994). Thus, William Krause (1900) wrote: "Disorders of the nervous system show selective inclination in regard to *age, sex* and *season* [emphasis in the original] to a greater degree than any other class of diseases.... It can be proven conclusively that certain neural disorders accompany and are a part of the different epochs in the life history of an individual and are not probable or even possible at different and remote periods" (641, 643).

If certain diseases occurred at certain ages, then diagnosis by exclusion became an important tool. Alzheimer adopted this exclusionary exercise when he initially expressed doubts that Frau Auguste D. could have SD. While her condition resembled SD, it could not be the same because it occurred at an inappropriately early age. By labeling the disorder dementia, earlier nosologists emphasized the time of life at which condition occurred and not its form. This label also contained an implicit etiology—that is, the very processes of growing old "caused" the dementia.

From the beginning, this association of old age, SD, and involutional changes in the brain would raise perplexing questions. One result was a semantic and practical challenge that inevitably influenced the concept of AD. What diagnosis should physicians affix on younger patients who exhibited patterns of symptoms and that were comparable but not identical to those of their older patients with SD? They were unable to solve the semantic problem by adopting the solution that is current today—that is, the position that their younger patients did not have SD, but rather that their older patients had SD. As a result, they encountered a gray area in which it is hard to decide whether similarities or differences should weigh most heavily (Fleck 1985 [1935]). They chose to focus on differences. The age assumptions that supported nosology permitted physicians to solve the problem of non-specificity without requiring a single dis
classification. They generally described AD a
early, accelerated, or atypical form of sen
without explaining those terms. Adopting a p
tion that highlighted diversity over unity, t
also emphasized the greater severity and o
unique features of the early-onset disease fo

The foregrounding of differences also kept
tions open for varied explanatory accou
Pathological signs, however similar, might h
different causes. By discovering *a* cause, they
lieved that they might not have discovered
causes. Thus, similar neuropathological a
even behavioral changes in older and youn
patients did not necessarily imply a compara
etiology. Confusion surrounding the diagnosi
mental disorders in old age reinforced the w
dom of this move. In addition to providing
clues to understanding the disorder, the term
nile dementia was used so broadly that it was h
to know what a specific diagnostic label mi
connote. There was little agreement on symp
matology and even less agreement about eti
ogy. In part because of this diagnostic agno
cism (see chapter 6 on the Rothschild period
other reasons), the belief that neuropatholo
caused behavioral changes was challenged
a time in midcentury. The seeming pleth
of mental ills that affected older people, of
loosely called organic brain syndrome, confus
efforts to understand AD and its etiology. Wi
out a clear diagnosis, studies that attempted
correlate pathology and symptoms were bound
be inconclusive. Given all the uncertainties,
seemed best to keep what appeared relativ
clear—AD in younger patients—separate fro
the diagnostic perplexity evidenced by SD.

One further aspect of the physician's conce
tual world reinforced their interpretation of t
cases they encountered and sought to classi
Most physicians held time-honored, though n
universally accepted, ideas about what caus
SD. Since many of these etiological factors cou
only be found in aging persons, it would

cult to assume that AD had the same causes SD. Signaling the continued belief that se- dementia's etiology originated in the aging cess, psychiatrist William Pickett (1904) wrote t "senile dementia is that mental impairment ich is a direct result of cerebral deterioration *n old age*" (81, emphasis added). He did not icate whether he believed this deterioration vitably accompanied old age, nor did he iden- specific factors associated with old age as ng responsible for the cerebral deterioration. ile generally supporting the etiologic con- tion between the processes of aging and SD, l not having a commonly accepted explana- n of those processes, physicians had wide pe for adapting traditional, or offering new, ex- natory frameworks. Even investigators like E. Southard, Harvard's Bullard Professor of uropathology, who were most committed to newest research strategies, often made em- ical leaps when their research did not demon- ate clinicopathologic correlations.

University of Pennsylvania professor Charles rr (1907) for example, suggested that senile de- entia in persons without diseased arteries "is netimes caused by a failure of the excretory or- ns of the body to fulfill properly their func- ns" or, if not that, perhaps the cause lay in me "perturbation of function of the ductless nds" (234). E. E. Southard (1910) asserted that he hypothesis is very near that some part of the ental picture must be related to these defects the distance receptors.... These may be the use, not the effect, of cerebral atrophy" (687). most thirty years later, Arthur Noyes (1939) served in a popular psychiatry textbook that here is much to suggest that the tissue deterio- tion [that occurs during the senile period] is e to an innate inadequacy in durability of neu- ns. Why senile psychoses occur in some per- ns and not in others is still unknown" (290).

In pursuing etiological explanations, the next neration of research (though not necessarily searchers) focused more specifically on three anatomical observations: brain atrophy; cerebral arteriosclerosis; and specific changes in the brain, such as senile plaques and neurofibrillary tangles. Primarily interested in establishing clinicopathologic correlations they easily returned to older, more speculative hypotheses when research techniques did not exhibit specific correlations. They could not, however, resolve a basic dilemma: Were the illnesses experienced by older people caused by age or by disease? In particular, was SD caused by age or by disease? This question persists.

MOVING TOWARD A CHANGED CONCEPTUAL FRAMEWORK

Systematic medical and biological research on the processes of aging began to fracture the link among perceptions of old age, common assumptions, and the tendency to classify disease on the basis of age. By 1930 demographic changes heightened awareness about aging. With funding from the Macy Foundation, Edmund V. Cowdry convened a conference on aging in Woods Hole, Massachusetts, in 1937. From that meeting emerged *Problems of Ageing* (1939), the first multidisciplinary text on aging and an important milestone in understanding old age. Some common questions that physicians asked about old age included: What changes in aging are individual? Which may be regarded with reasonable certainty as inevitable? What are the conditions superimposed on them. Should arteriosclerosis be regarded as "normal" or as a result of wear and tear, or may it be dependent mostly upon disease processes that can be prevented (Malamud 1941, 49, 39). To answer such questions, investigators studied what they called "normal" aging as the foundation for understanding abnormal aging (Lewis 1946; Rudd 1959).

Opening a 1957 conference on the Process of Aging in the Nervous System, Pearce Bailey, the Director of the National Institute on Neurological Diseases and Blindness remarked: "I suspect that much of our current information about the process of aging in the nervous system has accumulated by incidental observation and had not been deliberately sought. Perhaps the nature of the process should be explored much more thoroughly in the future than it has been in the past" (Bailey 1959, viii).

Investigators were concerned about structural alterations in the aging nervous system—baseline data for studying abnormal changes. By the 1950s, animal models of cellular and other changes, basic studies of the nervous system, specific studies of cerebral blood flow and oxygen consumption, studies of intelligence and memory, and investigations of EEG patterns and the aging brain were produced in growing numbers.

Such research only gradually modified understandings. Longitudinal studies of age-related changes required complex research designs and organization that were still new to medicine and the social sciences. Much research in this early period reflected individual ventures (Achenbaum 1995) which made studies that accounted for the simultaneous changes in all organ systems and in the older person's social world particularly difficult. Such research would also demand long-term financing and the commitment of research time. In addition to these practical problems, many physicians still shared society's pervasively negative attitudes toward old age. Some researchers, including Nascher, and some social reformers began to challenge prevailing assumptions that decline in old age was both inevitable and lodged in internal changes. Nascher, for example undertook a study of poverty in old age to buttress his belief that pathological conditions in the elderly were multicausal. Once the problems associated with old age were analyzed contextually—for example, by critiquing a society that failed to give older people a sense of security, observers could argue that it was no wonder that "ultimately social responsibility is lost and replaced by childish selfishness, a natural result of the instinct of self-preservation and unappreciated a (Reed and Stern 1942, 254). As gerontology a geriatrics emerged more visibly as fields of stu more attention was devoted to the social sou of physical and mental problems associated w old age. While often continuing to describe "n mal" senescence as dogmatic, inflexible, and tolerant of environmental changes, the new g eration of researchers and clinicians predic that change could occur if social and econo conditions were ameliorated. What physici once considered inevitable and generated by ternal cellular or other changes (which "bad" ing accelerated), seemed to become more s ceptible to remediation through social acti

While there was no agreement about mod of aging—that is, whether one adopted a mo conceptualized in terms of disease or in ter of "normal" change processes—there was so growing optimism that old age was subject amelioration if only one understood it enou Ironically, social reformers such as Abrah Rubloff generally adopted the profoundly ne tive views of aging that dominated society as platform on which to build reform efforts. Wh these views served noble ends—improving conditions of the elderly—the means to eff change were less certain. In addition, as ad cates worked to transform these negative ima of aging, the foundation that supported pub programs also seemed to evaporate.

By the 1950s efforts to define more precis the mental disorders that occurred in later l accelerated. In a highly regarded study, the p chiatrist Martin Roth (1955) defined senile p chosis as a condition with a history of gradual a continually progressive failure in common act ities of everyday life. In describing the clinic picture, he emphasized failures of memory a intellect and disorganization of personality wit out known causes such as infection, neoplas chronic intoxication, or cerebrovascular diseas He further argued that affective psychoses, la paraphrenia, and acute confusion were distin n the two main causes of progressive demen- in old age—senile and arteriosclerotic psy- ses. This research, which gave physicians ie basic tools with which to distinguish pro- ssive dementia of senile or arteriosclerotic ori- from affective disorders, did not, however, ckly transform the work of clinical geriatric chiatrists. The diagnostic label "senile de- ntia" continued in wide and loose usage oldman 1978; Wells 1978). As late as 1978, nmentators remarked that "organic brain syn- me," as used in *DSM-II*, was a poorly defined, chall diagnosis; however, it was still com- nly used in state mental hospitals where ysicians rarely sought to diagnose older pa- its differentially (Seltzer and Sherwin 1978,

The broad definitional boundaries for organic in disease meant that some writers considered) as a dementing process in old age that was as- iated with the histological changes of AD; ile at the same time, other writers considered nly a clinical syndrome without those patho- ical changes (Tomlinson, Blessed, and Roth 70). Furthermore physicians often classified ler people with slight deviations from the nor- al as having SD, and as a result, there was ich overdiagnosis (Wells 1972). Thus, classifi- tion continued to prove troublesome.

Investigators recognized the overlap between ysical and psychiatric disorders in their older tients and the frequent melding of "func- nal" and organic disorders. They understood e need for greater diagnostic rigor without hieving it. At a 1970 symposium sponsored by e Ciba Foundation, the British psychiatrist B. Tomlinson queried a presenter by saying, "We ust know whether the term senile dementia is ing used to refer to a clinical syndrome without y assumed pathological connotations, or to de- ribe dementia in old age with the pathological allmarks of Alzheimer's disease. If we don't get is agreed now, confusion will reign throughout ir seminar" (Tomlinson 1970, 33).

Nevertheless, by the mid-70s early longitudinal studies about mental functioning in old age stimulated popular as well as professional interest. Physician-researchers had become *public* advocates for a changed conception about old age, to be followed by a new understanding of AD. Robert Butler (1975) had a prepared audience when he affirmed that "intellectual abilities declined not as a consequence of the mysterious process of aging but *rather as the result of specific diseases*. Therefore, senility is not an inevitable outcome of aging" (899; emphasis added).

The interpretation of such studies served to narrow the gray area between normalcy and pathology. The corollary belief that what once was attributed to aging per se was now to be sought in medical disease, sociocultural effects, and personality factors was becoming an article of faith for many biogerontologists and other aging advocates. Changes of this sort supported what would become a dramatic reversal in the conceptualization of AD.

This work culminated in the establishment of the National Institute on Aging (NIA) in 1974 and facilitated resistance to "ageism," a term coined by Robert Butler in 1965. These moves sought to reposition the aged and present counterimages to former stereotypes. In this atmosphere, contemporary views about AD developed. Changing views about aging were only one aspect of the conceptual shift that facilitated the rethinking. It was only subsequent to these changes that an active campaign began to eliminate the word from the medical vocabulary. It has proved more difficult to remove it from popular thinking. Contemporary views of AD have both contributed to and benefited from this reconceptualization of aging and old age.

ESTABLISHING A UNIFIED DEFINITION

Anglo-American researchers unified SD and AD very quickly into an explicit disease category known variously as Senile Dementia of the Alzheimer type (SDAT), Dementia of the Alzheimer Type (DAT), or simply Alzheimer disease (AD) (see Fox 1989 and Chapter 12 in this volume for a fuller discussion of this period). Declaring that "aging is not a disease," they argued that the manifestations of biological aging were quite different than the common chronic diseases of the aged. AD in this view was explicitly *not* an extreme form of "normal" aging. This dichotomy prevails in gerontology, geriatrics, and, more generally in the medical sciences (Blumenthal 1993). Gubrium (1986) thus notes that by the late 1970s the "facts of aging" on the one hand, and the "facts of disease" on the other, were taken as givens, requiring no further analysis. Questions about disease versus age were "swept aside, unimportant for those who work on the concrete facts—the data of disease" (207, 209). In this model, a distinct border divides normal aging and disease; one is not the other. AD is a unified entity in a singular category, separate from aging (Gubrium 1986, 52).

T. Franklin Williams, then director of the National Institute on Aging, captured this view: "The advantage of trying to make a distinction between aging and disease is . . . that if one can identify a change in older people which is not universal or inevitable, there must be extrinsic causes and these may be preventable or modifiable. If they are inevitable, on the other hand, that is 'aging'" (1988, 48). In this view, aging itself results in few pathological conditions. Instead, there are many diseases that particularly beset older people.

Diseases imply the intrusion of an extrinsic or exogenous factor or factors that had been or would be identified. The recent focus on genetics enlarges this notion by shifting attention to intrinsic, molecular-level "causes." For investigators, it seems probable that these factors will prove to be the cause or causes of the qualitative differences that separate AD from normal or biological aging. AD thus resembles many forms of cancer—while it is more common in older than in younger people and so is age-dependent, not "caused" by "normal" age-related chan[ges]. These changes only make the person more [sus]ceptive to the disease process. Tacitly, both e[arly] twentieth-century researchers and their mod[ern] counterparts saw AD in ontological terms; disease existed apart from its embodiment in [ac]tual illnesses. In this way, it was easy to lose si[ght] of the features of the disease—especially m[any] behavioral factors that were linked to, but [not] necessarily directly caused by, the neuropat[ho]logical changes.

Although there are still dissenting voices (B[lu]menthal 1993; Huppert, Brayne, and O'Con[nor] 1994; Goodwin 1991), the dominant posit[ion] today is that SDAT is a disease in which exo[ge]nous and endogenous events cause pathologi[cal] changes in the brain. These changes, in turn, [re]sult in the signs that render a tentative diagno[sis] of AD probable. Without denying its a[ge-]dependent characteristics, key leaders have [in]sisted that AD represents more than a continu[ous] distribution of physiopathologic variables in as[so]ciation with specific risk factors.

The perceived "givenness" of this dise[ase] model, and the particular consequences th[at] flowed from it, are significant. Medicine, as a [so]cial enterprise, has developed what Goodw[in] (1991) called "an ideology of senility." It is a mo[del] that understands AD in classic disease terms with a specific etiology, visible signs and sym[p]toms, concrete structural alterations in the bra[in] and causing discomfort and suffering (Capl[an] 1981). It confirms the ontologically required sp[lit] between health and disease—or, in the langua[ge] that prevailed earlier in the century, between th[e] normal and the pathological. A corollary belief that the most effective response to a disease u[n]derstood in this way is through basic research d[e]signed to reveal its specific etiology, an importa[nt] step in the pursuit of interventions and, ul[ti]mately, cure.

It matters that a condition is called a diseas[e]. This acknowledgment generally implies actio[n:] a commitment to medical intervention and r

:ch to determine both cause and cure. It uences public attitudes and public policy, es- ially as the public investment in science and dical care accelerated in the twentieth cen- '. In the past century or more, it has also come nean coverage by health insurance and grant- privileges to the person with the disease that unavailable to the well (Reznek 1987; Engel- dt 1981). It can shape the patient's self-image l the family's expectations and behaviors. ner and in some ways equally important stakes, h as funding and research careers, were prag- tic. The development of a disease model was ential for obtaining resources for new re- rch. Thus, this view contributed to the con- iction of careers, the instruction of students, d the politicization of AD.

This model also fit well with the expectations a society that had recently identified ageism as prevailing social problem (Butler 1969) and allenged assumptions that had attributed to e conditions with the potential for remedia- n. It was important that AD became a disease fined by biological variables—which is, with v exceptions, the modern conception of AD. is age versus disease discussion assumes par- ular prominence when there are so many kes involved in addition to the altruistic goal of ducing pain and suffering. Earlier in the cen- ry, one must assume that physicians shared the truistic goals of medicine but were less troubled the uncertainty of the disease versus aging dis- iction since few interventions were possible d the ravages of old age were assumed; more- er, no research money was at stake. Whatever e remaining problems, the "diseasing" of AD is trenched today.

No single factor can explain the new pre- redness to think differently. Instead, several ctors prepared researchers to see one way and other (Fleck 1985 [1935], 64). Factors endemic both medicine and science joined cultural per- eptions about old age as a shifting subtext that odified the intellectual horizon within which searchers worked. For example, how physicians categorized symptoms influenced how they perceived similarities and differences between SD and AD. This cognitive activity was contextual, value laden, and conditioned by culture and history (Fleck 1985 [1935]).

While researchers were not yet prepared to focus on similarities between AD and SD, at some point roughly in the 1930s, it no longer seemed inevitable that the etiology of AD was rooted in a premature senility. The first shift, then, was simply, but importantly, the gradual distancing of AD from the poorly understood "processes of aging." Other causes began to appear more likely. That "senile" plaques became neuritic plaques implied a subtle shift in thinking. This move expanded etiologic possibilities without immediately resulting in changed ideas about either AD or SD. As the century advanced, new factors—advancements in technical capacities such as statistics and microscopy, basic understandings of the evolution of diagnostic techniques, the improvement in epidemiological and genetic research, and the development of specialty residency programs—further structured perceptual shifts about SD and AD. Later, the emergence of "big science" and the politicization of individual diseases through citizen action also influenced thinking.

CONCLUSION

The account I have just offered tells us something important about the negotiation of disease. If, as many believed, SD was rooted in the aging process itself, then investigators generally could interpret it in three ways. They could consider the mental changes associated with old age in its entirety as pathological; or, in contrast, they could view SD as a "normal" concomitant of aging. They could also adopt a continuum model in which the normal and the pathological blurred into one another. For the first half of the twentieth century, the view that aging processes were strongly, if not causally, implicated in the clinical manifestations of SD came the closest to medical understandings. Since social and individual expectations anticipated decline in old age, and since one implicit way of thinking about a disease was that it limited what was considered normal functioning, then SD would not be considered a disease. Even if statistical norms had been available, they could not have determined whether the behaviors associated with SD should be accepted as "normal" in old age. That is fundamentally a value question.

One could, theoretically, continue to believe that biologic and pathologic aging exist along a continuum—a quantitative distinction—and still consider SD a disease. For this shift to occur, a change in expectations about what was acceptable and what was unacceptable in old age would be required; this change would alter the norms. A pathological condition would violate norms of acceptable functioning in old age. It would also generally be linked to a quantitative distinction in brain pathology. A continuum model can be either behavioral or organic in its focus, but one will usually reinforce the other.

For most of this century, behavior patterns that had been normalized by cultural expectations were rarely interpreted as a disease. Commonly held notions about old age and the relationship of normal old age to pathology formed the cultural matrix within which symptoms of dementia were understood. More specifically, the culture of medicine reinforced more general cultural values through its classification of mental disorders on the basis of age and through its etiological views about both AD and SD.

Even more specifically, in part because their environment harbored so many uncertainties, most investigators tended to emphasize differences rather than similarities between the disorders. This choice preserved options for varied explanatory accounts. Pathological signs, however similar, might have different causes. Influenced by these views, physicians found it easier to see a "disease," in the ontological sense, in a young person. They accepted a disease label even if it were difficult to explain why brain patholo discovered in these younger people were so si lar to changes that occurred in old age. For older person, they were more likely to face a tr bling uncertainty—was the evident intensif tion of changes that occurred in "normal" agi even when the symptoms and neuropathol were quite similar to those in a younger perso disease or normal aging? Could the "same" c dition be a disease in the younger person "normal" in the older person? This dilemma rarely stated explicitly; however, its source is coverable in physicians' musings about the distinct line between the normal and the pat logical in old age. Disease is indeed a slipp concept.

The relatively loose classification of men disorders in old age also left wide areas of unc tainty. As a result, investigators had considera room for speculation and for developing inno tive ideas about SD. For example, if the bou aries between normal old age and SD w almost imperceptible, psychiatrists such as Ro schild could easily identify one or several ext nal life events that pushed the individual acr this gray line. In the same way, if the distinctic between various mental disorders of the seni were vague, researchers could test out differe treatment modalities and obtain positive resu Or they could assert, as did Rothschild that the were no, or at best rough, correlations betwe brain pathology and symptoms in senile p choses. That result would be expected if t clinical diagnosis were inconclusive. When co bined with the other uncertainties, this agnos cism with regard to differential diagnosis left gap that aged the thinking that flourished fro the 1930s onward.

Physicians in the first two-thirds of the twen eth century did not treat questions about no malcy versus pathology, or aging versus diseas lightly as they sought to understand early-ons and late-onset dementia. Attitudes toward old a and the clinical changes that seemed manifest period of life served to highlight age as an al-st insurmountable barrier to a common un-standing of SD and AD, thereby shaping their ceptions. It was not because they could not ceive of AD as an early or atypical senility, as contemporary writer suggests; after all, they just that for at least twenty years after Alzhei-r's first published paper (Fox 1989). While er making clear what they meant by the terms pical" or "early senility," they assumed the dition might have different causes than the ility of late life that would, in time, be re-led. After all, senility was little more than a gh and ready category for many changes that urred in old age.

Shifting views about AD and SD thus cannot explained solely by the processes of scientific covery. One encounters a text or text ana-gue—in this case, the brute data of brain pa-ology and memory loss, confusion, and other nptoms of dementia, which must be inter-ted. Our interpretative horizon is not unlim-d. It starts with prejudgments and is regularly ised to accommodate new information or his-ical shifts. In his presidential address to the nerican Psychiatric Association forty years ago, nneth Appel alerted his audience to this fea-e of research: "We are not outside observers of ternal neutral facts or things. Facts are con-uctions, aspirations of the exploring process hich are built up and organized by consensual ought" (1954, 12).

For the neurologists and psychiatrists who idied dementia, many changes, both internal d external to medicine and science, separately d together, molded the gestalt that became eir interpretive horizon. These changes in-rmed judgments at the same time that new ork helped modify previously held positions. s a medical anthropologist recently observed, Once medicine tries to explain, manipulate, or der some biological reality, a process of contex-alization takes place in which the dynamic re-tionship of biology with cultural values and the social order has to be considered. At each stage, biomedical conceptualizations were important, but they did not form in isolation. Social forces and interactive decision-making among key investigators shaped biological convictions" (Lock and Gordon 1988, 7).

Medical researchers negotiated disease categories within implicit boundaries shaped by culture, professional norms, technological possibilities, and intellectual context (Bechtel and Richardson 1993; Rosenberg and Golden 1992). In the case of AD and SD, different ways of explaining previously known phenomena slowly changed the way people thought about these disorders; as their horizons shifted and conceptual links loosened, new possibilities opened. These possibilities had been present, in some sense, from the very beginning. Dr. Solomon Fuller wrestled with uncertainty with each postmortem and then concluded that he had "found" a case of AD. Today, different genes are implicated in some cases of DAT; more might be found some day. Certainly genetics, which seems to represent the hope for remediation, is the dominant area of research (as other chapters in this volume suggest). Research on dementia is a major enterprise fueled by resources from both public and private sources.

How we think about any particular condition is important for another reason: it inevitably influences how we respond to patients who have the disorder and how they might think of themselves. For example, physicians who care for people with dementia describe their patients as "terrified." Terror itself is a cultural creation. In cultures where AD has not been politicized and staked out as an important area for research and funding, cultural conceptions of the condition (which may not even be labeled as AD) make it likely that it can be integrated into everyday life as just one of those "things" that happen to many older people. In Sawako Ariyoshi's (1987) novel *The Twilight Years*, as the old man Shigezo deepens into profound forgetfulness and incapacity, his daughter-in-law, Akiko, takes over his care. The primary problem that Ariyoshi addresses is not Shigezo's terror (he is actually rather calm as he deepens into his dementia); rather it is the slow transformation of her own busy life to care for her once ornery and even abusive father-in-law. Terror is simply not a part of the conversation.

Who is better served — Shigezo or the newly diagnosed patient at a major medical center? Have we done a disservice to patients and their families by the particular cultural construction of AD that is dominant in American society today? What does this construction suggest about American values, belief systems, and notions about old age? If culture shapes perceptions and understandings of disease, so does disease tell us something important about culture. Perhaps reflection about these interactions and their power is a worthy task for the twenty-first century.

REFERENCES

Achenbaum, A. 1995. *Crossing Frontiers: Gerontology Emerges as a Science*. New York: Cambridge University Press.

Appel, K. 1954. "Presidential Address: The Present Challenge of Psychiatry." *American Journal of Psychiatry* 111: 1–12.

Ariyoshi, S. 1987 [1972]. *The Twilight Years*. Trans. Mildred Tahara. Tokyo: Kodansha International.

Bailey, Pearce. 1959. "Foreword: Significance of the Process of Aging in the Nervous System." In *The Process of Aging in the Nervous System*, ed. James Biren and William Windle. Springfield, Ill.: Charles C. Thomas, vi–viii.

Beach, 1987. "The History of Alzheimer's Disease: Three Debates." *Journal of the History of Medicine and Allied Sciences* 42: 327–49.

Bechtel, W., and R. Richardson. 1993. *Discovering Complexity: Decomposition and Localization as Strategies in Scientific Research*. Princeton, N.J.: Princeton University Press.

Bick, K. 1994. "The Early Story of Alzheimer's Disease." In *Alzheimer's Disease*, ed. R. R. Katman and K. Bick. New York: Raven Press, 1–8.

Blumenthal, H. 1993. "The Aging-Disease chotomy Is Alive, But Is It Well?" *Journal of the Ar can Geriatrics Society* 41: 1272.

Burr, C. 1907. "Insanity in the Aged." *Internati Clinics* 17: 231–41.

Butler, R. 1969. "Ageism: Another Form of Bigo *Gerontologist* 9: 243–46.

———. 1975. "Psychiatry and the Elderly: Overview." *American Journal of Psychiatry* 132: 8 900.

Caplan, A. 1981. "The Unnaturalness of Agin Sickness unto Death." In *Concepts of Health and ease: Interdisciplinary Perspectives*, ed. Arthur Cap H.Tristram Engelhardt, and James McCartney. R ing, Mass.: Addison Wesley, 733.

Cole, T. 1991. *The Journey of Life: A Cultural His of Aging In America*. New York: Cambridge Unive Press.

Cowdry, E. 1939. *Problems in Ageing: Biological Medical Aspects*. Baltimore: Williams and Wilk

Critchley, M. 1939. "Ageing of the Nervous Syste In *Problems of Aging: Biological and Medical Aspe* ed. E.V. Cowdry. Baltimore: Williams and Wilk

Engelhardt, H. 1981. "The Disease of Masturbati Values and the Concept of Disease." In *Concept Health and Disease: Interdisciplinary Perspectives*, A. Caplan, T. Engelhardt, and J. McCartney. Readi Mass.: Addison Wesley, 267–80.

Eros, G. 1959. "The Aging Process — Physiologi and Pathological." *Diseases of the Nervous System* (Suppl.): 112–18.

Ferraro, A. 1959. "Senile Psychosis." In *Americ Handbook of Psychiatry*. New York: Basic Books, vol 1019–45.

Fleck, L. 1985 [1935]. *Genesis and Development o Scientific Fact*, ed. T. Tenn and R. Merton, trans. Bradless and T. Tenn. Chicago: University of Chica Press.

———. 1986. "Some Specific Features of the Medic Way of Thinking." In *Cognition and Fact: Materials Ludwik Fleck*, ed. Robert S. Cohen and Thom Schnelle. Dordrecht: D. Reidel.

Fox, P. 1989. "From Senility to Alzheimer's Diseas The Rise of the Alzheimer's Disease Movement." *M bank Quarterly*.

;oldman, R. 1978. "The Social Impact of the Or-c Dementias of the Aged." In *Dementia: A Bio-ical Approach*, ed. Kalidas Nandy. New York/Am-dam: Elsevier/North Holland Biomedical Press, .

;oodwin, J. 1991. "Geriatric Ideology: The Myth of ility." *Journal of the American Geriatrics Society* 39: –31.

;ubrium, J. 1986. *Old Timers and Alzheimer's Dis-: The Descriptive Organization of Senility*. Green-h, Conn.: JAI Press.

laber, C. 1983. *Beyond Sixty-Five: The Dilemma of Age in America's Past*. New York: Cambridge Uni-sity Press.

Holstein, M. 1996. "Negotiating Disease: Senile De-ntia and Alzheimer's Disease, 1900–1980." Ph.D. . University of Texas Medical Branch, Galveston.

Hughes, C. 1909. "Normal Senility and Dementia ilis: The Therapeutic Staying of Old Age." *Alienist l Neurologist* 30: 63–76.

Huppert, F., C. Brayne, and D. O'Connor. 1994. *mentia and Normal Aging*. Cambridge: Cambridge iversity Press.

Jellife, S. E., and W. A. White. 1923. *Diseases of the rvous System: A Text-Book of Neurology and Psychi-y*. Philadelphia and New York: Lea and Febiger.

Jones, H., and O. Kaplan. 1956. "Psychological As-cts of Mental Disorders in Later Life." In *Mental sorders of Later Life*, ed. O. Kaplan. Stanford, Calif.: anford University Press, 98–156.

Krause, W. 1900. "The Influence of Age upon the oduction of Nervous Disease." *Alienist and Neurolo-t* 21: 642–52.

Lewis, A. 1946. "Ageing and Senility: A Major Prob-n of Psychiatry." *Journal of Mental Science* 92: –70.

Lock, M., and D. Gordon, eds. 1988. *Biomedicine camined*. Dordrecht: Kluwer Academic Publishers.

Malamud, W. 1941. "Mental Disorders in the Aged: teriosclerotic and Senile Psychoses." *Public Health eports*, Suppl. 168. Washington, D.C.: United States ublic Health Service.

Nascher, I. J. 1911. "Senile Mentality." *International linics*, 2. 1st ser. 4: 48–49.

Neumann, M., and R. Cohn, 1953. "Incidence of Alzheimer's Disease in a Large Mental Hospital: Relation to Senile Psychosis with Cerebral Arteriosclerosis." *Archives of Neurology and Psychiatry* 69: 615–36.

Newton, R. D. 1948. "The Identity of Alzheimer's Disease and Senile Dementia and Their Relationship to Senility." *Journal of Medical Science* 94: 225–49.

Noyes, A. 1939. *Modern Clinical Psychiatry*, 2nd ed. Philadelphia and London: W. B. Saunders.

Palmer, H., F. Braceland, and D. Hastings. 1943. "Somatopsychic Disorders of Old Age." *American Journal of Psychiatry* 99: 856–63.

Pickett, W. 1904. "Senile Dementia: A Clinical Study of Two Hundred Cases with Particular Regard to Types of the Disease." *Journal of Nervous and Mental Disease* 31: 81–88.

Rabinbach, A. 1990. *The Human Motor: Energy, Fatigue, and the Origins of Modernity*. Berkeley: University of California Press.

Reed, G. M., and K. Stern. 1942. "The Treatment, Pathology, and Prevention of Mental Disorders in the Aged." *Canadian Medical Association Journal* 46: 249–54.

Reznek, L. 1987. *The Nature of Disease*. London: Routledge and Paul.

Rosenberg, C., and J. Golden. 1992. "Framing Disease: Illness, Society, and History." In *Framing Disease: Studies in Cultural History*, ed. C. Rosenberg and J. Golden. New Brunswick, N.J.: Rutgers University Press, xiii–xxvi.

Roth, M. 1955. "Natural History of Mental Disorders in Old Age." *Journal of Mental Science* 101: 282–301.

Rothschild, D. 1956. "Senile Psychoses and Psychoses with Cerebral Arteriosclerosis." In *Mental Disorders of Later Life*, 2nd ed., ed. Oscar Kaplan. Stanford, Calif.: Stanford University Press, 289–33.

Rothschild, D., and J. Kasanin. 1936. "A Clinicopathologic Study of Alzheimer's Disease: Relationship to Senile Conditions." *Archives of Neurology and Psychiatry* 36: 293–321.

Rudd, T. 1959. "Preventing Senile Dementia: The Need for a New Approach." *Journal of the American Geriatrics Society* 7: 322–26.

Seltzer, B., and I. Sherwin. 1978. "Organic Brain Syndrome: An Empirical Study and Critical Review." *American Journal of Psychiatry* 135: 13–21.

Southard, E. E. 1910. "Anatomical Findings in Senile Dementia: A Diagnostic Study Bearing Especially on the Group of Cerebral Atrophies." *American Journal of Insanity* 66: 673–707.

Tomlinson, B. E. 1970. "General Discussion." In *Alzheimer's Disease and Related Conditions*, ed. R. R. Terry, and K. L. Bick. New York: Raven Press.

Tomlinson, B. E., G. Blessed, and M. Roth. 1970. "Observations on the Brains of Demented Older People." *Journal of the Neurological Sciences* 11: 205–42.

Warthin, A. S. 1929. *Old Age, The Major Involution and Pathology of the Aging Process*. New York: Pau
Hoeber.

Wells, C. 1972. "Dementia Reconsidered." *Arch of General Psychiatry* 26: 385–88.

———. 1978. "Chronic Brain Disease: Overview." *American Journal of Psychiatry* 135:

Williams, T. Franklin. 1988. "Discussion: Ag and Disease." In *Research and Ageing Population*, David and Julie Whelan. Chichester, Great Brit John Wiley and Sons, 48.

PART IV

Normalcy, Genetic Disease, and Enhancement: The Future of the Concepts of Health and Disease

VARIOUS CONSTRUCTIONS OF health nd disease often rely on assumptions regarding what human conditions re "normal" or "abnormal." These assumptions are often challenged by ie power of new technologies, which can produce compelling evidence iat the accepted concepts of biological "normalcy" and genetic health nd disease are inadequate. For example, one result of technological adances in high-resolution diagnostics is that clearly distinguishing the healthy from the diseased is made more difficult. Advances in the domains of neuroscience and pharmacology have made the distinction between the need for treatment and the desirability of enhancement difficult, if not impossible, to describe. Physical conditions that might once have proven fatal or disabling—such as diabetes or deafness—challenge the constructions of normal or abnormal and call for an analysis that is more continuum based and less dogmatic.

Indeed, "normal" may not be a good state to be in! Sander Gilman, in the first chapter of this section, shows how cosmetic surgery is not simply a form of aesthetic enhancement but may also restore a degree of mental health (i.e., it is also a treatment) to those unhappy with their appearance. Historically, alterations to one's body were done within the confines of religious ritual or as other nonmedical procedures such as tattooing or body piercing. Now, Gilman asserts, such bodily alteration has moved into the ultimate secular sphere—medicine and science. Cosmetic surgery and accounts by patients and practitioners point to the connection between the concepts of "beauty" and "health," "ugliness" and "disease."

Part IV highlights many of the tensions that current advances in biomedical science and technology are creating in our understanding of health and disease. Renowned evolutionary biologist George C. Williams claims that notions of health and disease linked to statistical views of medical normalcy are useless concepts and that the evolutionary concept of adaptation can better capture the relationship between health and disease. In his description of various adaptations that are taken for granted, Williams suggests that the concept of medical normalcy may actually be harmful. This is so because it encourages medical interventions directed to eliminate proximate causational factors (in the case of a pathogen), which may jeopardize more fundamental and thus more important evolutionary mechanisms. One need only think of the significant problem of the increase in number of antibiotic-resistant bacteria to lend credence to his a ment. Williams goes further to show in surpris ways that the classic homeostatic model of o mum health developed by Walter Canno fraught with problems resulting from anatom and physiological "design flaws" that are only ognizable when health is analyzed in the con of adaptation and natural selection.

David Magnus and Eric Juengst desc how genetic diseases have been characteri the problems with those characterizations, what the potential upshot of these character tions of health and disease will be for the gen practice of medicine. One potential probl Juengst identifies is "genetic imperialism." Un this rubric, diseases may be oversimplified, be reduced to "bad" or "flawed" genes. Despite w genomic science has shown us about the inte lationship between genes and environment, basic concepts of Mendelian genetics (what Harvard biologist Ernst Mayr called "beanb genetics) have been and continue to be a driving force in clinical genetic medici Juengst identifies genetic reductionism, gene determinism, and their familial implications being three important consequences of a new netic concept of disease.

Moving from heredity-based diseases to a m contemporary view of environmentally cau discrete molecular anomalies, Magnus sho that the concept of genetic disease has traverse number of stages on its way to the broad conc tion of genetic disease popular at this time. T manner in which the concept of genetic disea is framed and the language by which it is pressed has a profound impact on very practic matters. From decisions regarding which patie gets treated to which researcher gets funding, t relevance of the concept of genetic disease is u deniable. In regard to normalcy—as the conce of genetic disease expands, we will, ironical find that we are all genetically diseased.

In their discussion of cognitive enhancemen Peter J. Whitehouse, Eric Juengst, Maxwe

HLMAN, and THOMAS H. MURRAY describe a ımon set of ethical concerns found across st of the selections in this section: from the ential inequities in providing enhancement nnologies to understanding how the notion of henticity (or inauthenticity) and the human lf" will change in response to the possibility of ıancing human functions.

After reviewing the enhancement/treatment ıtion offered by Norman Daniels, PAUL ROOT ›LPE raises three key questions that emerge m the use of various neuroenhancements. ese questions are basic to this section and re- d medical coverage, public policy perspec- s, and social mores about the use or misuse 'enhancement." Going further, Wolpe uses a mber of examples, particularly the compound ›dafinil, and he unpacks various arguments out enhancement of the human mind that y rely on ultimately incommensurable visions human life.

ARTHUR L. CAPLAN raises a set of ethical concerns regarding eugenics. He acknowledges the importance of the horrors committed in the past in the name of eugenics, but argues that these older forms of eugenics rest on coercive and population-based approaches that do not meet the emerging interest in trying to improve one's own genes or the genes of one's offspring. Noticing that eugenics movements may take may differing routes toward their goal, not simply as a totalitarian regime's goal, Caplan suggests we understand that in some cases, what might be considered eugenics may in fact be morally permissible (e.g., individual eugenics done to avoid giving birth to a child with cystic fibrosis, or using preimplantation diagnosis of an embryo to avoid creating a child with Huntington's Disease). But again, this decision relies upon the way in which society defines the core concepts of health, disease and illness and how the goals of medicine are met.

CHAPTER 21

The Medicalization of Aesthetic Surgery

SANDER GILMAN *[From* Creating Beauty to Cure the Soul: Race and Psychology in the Shaping of Aesthetic Surgery*]*

MODERN AESTHETIC SURGERY began
Europe, specifically Germany, France, and the United Kingdom, and in
e United States during the latter decades of the nineteenth century.
rom there it spread into every culture in the world, following paths of
olonial and economic expansion and the domination of Western medical
eory and practice. It followed the same path as the rise and spread of psy-
hoanalysis. To examine the broader culture of aesthetic surgery we need
recreate the inner fantasies of such cultures as they constructed the medal reality of the "aesthetic body" and the "happy psyche" in Western Eu-
ope (Germany, France, Great Britain), North America (the United States
nd Canada), and somewhat later South America (Brazil and Argentina).

To do so one must assume that there are shared cultural fantasies among nations with shared histories. In the West, the beautiful and the healthy (and the ugly and the diseased) are interchangeable concepts. Beauty surgery is understood as surgery to restore mental health, yet the understanding of what constitutes the "beautiful" and what constitutes the "healthy" shifts from culture to culture and from time to time. Only the relationship between the two remains constant. Making the body beautiful through aesthetic surgery is a means of restoring (mental) health. The power of the images of beauty and health in this tradition and its globalization has meant that models of aesthetic surgery with their origin in the European-American tradition have come to serve as the primary references for the development of aesthetic surgery in colonial as well as postcolonial cultures in South America, Africa, and Asia.

The globalization of both the procedures and the psychology of aesthetic surgery can be measured, for example, in the flourishing of aesthetic surgery by American- and European-trained surgeons in contemporary Argentina where "medical insurers say they have noticed an upsurge in claims for 'essential' nose jobs, while private clinics tout liposuction on the installment plan." This is seen as psychic improvement following the traditional model: "Argentines have long had a penchant for spending big on psychiatry and other forms of self-improvement. 'People have the feeling they can't control their own future; that working hard and being a good citizen won't get you anywhere,' suggests psychiatrist Marcel Hernandez, 'That's why beauty has become the main value in the market.'"[1] The cultural concept of the "beautiful" includes standards of male as well as female beauty, but we shall see that the term "beautiful" is not a simple one—even within seemingly related and seemingly homogenous cultures.

To write the history of psychology within aesthetic surgery is to write an account of the aesthetic alteration of the mind and the body wi
the public sphere of medicine. It is their ins
tional as well as their cultural base that ena
surgeons aesthetically to change the body. O
physical interventions into the body from
weaving to tattooing and body piercing had b
done throughout time and are in many ways
lated to aesthetic surgery. What changes in
late nineteenth century is the context in wh
these procedures are performed. Practices
tattooing have as their intent the creation of a
hort, all of whom bear identical physical fo
These procedures are culturally ubiquitous
have a specifically modern form. In the Enlig
enment, the desire to efface individual differe
came to be part of the creation of a "public" fa
and it slowly became the task of the physician a
the surgeon to address this need to efface dif
ence. As Richard Sennett notes, "Nowhere
the attempt to blot out the individual characte
a person more evident than in the treatment
the face. Both men and women used face pa
either red or white, to conceal the natural colo
the skin and any blemishes it might have."[2] W
Sennett does not address is that the disguise
"blemishes" was the attempt to mask the real
imagined signs of syphilis, which were seen
written upon the face. Cosmetics becomes
adjunct of the treatment (or at least the disgui
of illness. It was the syphilitic who demand
that the missing nose or ulcerous lesion
masked in such a way as to render him or h
(in)visible as one suffering from a stigmatizing i
ness. This demand was the basis for many of t
technical innovations in aesthetic surgery fro
the sixteenth century to the nineteenth centu
The expansion of the use of "cosmetics" is relat
to the creation of a cohort "seen" as acceptab
Aesthetic surgery, which has its modern origi
in the Enlightenment, can be seen as the "mo
ern" equivalent of such procedures. Indee
the more common term "cosmetic surger
has its origin in the late-nineteenth-century su
specialty of "medical cosmetics" in which th

guise of the syphilitic's symptoms was paramount.

The insightful cultural critic Lewis Mumford erved that "the structure of the human body, less than its functions and its excreta, called h early efforts at medication. The cutting or ting together of the hair, the removal of the le foreskin, the piercing of the penis, the extirion of the testicles, even the trepanning of the ll were among the many ingenious experints man first made on himself."[3] Charles Dar-n (1809–1882) had already claimed "that the ne fashions in modifying the shape of the ad, in ornamenting the hair, in painting, tating, perforating the nose, lips, or ears, in reving or filing teeth, etc., now prevail and have g prevailed in the most distant quarters of the th. They rather indicate the close similarity of mind of man, to what ever race he may beg."[4] These were signs of the universality of the man being in the collective modification of body as understood from the perspective of Enlightenment. But Anthony Giddens has mmented that "in [traditional cultures], where ings stayed more or less the same from generan to generation on the level of the collectivity, changed identity was clearly staked out—as ien an individual moved from adolescence to ulthood."[5] This would be marked by the ritual teration of the body. Giddens continues, "In e settings of modernity, by contrast, the altered lf has to be explored and constructed as part of eflexive process of connecting personal and soal change." All of the changes in "traditional soety" were seen as part of ritual and religion, aling with the inner world of the spirit as well with the world of the flesh. Unlike religious rital, aesthetic surgery demands the putative aunomy of the individual inherent to the modern the grounding for any choice as to how his or er body is to be altered. No such autonomy is ossible within religious practice except where it ternalizes secular norms that are not related to e body as such, as we shall see later in this book. Like body building, which also arises at the close of the nineteenth century, aesthetic surgery is a secular restructuring of body modification.[6] It arises, however, within that most radically secular of the institutions of modernity, the world of science and medicine.

Older, nonmedical procedures merge seamlessly into the practice of aesthetic surgery. The use of tattooing to create "the so-called 'Cupid's Bow' of the upper lip" before World War I is paralleled by the use of such tattooing for similar purposes (permanent eye liner) at the end of the century.[7] And, indeed, in the 1990's the removal of tattoos through laser surgery has become a booming industry among aesthetic surgeons. Yet the meaning of "tattooing" seems to be quite different from the use of tattoos within religious ritual and its use within the autonomous culture of aesthetic surgery. That the medical meaning of tattooing parallels the rise of a culture of tattooing in the nineteenth and twentieth centuries is further proof of the potential for the parallel existence of similar practices within different social environments and with quite different meanings.

The movement of such actions as tattooing (often quite literally) into the public and cultural sphere of medicine gives them a quality of the "modern." The desire and need to transform the body, which are labeled as "universal," are present, but additional techniques in reforming the body evolve out of and become part of the culture of medicine. They move from signs of belief that mark and identify the body, to being seen as the means of masking the body, of making it (in)visible. In both cases they link the internal life of the individual to cultural institutions (ranging from circumcision societies to medical schools) devoted to altering the body.

NOTES

1. Jonathan Friedland, "Argentina Is a Land of Many Faces, Fixed by Plastic Surgeons," *Wall Street Journal* (February 2, 1996): I.

2. Richard Sennett, *The Fall of Public Man* (New York: Norton, 1974), p. 70.

3. Lewis Mumford, *The Myth of the Machine: Techniques and Human Development* (New York: Harcourt, Brace, and World, 1967), p. 109.

4. Charles Darwin, *The Descent of Man and Selection in Relation to Sex* (New York: D. Appleton, 1897), p. 575.

5. Philip Cassell, ed., *The Giddens Reader* (Stanf Calif.: Stanford University Press, 1993), p. 304.

6. Christopher Derek Kenway, "Kraft und Scl heit: Regeneration and Racial Theory in the Ger Physical Culture Movement, 1895–1920." Ph.D. d University of California at Los Angeles, 1996.

7. Frederick Strange Kolle, *Plastic and Cosm Surgery* (New York: D. Appleton, 1911), pp. 190–91.

CHAPTER 22

The Quest for Medical Normalcy—Who Needs It?

GEORGE C. WILLIAMS

MEDICINE DEALS WITH conflicts, and its ain function is to intervene on the side of one of the contenders, the pa- ent. The conflict may be between patient and neoplasm, between patient nd pathogen, between a plant that made a defensive toxin and a patient ho ingested it, between patient and patient, as in the maternal-fetal onflict analyzed by Haig (1993). Even the victim of a mechanical injury r sunburn or hypothermia may usefully be recognized as taking part in a ontest, just as, in behavioral ecology, it is routine to use a payoff matrix to redict an individual's ploys against nature when there is no identifiable or- anism with conflicting interests. Patients can always be regarded as using eir own adaptations to win a struggle against whatever caused a current medical problem. Surely, then, it must be helpful for medicine to make use of the insights of modern evolutionary biology that deal explicitly with the nature and limitations of adaptations in general, with much recent emphasis on their use in contests.

Unfortunately, it does not. Physicians no doubt think of their patients as engaged in contests, especially when it is pathogens that cause illness, but they do so in a naive and intuitive manner, with no benefit from formal training in the use of the biological concept of adaptation. Unfortunately also, such casual use of the adaptation idea can lead to serious mistakes from common but erroneous views of what natural selection can or normally does accomplish. People often underestimate the power of this process in optimizing quantitative variables or producing mechanisms of great subtlety and complexity. At the same time, they fail to appreciate its important limitations. It can optimize quantitative aspects of complex mechanisms but cannot generate qualitatively new designs. Thus, it keeps marine mammals swimming by vertical undulations and crocodiles by horizontal ones for purely historical rather than functional reasons. Both are normal for their respective groups, and one way of swimming is as good as the other. Such functional equivalence is not always true; what has evolved need not be as good as what might have evolved. In this essay, some of evolution's impressive accomplishments, and also some functionally arbitrary and dysfunctional features, as manifest in our own species, are briefly discussed.

HUMAN ADAPTATIONS OF MEDICAL INTEREST

"Let nature take its course" is advice often offered to the sick. Physicians have been advised, "Don't just do something, stand there" (Silverman 1993). Either statement implies faith in a high level of competence of evolved adaptations in dealing with the challenge of disease, and doubts about the effectiveness of medical intervent
The evolved adaptations are indeed impress
As a distinguished invertebrate physiologist o
observed, "The cells and organs that make
possible had better be well designed, because
job of living is formidable" (Liles, 1988, p. 13).
was led to this conclusion by a study of the se
ingly easy hydrodynamic problem a clam ha
maintaining a stream of water through its f
filtering apparatus. This is a simple task c
pared to that of meeting medical challen
posed by pathogens or toxins or even minor
chanical injuries. Medical problems can be s
ous, and effective intervention needed, desp
well-designed adaptations. Any infectious
ease is a contest between the host's adaptati
and those of a pathogen. The first thing y
would want to know in viewing such a contes
which of the phenomena (departures from n
malcy) represent the host's adaptations, wh
the pathogen's, and which just incidental con
quences or unavoidable costs (see Table 1). T
observational categories are meant to be qu
general. Any sort of body care behavior wo
probably fit in the first category: avoidance
foods that do not smell quite right, and so on. A
of the great arsenal of host defenses would go
the second category, including the simple m
chanical properties of the human skin. It is
tough armor that is difficult to get through, a
any toxin or incipient infection is soon shed a
result of the constant wearing away of outer e
dermal cells and their replacement from belo
There is an interesting historical question abo
Table 1. When do you think these really eleme
tary and important ideas were first recognize
Early in this century, the complex life histories
many parasites had been worked out, the ger
theory of disease well established for bacteri
and viral infections, and people had known abo
evolution by natural selection for many years.
fact, the ideas used for this table were first e
pressed by Ewald (1980) in a brief article, ar
they are still largely missing from medical educ
tion. As a result, it must undoubtedly be true th

BLE I. *Host and pathogen adaptations and beneficiary of the adaptive process*

SERVATION	EXAMPLES	BENEFICIARY
;ienic behavior	Kill mosquitoes; avoid sick neighbors	Host
st defenses	Fever, sneezing, immune response	Host
)air of damage	Tissue regeneration	Host
mpensation for damage	Chewing on left with tooth pain on right	Host
mage to host	Destruction of infected liver tissue	Neither
st impairment	Reduced detoxification by liver	Neither
ısion of defenses	Molecular mimicry, changing antigens	Pathogen
ack on defenses	Destruction of immune cells by HIV	Pathogen
hogen growth	Higher trypanosome counts	Pathogen
hogen dispersal	Mosquito puts *Plasmodium* into new host	Pathogen
st manipulation	Exaggerated diarrhea (or sneezing?)	Pathogen

er Nesse and Williams, 1994.

ıch of what is called medical treatment is unterproductive for anyone whose main goal is quickest and most reliable victory of host over thogen.

If the pathogen causes a respiratory infection, mptoms are likely to include fever, sore throat, adache, anemia, sneezing, coughing, malaise, d impaired speech. Do any of these abnormales arise from patient adaptations? Yes, all of em, except impaired speech. Pharmaceutical lief of the other symptoms could well delay revery and increase the likelihood of secondary fections. The symptoms are unpleasant, but so e those from a firefighter squirting water on a ɔuse. Most people with burning houses probay recognize that the firefighters are acting in e residents' interest and would not attack them. Iost with respiratory infections do not recognize at fever, iron sequestration, mucus secretions, nd the inactivity favored by pain may speed their covery from the infection.

Consideration of a long list of symptoms is beɔnd the scope of this article. Only fever will be riefly discussed. The defensive importance of a igher temperature has been known since the pineering work of Kluger (1979, 1991). Even coldblooded animals with infections routinely seek warmer habitats to keep their body temperatures higher than they would normally. Infected mammals raise the set point of temperature control, presumably to an optimum based on tradeoffs between the benefits of fever-enhanced defenses and associated metabolic costs and tissue stresses. This sort of optimization is what natural selection is especially good at. Temperature is a continuous variable, the sort of thing that ought to be subject to quantitative genetic variation and continuous facultative control. Selection should normally set such variables at close to ideal values (see Fig. 1).

Random processes such as recombination and drift and mutation are constantly increasing variability, while selection constantly weeds out the extremes and keeps the mean close to the optimum. This is an extremely simplified picture of natural selection, and many complications arise in real life. The distribution of fitness may be asymmetrical, with a deviation in one direction decreasing fitness more than the same deviation in the other direction. This causes interesting effects, medical problems among them. If fever a degree too low might possibly have a much greater cost, such as death, than if it were a degree

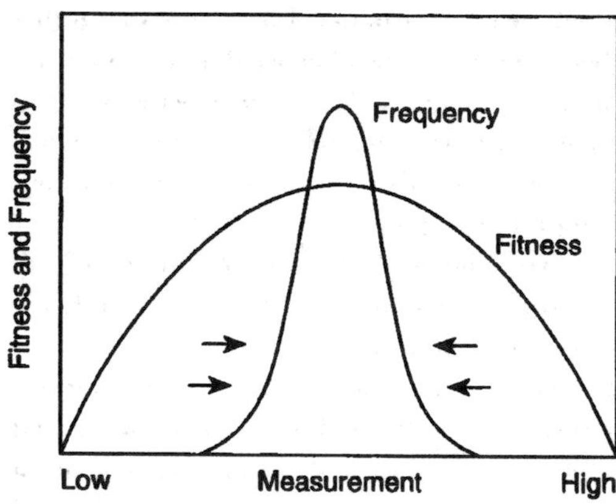

Fig. 1. First-approach model of the action of natural selection on a polygenic quantitative trait, such as body temperature.

too high, the fever-regulating mechanisms should be calibrated so as to make the cheap kind of mistake more often than the expensive. Most real-life fevers might be excessive. Nesse and Williams (1994) have called this the *smoke-detector* principle. Your smoke detector is set to give false alarms more often than it fails to tell you your house is burning down. It should be realized that patients with throat infections are not merely contestants in contests with bacterial or viral pathogens. They are complex entities engaged in many other contests. Freedom from a minor infection must not be purchased at too great a cost to a patient's financial security, success in raising children, or enjoyment of life. It is not the purpose of medicine to uncritically assist patients' biological adaptations. Like all other real-world mechanisms, defenses against pathogens can malfunction, just as a firefighter may spray water on the wrong house. Another serious problem is that host mechanisms are subject to manipulation by pathogens. It might be assumed that the coughing done by a patient may be optimally adjusted for ridding the throat of pathogens, but that need not be true. Perhaps the pathogens depend on that host defense for dispersing propagules to new hosts. Might they not secrete a special stimulant with the ideal molecular configuration for setting off the cough reflex? The cough may then be far more frequent and intense t what would be best for the patient. Amazingly tle research effort has been devoted to possi ties of manipulation by pathogens. What litt known is discussed by Ewald (1994) and N and Williams (1994). If there are such manip tive secretions by pathogens, would it not be w to identify them and devise countermeasure the form of cough syrups or nasal sprays would denature them? More frequent attent to possible mechanisms of manipulation pathogens is one of many examples of import kinds of research that would be stimulated b consistent adaptationist approach to disease, is not likely to occur with concern only for sh term proximate causation.

In fact, an enormous accumulation of kno edge about the adaptations of organisms and human medical adaptations in particular is av able. One of the main intellectual difficult that inhibit the appreciation of these mec nisms is a contempt bred of familiarity. The m velous protection provided by human skin is normally marveled at, but merely taken granted. It is surprising to learn that a person h cancer when what should really surprise us is fact that so many do not. Cancer is merely ce reproducing, what all their ancestral cells have ways done back to the earliest cells billions years ago. Now for the first time they are assign a servile role and called upon to stop dividing, to do so only in the special conditions that enl them for the repair of injury or replacement parts not worth maintaining. Freedom from ca cer is made possible by layer after layer of an cancer mechanisms arrayed so that when o fails another will come into play.

One of the immensely important adaptatio is the immune system, which is, among ma other things, one of the layers of defense again cancer. Incipient maladaptive growths that ha escaped earlier safeguards are attacked by leuc cytes and usually destroyed. The profoundly i teresting aspect of this and related phenomena t such cells know what to attack and what to ve in peace. Basic immunological research ay is largely directed at the question: How s the immune system so reliably conduct war- against enemies and show benign tolerance ard friends? At the moment, the only reliable nclusion is that the answer is much more com- cated than the traditional idea that the im- ne system merely distinguishes self from non- . A related and directly medical question is: ny does the immune system (rarely) make a stake and attack normal human tissue and use autoimmune diseases such as lupus? A re- t of current research is an awareness of the im- nse complexity of the problems that the im- ne system must, and usually does, solve iably.

There is a related problem in the adaptive roles the immunoglobulin-E (IgE) system. This all minority of immune cells triggers local nergencies by releasing stimulants for other lls. The result is local inflammation and in- eased activity by other immune cells. The main oblem is that, in modern societies at least, IgE lls seem to have no function other than causing ergy. Here is an elaborate cellular mechanism parently evolved to punish arbitrarily selected ople for using some common laundry deter- nt or inhaling during August. Substances re- ased by a pollen grain have no effect on most ople but trigger emergency measures in a few.

This is a common kind of adaptationist prob- m: an organism sports a complex mechanism r which evolutionary theory would predict pid degeneration and loss if it were not making important contribution to fitness. Yet it is not vious what this contribution might be. When ch a problem arises in a field steeped in Dar- inism, for instance in ichthyology, it stimulates vigorous effort to answer the question: What is is mechanism for? Thus ichthyologists were otivated to identify the normal function of the mpullae of Lorenzini in the noses of sharks. uch complex and reliably developed organs ust be good for something, and after a number of false leads researchers finally discovered that they were amazingly effective devices for detecting exceedingly weak electrical fields, such as emanate from the heartbeat and gill aeration of a flounder hidden in the sand (Bone, Marshall, and Blaxter, 1995).

What is the medical research community's reaction to the question: What good is the IgE system? Widespread apathy! A few immunologists have noted that the IgE system sometimes reacts to secretions of attached ectoparasites or internal helminthes, and suggested that IgE cells are a defensive response to such parasites (Capron and Dessaint, 1990). The rapid increase in allergy in recent years is perhaps attributable to the extraordinary freedom from such parasites. The IgE system, having nothing else to do, triggers reactions to innocent substances instead of the missing worms and lice.

The most serious attempt to explain the existence of IgE cells is that of Profet (1991), who is very much outside the medical establishment. She criticized the antiparasite idea and proposed that IgE is a backup defense against environmental toxins, especially those elaborated by plants to discourage herbivores. There is an impressive array of detoxification enzymes that enabled our ancestors to manipulate vegetation and to eat a limited quantity of a selection of wild plant products. This detoxification system, like all other real-world mechanisms, is not likely to be uniform or perfect. Some individuals may be genetically deficient in some key enzyme, and exposure to a toxin that most people can handle effectively is potentially harmful to the genetically deprived minority. For them, the IgE system steps in and invokes backup defenses (sneezing, diarrhea, epidermal eruptions, and other adaptive abnormalities) to get rid of the toxin mechanically rather than by the more common chemical denaturation. Profet (1991) supported her theory with an extensive review of published evidence. Although worthy of serious consideration, the explanation is no more convincing than the antiparasite theory. Neither pollen chemistry nor human detoxification capabilities have changed much during this century. Something environmental must have changed to account for the allergy increase, and a search for this cause must become a major concern of the medical research community. The immune system is of central importance in medicine, but obviously just one of a long list of human adaptations, any one of which would have been worthy of lengthy discussion. For support of this proposition, take note that you have been living for a long time and perhaps expect to go on doing so through the near future. Try making a list of the absolutely essential items of bodily machinery on which your everyday life depends. The fact that you continue to live is a magnificent accomplishment. In Liles' (1988) terminology, you are, indeed, well designed.

THE STUPIDITY OF THE BODY

In 1932, Canon published his classic work, *The Wisdom of the Body.* It was an adaptationist treatment of human physiology and emphasized the concept of *homeostasis,* the control of the internal environment's temperature and its ionic and chemical composition, despite great fluctuations in the external environment. The immune system, discussed above, is very much a part of the machinery that maintains this internal control. The validity of Canon's argument, and of his use of the term *Wisdom,* and of Liles' (1988) point that the body is well designed is accepted. I will now consider a few of the many ways in which the design is functionally stupid as a result of its production by the shortsighted, trial-and-error process of natural selection rather than by rational planning. There are many ways in which normalcy can be a serious handicap.

For a start, the normal human skeleton has many dysfunctional features. Note the ring of bone that forms the pelvis. In order to get born, most people had to squeeze through that space. Various nerves, tendons, and blood vessels, the wall of the vagina, and the exits to the digestive and excretory systems all crowd through that sa narrow ring of bone. For purely historical reas in vertebrates, the exits to all these systems through a bony pelvic ring, but for most the plenty of room. A fish egg is typically about a limeter in diameter, and even in mammals n newborns are proportionately smaller tha full-term human infant and have much sma heads. The narrowness of this passage relate the need to keep the pelvis effective for the b and muscle attachments for operating the and trunk, and the resulting narrowness of birth passage may account for the really ea stage of development at which human birth m take place.

The normal routing of the human vagina is functionally explicable. Functionally, the vagi should exit above the pubic symphysis, where viously there is plenty of room. The routing of vagina has a historical, not a functional exp nation. It is a legacy of an evolutionary devel ment in the remote past that was no doubt ad tive for the circumstances of the time. Now burdens us with a more difficult birthing proc than if evolution were guided by something b ter than short-term trial and error. There can b traumatic surgical fix for this evolutionary m take (i.e., cesarean birth) and the fix is sometim worth the trauma.

The male reproductive system likewise has d sign flaws, and one example is the relationsh between sperm ducts and ureters. The testic moved from well forward in the abdomen to ever more posterior position and, in most ma mals, ended up in an external scrotum. This tr took the testicles ever closer to the point at whic their products exit the body. So shorter tubin you might think, would be needed to convey th semen. If so it is because you are being functio ally rational, not evolutionary. The testicles ju happened to go dorsal to the ureters, which dra the kidneys into the bladder, even though th sperm ducts went ventral to them (see Fig. 2 The reproductive tubing got hung up on that the excretory system, and as the testicles move closer to the exit, the tubing had to get longer er than shorter. This is a clear illustration of short-sightedness of the evolutionary process. he last example is the rather different one of tionally onerous limitations on numbers of s. An ancient commitment to bilateral sym- ry limited many structures to even numbers, minimum being a single pair. We have 26 eight premolars, four limbs, two eyes, and ears. Some of these are serious constraints on tive evolution. Two eyes are surely better one; they permit stereoscopic vision that s us three-dimensional information about by objects, but that capability is achieved by ificing the breadth of our visual fields. Most ebrates have the eyes more towards the side of head, so that they have a wider range of pe- eral vision, but less stereoscopic capability. h three eyes we could have more of both ad- tages. We could have stereoscopic vision of t lies ahead and also check on what may be king up behind. Likewise, having two ears bles us to tell the horizontal direction of a nd source, but three would be better. We ht have better vertical directional sense and ld theoretically analyze not only the direction the curvature of soundwaves. This would pro- valuable distance cues. We could hear in e dimensions, rather than just two.

eing restricted to four limbs must give verte- es a serious disadvantage compared to in- s. A preying mantis uses its first pair of limbs eapons for seizing prey, but can still perform e adequate four-footed locomotion. And then e are the insects' two pairs of wings. Think of seriously constrained birds are. Having con- ed one pair of limbs into wings, they have to gate many other jobs to the one remaining . A hawk or owl has to grab prey with its hind . Artists in many cultures throughout history e been smarter than evolution and have not mitted to the constraint of four-limbed nor- cy. Angels have big bird-like wings in addi- to human arms and legs! Then there are cen- s, with perfectly human torsos with arms and

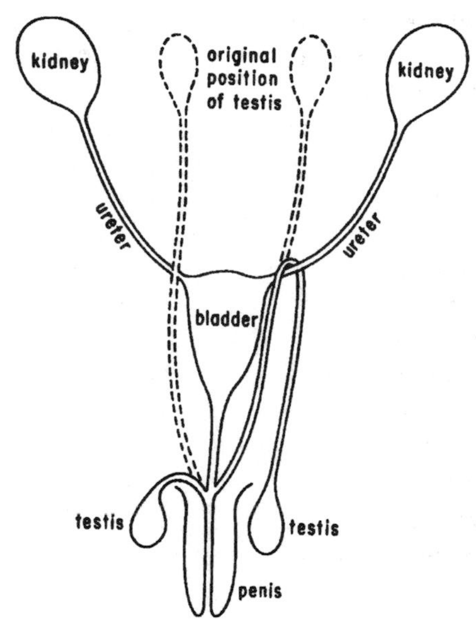

Fig. 2. Diagrammatic representation of the human male reproductive system, as it logically ought to be (left), and as it really is (right).

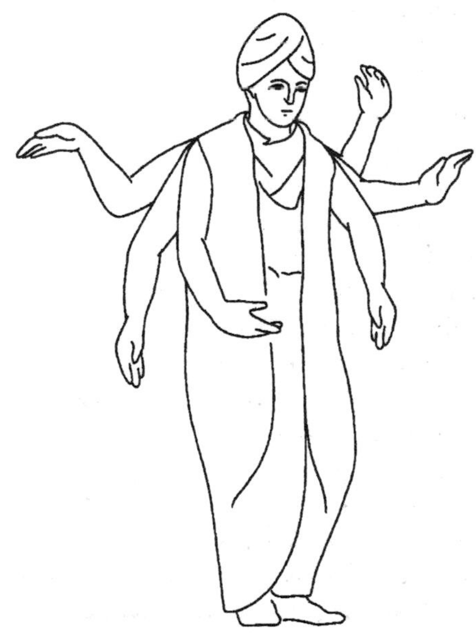

Fig. 3. The Indian god Vishnu, who is not cursed with human normalcy.

hands, but with four hooves on which to gallop. The multiple-armed Hindu deities are a favorite example (see Fig. 3). Imagine having the manipulative capabilities of the god Vishnu at one of those stand-up parties where you have a plate of food in one hand and a glass of wine in the other. You could use your third and fourth to operate a knife and fork and maybe hold a cup of coffee with your fifth and keep the other for eloquent gestures in your conversations. Unfortunately none of this is possible as long as we retain our human normalcy.

REFERENCES

Bone, Q., N. B. Marshall, and J. H. S. Blaxter. 1995. *Biology of Fishes.* 2nd ed. London: Blackie Academic & Professional.

Capron, A., and J.-P. Dessaint. 1990. "From Protective Immunity to Allergy: The Cellular Partners of IgE." *Chem Immunol* 49:236–44.

Ewald, P. W. 1980. "Evolutionary Biology and the Treatment of Signs and Symptoms of Infectious ease." *J Theor Biol* 86:169–76.

———. 1994. *Evolution of Infectious Disease.* ford: Oxford University Press.

Haig, D. 1993. "Genetic Conflicts in Human P nancy." *Q R Biol* 68:495–632.

Kluger, M. J. 1979. *Fever, Its Biology, Evolution, Function.* Princeton, N.J.: Princeton University P

———. 1991. "The Adaptive Value of Fever." In Mackowiac, editor. *Fever: Basic Mechanisms and M agement.* New York: Raven Press, pp. 105–24.

Liles, G. 1988. "Why Is Life So Complex?" *M Science* 3:9–13.

Nesse, R. M., and G. C. Williams. 1994. *Evolu and Healing: The New Science of Darwinian Medic* London: Weidenfeld & Nichoson. [Published as W *We Get Sick.* New York: Times Books, 1995.]

Profet, M. 1991. "The Function of Allergy: munological Defense against Toxins." *Q Rev B* 66:23–62.

Silverman, W. A. 1993. "Doing More Good Th Harm." *Ann N Y Acad Sci* 703:5–11.

CHAPTER 23

The Concept of Genetic Disease

DAVID MAGNUS

AT A VERY BASIC LEVEL, concepts of disease (and health) are important. They tell us something about what sorts of things we believe should be treated, what the goals of medicine are, and what values we hold about various states and conditions. As we shall see, our concepts can carry important commitments that have policy implications. As Caplan has claimed

It may strain credulity to believe that the analysis of concepts such as "health," "disease" or "normality" can shed light on the ethical and policy issues associated with the vast amounts of new knowledge being generated by the human genome project and related inquiries in biomedicine. However, credulity must be strained. The focus of attention *qua* philosophy tends to be on who owns the

> genome or whether an insurance company can boot you off the rolls if you are at risk of succumbing to a costly disease. But this is not really where the ethical and philosophical action is with respect to the ongoing revolution in genetics. (Caplan 1992, 128)

The concept of "genetic disease" is doubly difficult. Not only does it have the difficulties that seem to be inherent with deciding what is meant by labeling something a "disease," but the additional difficulties of selecting which diseases will count as "genetic." In light of the various meanings of "gene" and "genetic" that have occurred, it will be unsurprising that the meaning of "genetic disease" is a complex one.

Before launching into the meaning of genetic disease, it will be helpful to review briefly the most prominent perspectives on the meaning of "disease." There are essentially two approaches to disease. One approach claims simply that diseases are ontologically real entities that can be identified without appeal to values. This view is best exemplified by diseases that are identified with specific, particular pathogens. The alternative view claims that the concept of disease is inherently normative. Diseases are socially constructed and reflect our social values. The concept of genetic disease brings up these issues and more. The status of genetic disease (real or constructed) will depend on the meaning of the concept and how it is used.

COMPETING CONCEPTS OF GENETIC DISEASE

What does it mean to call something a "genetic" disease? It is clear that at least part of that judgment rests on some kind of causal assessment. If a disease is genetic, it is caused by one or more of an organism's genes. Indeed, this seems to fit a more general concept of disease, in which the causal basis of disease is incorporated into our nosologies. As Richard Hull has explained, "In its efforts to understand, control, and avoid dis modern medicine has incorporated into the identification of a disease the notion of the c of the syndrome. This permits the individua of similar syndromes with distinct causes int ferent diseases" (1979, 61).

There is a fairly obvious problem with this way of distinguishing between genetic and ep netic diseases. That is because there are ger and nongenetic factors that are causally rele to every trait, a fact recognized by virtuall commentators on the concept of genetic dis (see, e.g., Gifford 1990; Hull 1979). So the issue in deciding that something is a genetic ease, is whether the causal factors that are ger are the most important causes. I will call this "selection problem." How do we decide whe genetic factors or environmental factors are n important in the production of various disea In response to the selection problem, a num of solutions have been proposed. These ca grouped into a few major categories.

One approach is to try to tease out a notio genes as "direct" causes of disease. Gifford (1 tries to capture this notion in one of his two nitions: "The trait must be the specific effe some genetic cause, that the trait must be scribed or individuated in such a way that properly matched to what the gene causes cifically" (1990, 329). This approach, howe seems hopeless in the face of the actual comp ity of development. Quite simply, this defini probably does not identify any diseases or t as "genetic." As Smith has argued, "Gene not directly cause anything of immediate ph typic significance" (1990, 338). If this approa abandoned—and I am giving it short shrift cause it seems impossible to develop a work notion of genes directly causing effects—t are still several other ways of solving the selec problem.

Perhaps the most obvious and promising proach is to try a statistical approach. A num of variants on this have been attempted.

st straightforward statement of a statistical inition makes its virtues clear. Again, Gifford ers a clear explication: "The first and central se of 'genetic' is this: a trait is genetic if genetic *erences* in a given population account for phenotypic *differences* in the trait-variable ongst members of that population" (1990). is seems to exactly capture at least something portant about our concept of genetic disease. an be put perhaps more precisely in terms of variance. When we pick out some trait as genetic, we are claiming that, in that population, covariance of the trait with some genetic fac(s) is greater than the covariance of the trait th other (nongenetic) factors. This solves the ection problem neatly by allowing us to pick t which causal factors are irrelevant (the ones at are fixed) and highlight the important ones e ones that *make the difference*). In one of the nonical examples of causality, we are inclined say that the lighting of a match (under normal cumstances) was the cause of the fire, whereas e presence of oxygen (while a contributing usal factor) was not. In contrast, in an environent where fire was normally present and oxyn was not, we might well pick out the (unusual) esence of oxygen as the cause of a fire.

There are several advantages to this approach the selection problem. First, it corresponds the use of analysis of variance that is used by ologists to measure the causal contribution of reditary and environmental factors in a population. Second, it is capable of clear explication. hird, it has at least some intuitive support. onetheless, it is inadequate as analysis of common usage of the concept of genetic disease. here are several problems.

First, as Sober (1988) has pointed out, an analys in terms of variance only applies to populaons, not individuals. Yet in the case of disease, it typically the individual that we are concerned ith. Indeed, a nominalist position is sometimes eld toward disease states—there are no diseases, nly sick patients. Though nominalism presents a general problem for the concept of genetic disease, it is especially problematic for a statistical approach to defining genetic disease.

A perhaps more serious problem can be brought out by the following example. Suppose a significant portion (say 50 percent) of the people in a village suddenly become violently ill with cramping, diarrhea, and subsequent dehydration problems. A team of health experts and scientists are dispatched to the area to determine the cause. In the end, it is discovered that the water supply for the village has been contaminated. It is clear that we would be likely to identify the contaminated supply water (or the contaminant) as the cause of the disease. But note that, even though 100 percent of the villagers were exposed to the water, only 50 percent became ill. If this is because of genetic factors that make some of the villagers more resistant to this particular pathogen, then the statistical analysis will give the wrong solution to the selection problem. The covariance of the genetic factors with the disease in the village may be close to 1, while the covariance between the disease and the presence of the pathogen is 0.5.

One way of defending this type of analysis would be to claim that it is a mistake to identify the population in the analysis with the villagers. If the population was taken to be the entire planet, or other nearby villages, the analysis in terms of variance might work. Indeed, Hesslow (1983, 1984) has argued that all claims that pick out one among many causes as "the most important" must do so by implicitly referring to a contrast class. These contrasts can vary quite widely, but there is always a way of identifying a population within which it really is the desired causal factor that "makes the difference."

This defense is clearly inadequate. The original selection problem was deciding the grounds upon which one cause from many could be picked out as most important. At best, this new approach pushes the problem back a level; instead of having to select among causes, we now have to select among populations or contrast classes. If we take the relevant population to be the village, the statistical approach would define our hypothetical disease as genetic. If we take a population with healthy people who are not exposed to the same pathogen as the contrast, it is the pathogen that is the cause of the illness. In fact, something more fundamental is missed by this analysis. In this case, our hypothetical team of medical experts and scientists could not, in advance, tell what population would be relevant for the statistical analysis to work. Presumably, in a village where roughly half the members became ill, trying to find out what the difference was between those in the village who were ill and those who were not is a plausible initial approach to take. It is only after it is discovered that the water contains a pathogen (and it is identified as the cause) that the defender of the statistical approach would be able to appeal to a broader population that would salvage the analysis.

The shortcomings of the statistical approach to the selection problem point to another solution that has been proposed. The reason that we are inclined to identify the most important cause of the illness in the village as the water-borne pathogen is because it is the obvious locus of activity with respect to eliminating the problem. Collingwood (1940) has claimed on quite general grounds that the way we pick out the most important cause is in terms of the manipulability of the various factors. Whatever the general virtues of this approach, it is promising when it comes to medicine. In the natural sciences, it could be argued that there is a strong interest in prediction and explanation. In contrast, it has been argued that the medical realm is more concerned with the prevention and treatment of disease than with explanation (Engelhardt 1984; Wulf 1984). Instrumentalist interests play a much more central role in medical practice than in science. Hence, the appropriate solution to the selection problem can be formulated in terms of manipulability. The most important cause is the one that is identi as the most easily manipulated to prevent or t disease. A disease is genetic if it is genes that p this role and epigenetic if it is nongenetic fac that are most easily manipulated.

Like the statistical definition, the manip bility definition captures something import about our usage of the term. In addition, i often an implicit aspect of the justification for extension of the concept of genetic disease new cases (see Englehardt 1981, 14). There a however, some problems with this approach well. The obvious problem seems to be that this analysis, no disease could be classified as netic. After all, it is not clear that any gene th apy has been successful, and there is no thera for many of the paradigm examples of genetic d ease (such as Huntington's disease [HD]).

This criticism is perhaps unfair. Althou gene therapy is lagging far behind, the techn ogy that perhaps most exemplifies the gene zation of medicine is genetic testing. The hu fights over patent rights and the race to devel test procedures are already having an impact the way medicine is practiced. And genetic te ing *can* provide a basis for the prevention of d ease. It is at least possible for someone at risk avoid bringing a child with HD into the wor Although testing and abortion may seem li a crude preventative measure, it is also an i creasingly important one to many prospecti parents. Moreover, as we shall see, there is an i portant historical connection between gene testing and selection as a therapeutic approa and the development of the concept of gene disease.

Even if we accept this defense, the manipu bility approach will not work. Many of the par digm genetic diseases (phenylketonuria [PKU or cystic fibrosis [CF]) involve treatments th are not molecular. Indeed, in the case of PK the standard treatment involves a change in die At the same time, the tests for PKU were deve d before the actual mutation responsible for disease had been identified. It is impossible to ere to the manipulability definition and ac- ot that PKU is a genetic disease. This seems to a fatal flaw in the manipulability definition. In lition, it is not true that biomedical science is ays instrumentally oriented. A great deal of ef- t is aimed not just at treating and preventing ease, but also at understanding it. This may d to a conflict over which causal factor is most portant—the factor most easily manipulated treating or preventing a disease may not be the ost revealing for our interests in understanding isease.

It is worth noting that both the statistical ap- oaches and the manipulability approaches em to imply a relativity in the concept of ge- tic disease. In the case of the statistical notion, nething will or will not count as a genetic dis- se depending on the population it is a part of. e manipulability definition implies that tech- logical advances will affect what counts as a netic disease as the "reach" of our technology extended. Yet, this result seems to be incom- tible with an ontological conception of dis- se. If diseases are real entities (and indepen- nt of values), the solution to the selection oblem should not depend on factors outside of e organism (Boorse 1981). Thus, the norma- ist or constructivist position on disease seems be supported by these analyses (however inad- uate they are as a general account).

All analyses of the concept fail in the end. here is no general solution to the selection oblem. This is not just a function of the limita- on of conceptual analysis. It reflects the fact that its core there are conflicting aspects of the sage of the concept. Moreover, all of these ap- roaches are essentially static. They are not ade- uate precisely because the concept of genetic isease changes over time and is used differently y different actors—something that would not be ossible if any of these analyses were correct.

THE HISTORICAL DEVELOPMENT OF THE CONCEPT OF GENETIC DISEASE

The concept of genetic disease has passed through many stages, just as the concept of the "gene" has. Before the twentieth century, people understood the idea of diseases running in families; by the late nineteenth century several had been identified and named (e.g., HD). In the early decades of the twentieth century, Mendelism gave a new meaning to the concept of genetic disease. A disease was genetic if it was inherited and followed a Mendelian pattern. Many genetic diseases became exemplars that would last until today, including HD, CF, and PKU. There were attempts to put much more complex traits into the simple structure of the two alleles at a single locus—particularly egregious was the work of many eugenicists; however, the results of these attempts failed to stand up to the test of time. By the 1930s, the earliest work on genetics—by scientists such as C. B. Davenport—had been exposed to serious criticism, while the work on the exemplars survived (Paul 1999; Kevles 1998; Allen 1986). By the middle of the twentieth century, the general molecularization of biology that had begun to take place allowed for a link between the Mendelian concept of genetic disease and the new molecular understanding of the pathways responsible for traits. The "golden spike" turned out to be sickle cell anemia (Strasser 1999; Conley 1980). Indeed, historians have identified the 1949 paper by Pauling et al. ("Sickle Cell Anemia: A Molecular Disease") as the first clear identification of a genetic disease, in the modern sense. That article pointed the way toward the second concept of genetic disease. This concept tied the Mendelian concept to an understanding of the molecular basis of the disease, and raised the hope of an eventual identification of the underlying structure, which eventually came to be understood as the particular set of DNA sequences associated with the disease. This new conception made use of the same exemplars as the Mendelian conception. But, now, we would strive to understand the underlying mechanisms and eventually identify the sequences seen as responsible for HD, CF, and PKU as well as other easily identifiable "Mendelian" diseases, though these projects were not to be completed for several decades. At the same time, Pauling et al. (1949) identified several ways in which the identification of the disease as genetic could be useful for therapeutic and preventive purposes. This partly involved foreseeing a future in which genetic knowledge could lead to direct therapies, but especially appealed to eugenic methods (or, in less-charged language, genetic counseling) to prevent the occurrence of disease. Thus, genetic testing would be the principal therapeutic outcome, at least initially.[1]

By the 1960s several things had changed. One development was the restriction of the cultural importance of genetics as determinants of who people are and what they do (Keller 2000; Nelkin and Lindee 1995). This helped to reinforce the exemplars within a narrow conception of genetic disease. At the same time, developments in the clinical setting were already setting the stage for an expansion of the concept. The development of tests for chromosomal abnormalities was often carried out by geneticists and helped create a new medical specialty in clinical genetics (Coventry and Pickstone 1999). It should be noted, however, that these diseases and disorders were often congenital, rather than inherited. This was the first hint of a significant expansion in the concept, though the only implication at the time was a bifurcated notion of genetic disease—the exemplars, plus the chromosomal abnormalities identified by testing by clinical geneticists.

During the 1970s and 1980s, the gene again became the unit of choice for explaining more and more of who we are and what we do. The genome became the "holy grail" for our culture (Keller 2000; Nelkin and Lindee 1995). As part of process the concept of genetic disease bega change. Although the broader cultural and so changes are a significant part of the story, th was also an accumulation of information on heritable contribution to traits and diseases were much more complex than the simple emplar genetic diseases. The expansion initi included traits such as diabetes and gout (Ed 1984). It was fairly clear that there was a sigr cant genetic component to these diseases, they were likely influenced by many genes, a there was far less than 100 percent penetrance well as a strong environmental component). T increasing enthusiasm for genetic explanatio eventually gave rise to an expanding conce even when it was less clear that there was good idence for the heritability of a disease. Just as telligence came to be seen by many as a gene trait, so too did alcoholism, schizophrenia, a other behavioral "diseases" (Edlin 1984). T medicalization of many traits into diseases a contributed to this expansion (Caplan, Eng hardt, and McCartney 1981).

More recently, several developments ha given rise to a new expansion of the concept genetic disease. First, there is the growing sen that genes are always relevant to what happe When exposed to the same pathogens, some pe ple get sick and others do not. That is in pa a function of their genetic makeup. As was not in the last section, there is a sense in whi genes are *always* causally relevant. This conce tual point has come to be seen as very significa by clinicians, scientists, and the public. As redu tionism has gained cultural and scientific dom nance, the claim that genes are causally releva is transformed into the claim that genes are central explanatory importance (Juengst 2000 Second, there has been an increase in our un derstanding of the role of different genes in *no inherited* diseases. This has been particularly no ticeable in cancer research, where a tremendou amount is now known about the role that variou es play in (often environmentally induced) eases. And third, the hope and promise of gene rapy is influencing the way we look at genetic ease. The gene therapies that are among the st promising in terms of their likely impact on dicine are those that are aimed at noninher- l diseases (again, most notably, cancer). These rapies involve ways of genetically manipulat- cells so that they are targeted for destruction, ier by the immune system, or by other, com- mentary drugs. Many scientists and clinicians licitly appeal to the manipulability definition discussing the implications of the develop- nt of these therapies.[2] They claim that these rapies show that these diseases are genetic. er all, if the key to treating a disease turns out be a gene therapy, then it is a genetic disease.

These three developments have expanded the ncept of genetic disease in important ways. st, the concept is becoming disentangled from earlier tie to heredity. A disease does not have be inherited to be genetic. There are refer ces to environmentally caused, genetic dis- ses. Cancer, in particular, has been reconcep- alized to be seen as a genetic disease (even ough it is also acknowledge as often caused by vironmental or behavioral factors). Second, e concept of genetic disease has greatly ex- nded. The combination of disentangling the ncept from any notion of heredity and the re- ictionist move toward seeing any causal rele- nce as establishing a disease as genetic results a complete transformation of our categories. irtually all disease becomes genetic disease. In- eed, a host of prominent scientists, clinicians, nd journalists have concluded that "all disease genetic disease" (Magnus 2001; Juengst 2000). his expansion of the concept of genetic disease xplicitly ties together issues of understanding nd treating disease. Francis Collins, director of e Human Genome Project, has claimed, "Be- ond the development of new genetic tests and eatment strategies, my long-term dream is for cientists to figure out how diseases work and cure them in advance. In two or three decades, we hope to be able to find out what genetic disease a person is at risk for and fix it by putting in a gene that has the appropriate sequence" (see also Juengst 2000; Caskey 1992; Baird 1990).

A REEXAMINATION OF THE EXEMPLARS

At the same time that the role genes play in noninherited disorders is being elucidated, much more information about the exemplar genetic diseases is coming to light. The result of this work is rather surprising. The advantage of the exemplars was their simplicity. They seemed to be straightforward diseases, with 100 percent penetrance. Yet increased study of CF and HD has yielded surprising complexity. In the case of CF, rather than a single mutation, there are perhaps hundreds of mutations that can produce the disease. Moreover, some of these mutations appear to have far less severe effects than other mutations. And some of these "mild" mutations appear to be dominant over "severe" mutations. Further complicating the picture is the discovery of individuals who are homozygous for the most common (and lethal) mutation (DF508), who do test positive on a sweat chloride test ("the gold standard"), but who nonetheless exhibit few or none of the symptoms of CF. What all of this means is unclear. But it seems to follow that CF is not 100 percent penetrant, that there is no one sequence that is the allele for CF, and that environmental factors (including perhaps other genes) play some role in the expression of CF. Similarly, our understanding of HD is much more complicated. The discovery that HD results from too many CAG repeats in a section of chromosome 4 would seem on its surface to fit the traditional model of genetic disease envisioned by Pauling et al. (1949). Yet there have been some surprising developments. Individuals with more than forty CAG repeats all seem to come down with the dreaded, fatal disease (if they live long enough). Most people have fewer than thirty CAG repeats and never show any symptoms of HD. But, in individuals with between thirty and forty CAG repeats, it is not clear whether they will develop the disease or not (nor even what the chances are). So a disease that was previously thought to be 100 percent penetrant, with no gray area, now has a gray area. Moreover, there is speculation that the fewer than thirty CAG repeats that most people carry may well produce HD if people lived long enough. The difference is that the age at onset is beyond a human life span. But if that is true, there is a sense in which we all have HD—and the meaning of the disease becomes unclear.

The implication of this work is that diseases that seemed to be very simple when we did not know much about their genetic basis have turned out to be much more complicated. HD and CF have been exemplars of genetic diseases for decades. Yet the textbook stories about these diseases are inadequate. And the more we learn about these diseases, the more we discover room for epigenetic factors in the production of the phenotypes even in the case of paradigm genetic diseases.

THE USES OF THE CONCEPT OF GENETIC DISEASE

In light of both the changing nature of the concept of genetic disease and the failure of any conceptual analysis to yield a definitive explication that is descriptively adequate, it is important to consider the way the concept is used and what assumptions are being made in that usage. In view of the fact that both genetic factors and epigenetic factors are nearly always relevant, what does it mean when someone identifies a disease as genetic? "The application of the term 'genetic' reflects a choice having been made to emphasize, among the causal factors, the genetic component and de-emphasize the environmental one" (Hull 1979, 59).

The fact that the competing analyses of
concept of genetic disease seem to imply a r
tivity that is incompatible with an ontolog
view of disease supports a normative approac
disease. Thus, we would be well served by c
sidering the values inherent in the classificati
that are adopted, both now and in the past.
though the therapeutic value of genetic in
vention is often appealed to as a justification
clinicians and scientists—and hence an impl
endorsement of the manipulability definitior
genetic disease—it may be more insightful to
the situation the other way around. By examin
the classification system and the language u
by contemporary biomedicine we can see
commitments of practitioners to certain ways
gaining knowledge, and treating and preventi
disease. In essence, labeling a disease as "
netic" is to make an implicit claim that, for t
disease, understanding and therapy will b
come about through research at the gene
level. In other words, smuggled into the very co
ceptual classification is a set of commitme
about the best way to allocate resources and t
best way to do good science and medicine. T
commitment to a reductionist approach to me
cine would not be objectionable if it represent
the best way to achieve the goals of biomedic
science. But there is little or no evidence that th
is the case. In fact, very little empirical researc
is done to examine the success of various a
proaches to biomedical practice and what the
influence is (e.g., on the health of populations
Yet, in the absence of such evidence the expa
sion of the concept of genetic disease represen
an unjustified commitment. "[T]he strong em
phasis on genes and heredity in disorders suc
as allergies, sociopathy, suicide, alcoholism, d
pression, obesity and others is both scientifical
unjustified and ethically questionable. More
over, the increased overemphasis on 'genetic fa
tors' and 'genetic tendencies' in human disorde
has serious consequences in allocating federal r
search funds and in formulating public healt
policies" (Edlin 1984, 48).

There are several ways in which this focus on etic determinants of health is important. First, ndicated, there is an influence on allocation research dollars. "To build one causal factor o the very conception of a disease and thereby prefer one causal hypothesis over others is to ite stagnation of research and treatment and tortion of funding priorities" (Hull 1979, 64). Second, it seems to follow that education eds to be altered. As Collins claimed (shortly er distributing a promissory note on how derstanding the genetic basis of disease will nsform medicine), "Unfortunately, medical ining is lagging far behind these scientific vances. Most medical schools are not yet phasizing the genetics courses so vital to medl education, and many physicians in practice day have had no genetics training at all. This uation will have to change dramatically if medl science is to keep up with and make use of e rapid and extremely valuable discoveries that n affect so many lives" (Collins 1999, 000).

Third, the classification of a disease as genetic n have an influence on the public health polies we develop. As agencies such as the Centers r Disease Control struggle to develop a genetic blic health policy, which diseases fall within e purview of the policy is likely to be determined by the language we use. A genetic disease ems to require a genetic policy.

Fourth, the identification of diseases with their uses and identifying genes as the causes of disase seem to imply that to have a certain gene .g., for HD, CF or breast cancer) is to have the sease. Thus, even healthy (presymptomatic) atients will become "diseased" on this analysis. his move is being hotly contested by different atient advocacy groups, but the dominant coneptualization of disease seems to require the exansion of the diseased population as it expands e concept of genetic disease (Juengst 2000). It is kely that we are all genetically diseased.

In each of these considerations, what is missng is adequate recognition of the important role hat nongenetic factors play in disease. What is needed is more empirical evidence that could be brought to bear on deciding exactly which areas of research and which diseases would be most profitably treated as genetic and as nongenetic. And, in the absence of that information, we should recognize that every genetic disease—which may be all disease—is also an epigenetic disease.

NOTES

1. It is worth noting that genetic testing in this sense could not have required the identification of the DNA sequence. Ambiguity in the concept of genetic testing mirrors ambiguity in the concepts of genetic disease and the concept of a gene. This ambiguity in the case of testing is particularly troubling for legislation dealing with discrimination by insurance companies and employers on the basis of genetic testing. Different states define the concept very differently and it is often left vague. See Magnus (2001).

2. Sometimes this appeal is straightforward. Khoury (2003) has argued that the range of impact of genetic technology will change our conception of genetic disease. Sometimes the appeal to manipulability is more subtle, emphasizing both the central role that genes play, and how that will lead to (often unspecified) changes in the way we treat disease. See, e.g., Collins (1999).

REFERENCES

Allen, G. E. 1986. "The Eugenics Record Office at Cold Spring Harbor, 1910–1940: An Essay in Institutional History." *OSIRIS* 2nd series vol. 2: 225–64.

Baird, Patricia. 1990. "Genetics and Health Care: A Paradigm Shift." *Perspectives in Biology and Medicine* 33: 203–13.

Boorse, Christopher. 1981. "On the Distinction of Disease and Illness." In *Concepts of Health and Disease: Interdisciplinary Perspectives.* Edited by Arthur Caplan, H. Tristram Engelhardt, Jr., and James J. McCartney. Reading, Mass.: Addison-Wesley.

Caplan, Arthur. 1992. "If Gene Therapy Is the Cure, What Is the Disease?" In *Gene Mapping: Using*

Law and Ethics as Guides, edited by George J. Annas and Sherman Elias. New York: Oxford University Press, 128–41.

Caplan, Arthur, H. Tristram Engelhardt, Jr., and James J. McCartney, eds. 1981. *Concepts of Health and Disease: Interdisciplinary Perspectives.* Reading, Mass.: Addison-Wesley.

Caskey, C. Thomas. 1992. "DNA-Based Medicine in the Twenty-First Century." In *The Code of Codes*, edited by Daniel Kelves and Leroy Hood. Cambridge, Mass.: Harvard University Press, 112–35.

Collingwood, R. G. 1940. *An Essay on Metaphysics.* Oxford: Clarendon Press.

Collins, F. S. 1999. "Medical and Societal Consequences of the Human Genome Project" (Shattuck Lecture). *New England Journal of Medicine* 341: 28–37.

Conley, C. L. 1980. "Sickle Cell Anemia: The First Molecular Disease." In *Blood, Pure and Eloquent*, edited by M. M. Wintrobe. New York: McGraw-Hill, 319–71.

Coventry, Peter, and John Pickstone. 1999. "From What and Why Did Genetics Emerge as a Medical Specialism in the 1970s in the UK? A Case-History of Research, Policy and Services in the Manchester Region of the NHS." *Social Science and Medicine* 49: 1227–38.

Edlin, G. 1984. *Genetic Principles: Human and Social Consequences.* Boston: Jones and Bartlett.

Engelhardt, Jr., H. Tristram. 1981. "The Concepts of Health and Disease." In *Concepts of Health and Disease: Interdisciplinary Perspectives*, edited by Arthur Caplan, H. Tristram Engelhardt, Jr., and James J. McCartney. Reading, Mass.: Addison-Wesley, 3–31.

Gifford, Fred. 1990. "Genetic Traits." *Biology and Philosophy* 5, no. 3 (July): 327–47.

Hesslow, G. 1984. "What Is a Genetic Disease? On the Relative Importance of Causes." In *Health, Disease, and Causal Explanation in Medicine*, edited by L. Nordernfelt and B. I. B. Lindahl. Dordrecht: Reidel.

———. 1983. "Explaining Differences and Weighting Causes." *Theoria* 49: 87–111.

Hull, Richard. 1979. "Why Genetic Disease?'" In *Genetic Counseling: Facts, Values and Norms*, e by Alexander M. Capron, Marc Lappé, Robert F. ray, Jr., Tabitha M. Powledge, and Sumner B. T New York: National Foundation March of Dimes Defects Original Article Series, 57–69.

Juengst, Eric. 2000. "Concepts of Disease afte Human Genome Project." In *Ethical Issues in He care on the Frontiers of the 21st Century*, edite Steven Wear, James Bono, Gerald Logue, and Ac McEvoy. Philosophy and Medicine Series. Bo Kluwer, 125–52.

Keller, Evelyn Fox. 2000. *The Century of the G* Cambridge, Mass.: Harvard University Press.

Kevles, Daniel. 1998. *In the Name of Euge* Cambridge, Mass.: Harvard University Press.

Khoury, Muin. 2003. "Genetics and Genomi Practice: The Continuum from Genetic Disea Genetic Information in Health and Disease." *Gen in Medicine* 5: 261–68.

Magnus, David. 2001. Review of Peter Beu R. Falk, H.-J. Rheinberger, "The Concept of the C in Development and Evolution." *Journal of the Hi of Biology* 34: 406–07.

Nelkin, Dorothy, and Lindee, M. Susan. 1995. *DNA Mystique.* New York: W. H. Freeman.

Paul, Diane. 1999. *Controlling Human Here 1865 to the Present.* Amherst, N.Y: Humanity Bc

Pauling, Linus, H. Itano, S. J. Singer, and Wells. 1949. "Sickle Cell Anemia: A Molecular ease." *Science* 110: 543–48.

Smith, K. 1990. "Genetic Disease, Genetic Tes and the Clinician." *MSJAMA* 285: 327–47.

Sober, Elliott. 1988. "Apportioning Causal Res sibility." *Journal of Philosophy* 85, no. 6 (June): 30

Strasser, B. J. 1999. "Sickle Cell Anemia: A Mol lar Disease." *Science* 268: 1488–90.

Wulff, Henrik. 1984. "The Causal Basis of the rent Disease Classification." In *Health, Disease, Causal Explanation in Medicine*, edited by L. Nord felt and B. I. B. Lindahl. Dordrecht: Reidel, 169

CHAPTER 24

Concepts of Disease after the Human Genome Project

ERIC T. JUENGST

IN AN ARTICLE WRITTEN IN 1990 at the awn of the U.S. Human Genome Project, James Watson and Robert ;ook-Deegan wrote something guaranteed to catch the eye of a philoso- her of medicine. They said that "The major impact of the genome proj- ct will be a slow but steady conceptual evolution—a change in the way ıat we think about disease and normal physiology" (Watson and Cook-)eegan, p. 3322). The concepts that frame the way we think about disease nd health, of course, are central to the philosophical task of attempting to larify and explain the dynamics of medical reasoning. They also play im- ortant roles in quite practical matters of health policy and medical prac- ice: significant changes in our disease concepts will affect both what we count as legitimate medical problems and how we assign the social responsibilities and roles that attend such problems. For example, recall the way that the germ theory helped highlight the problem of the infected, but symptomless, "carrier" of disease for turn of the century medicine, and the social authority that problem gave to public health initiatives designed to control the behavior of those cast in the "Typhoid Mary" role (Brandt 1987). If the major effect of the Human Genome Project is going to be a change of this sort, it will be important for both medical epistemology and medical ethics to understand that change as clearly as possible, since both the logic and norms of medicine could show the consequences.

Watson and Cook-Deegan go on to suggest the direction in which they think the Human Genome Project will take our thinking about disease:

> A century ago, a revolution in medicine was in full stride following the discovery of infectious organisms and the dawn of bacteriology. Over the course of the century, the conceptual base of medicine has broadened from gross anatomy of organs to cellular biology to dissection of biochemical pathways. The next step is to study the most fundamental elements in biology—Mendel's hereditary factors, now known as "genes." This will not replace population biology, organismal biology, cellular physiology, or biochemistry, but will supplement them with a new and powerful foundation of knowledge.... Once this foundation is solid, the next stage will be to use the masses of information and new analytical techniques to understand disease and normal biology (Watson and Cooke-Deegan 1990, pp. 3322, 3324).

This is, in fact, a reasonable thumbnail sketch of how many genome scientists see their place in history: as laying the groundwork for the final flowering of the search for "specific causes" of disease that revolutionized medicine a century ago, by focusing our understanding of disease genes and their dynamics.[1] Having made t claim, however, Watson and Cook-Deegan go to describe the Human Genome Project itsel more detail, and leave the conceptual and so implications of their prediction unaddress This poses a challenge for the philosophy of m icine: What might it mean to use our knowle of genes as a new foundation for understand health and disease?

My goal in this essay is to take one first step addressing this challenge, by exploring three s of shorter-range implications of the concept sea-change that Watson and Cook-Deegan fo cast for medicine that one can already detect the medical genetic literature. The first set the implications of what I call "genetic imperi ism": the view that, since genes are foundatio to understanding disease, all diseases are b conceptualized as "genetic diseases." The se ond set are the implications of what I call " netic contagionism": the view that conceptual ing health problems as genetic diseases mea understanding the genes themselves as t specific causes of the problem, much as the ger theory isolated microbes as the pathogens for i fectious disease. The third set are the implic tions of what I call "genetic humoralism": th view that the frank health problems caused genes are also just extreme examples of the influence, which really ranges across the spe trum of human traits from pathological healthy.

To look ahead, my conclusion in examinin these three sets of implications will be that unle we can use genomics to effect a genuine concep tual *revolution* in the way we think about diseas the principal effect of the conceptual *evolutio* that Watson and Cook-Deegan anticipate will b an increase in the incidence of genetic healt problems in our society. Specifically, I argue tha unless we can finally replace two strains of nine teenth-century thinking that still run strong i modern genetic medicine, the doctrine of spe c causation and the tradition of constitutional nology, the principal effect of the Human nome Project may well be that more health blems will be understood as genetic health blems, more people will be identified as sufng from those genetic health problems, and re genetic differences will be reinterpreted as etic health problems. In the next three secns I try to explain each of these overlapping ims in turn, and to point out some of the pracl consequences that each kind of conceptual nge would produce.

GENETIC IMPERIALISM: ARE ALL DISEASES REALLY "GENETIC DISEASES"?

s becoming commonplace for proponents of nome research to point out that, to the extent t all our physiological responses to the envinment and its insults are products of our genes, ll disease is genetic disease," and to back that up th lists of recent findings that suggest that "curnt research in human genetics is providing, at nost a weekly pace, more and more examples the central role that genes play in human alth" (Guyer and Collins 1993, p. 1145). But it one thing to acknowledge that genes constitute rt of the background conditions against which alth problems occur, and another to give them e central role in the process. The former claim true by definition, and does little to threaten edicine's existing nosological taxonomy. The undaries between "infectious diseases," "canrs," and "genetic diseases" can still be procted by the doctrine that amongst all the co-facrs involved in any disease there are identifiable pecific causes" that are more definitive than the st. In the context of this same doctrine, howver, giving genes "the central role" in health and isease makes quite a different claim. It suggests at the genetic influences on the expression of isease should be counted as their specific auses, and that every disease that can be shown to be so influenced should be subsumed into the category of genetic diseases (Hesslow 1984). The result of these reclassifications, of course, is a remarkable increase in the number of diagnoses from this domain, and a corresponding rise in the population incidence of "genetic disease."

It is easy to find the signs of this nosological expansion in the biomedical literature over the last decade. It was forecast in the early discussions of the Human Genome Project by those who argued that the project's main accomplishment would be:

> to markedly increase the number of human diseases that we recognize to have major genetic components. We already understand that genetic diseases are not rare medical curiosities with negligible societal impact, but rather constitute a wide spectrum of both rare and extremely common diseases responsible for an immense amount of suffering in all human societies. The characterization of the human genome will lead to the identification of genetic factors in many more human diseases, even those that now seem to be multifactoral or polygenic for ready understanding (Friedman 1990, p. 413).

At the same time, such "genetic imperialism" was repudiated by those biomedical scientists afraid that the Human Genome Project would divert needed funding from their (non-genomic) research programs (Cook-Deegan 1994), and by philosophers who argued that the genome research simply amounted to "blind reductionism gone too far" (Tauber and Sarkar 1992). By setting out to explicate the ways in which particular genes condition the natural histories of medicine's whole suite of diseases, the critics argued, human genome research would inevitably encourage us to discuss those diseases in genetic terms, regardless of the genes' actual etiologic significance and at the expense of more manipulable causes (Hubbard and Wald 1993; Strohman 1993).

Of course, those exploiting the genetic strategy are quick to admit that the etiologies of most diseases are more complex than simple Mendelian "single gene" disorders; but there is plenty of room within the traditional nosology of medical genetics for "multi-factoral" and "polygenic" disorders as well. More important to successfully annexing new diseases into genetic medicine is to promise the practical benefits of the new orientation for clinical medicine: e. g., to identify the new therapeutic and prophylactic interventions it makes possible. Thus, proponents of genome research argued that, because "the benefits of public health and good nutrition in Western societies have led to a remarkable decrease in those diseases with a primarily external cause," it is time to give attention to the "internal causes" of disease:

> As a society we need to change our view of disease as an outside enemy and find a new way of thinking about illness.... This new way of thinking about what determines health or disease will be fueled by our increasing knowledge in genetics. This is giving us a new concept of cause and pathogenesis of disease and helping to explain the variations seen in particular diagnostic categories by showing interaction of nature and nurture for common diseases. Genetics will increasingly allow us to interfere earlier in the cascade of events leading to overt disease and clinical manifestation (Baird 1990, p. 205).

Thus, most who hail the "new era of molecular medicine" promised by genome research explain their enthusiasm in terms of the clinical purchase that genes might give us on medicine's remaining challenges, simply as a newly visible element of a complicated process. They write that "the ability to detect individuals at risk for a disease prior to any pathologic evidence for the disease theoretically offers medicine a new strategy—anticipation of disease and pre-emptive therapy" (Caskey 1993, p. 48).

Clearly, the clinical benefits of geneticizing disease categories are still mostly promissory. However, that promise is already enough to begin to shift our understanding of diseases like car or Alzheimer Disease to the point that testing their (quite marginal) genetic factors is alre being called both "presymptomatic" and "d nostic," as if their presence were indicative of ease (Caskey 1993; Brandt 1989; Malkin et 1990). In fact, the increasing genetic reorie tion of biomedical research all across the no logical spectrum has already encouraged the rector of the NIH's genome research effort declare a conceptual victory by claiming th

> The Human Genome Project is arguably the s gle most important organized research projec the history of biomedicine. Through this inter tional research effort, we will obtain the sou book for biomedical research in the 21st cent and beyond.... We will gain unprecedented sight into the manifold ways in which organism dysfunction can arise and how this can result disease, and we will elucidate many new ways altering such situations. From this informati will come new therapy and, perhaps more i portant, new strategies for prevention based understanding individual risk and how to avo illness (Guyer and Collins 1993, p. 1145).

The apparent continuing success of gene medicine's conceptual imperialism is a tes ment to the power that Collingwood's "manip lability theory" of causation exerts in medical re soning (Collingwood 1974; Juengst 1993). In th case, just the increasing visibility of genes causal factors, in the wake of genome researc and the sheer promise that their contributio will become the most susceptible (of all th possible causal factors in complex diseases) human control, seems enough to promote the to the status of today's "specific causes" of diseas However, the promotion of genes to the status pathognomic specific causes does have impo tant epistemic and ethical implications.

First of all, casting genes in the role of specifi causes for disease requires disregarding a good b of what genome research is itself teaching u ut genes and their dynamics. In fact, it re-res holding onto a strikingly old-fashioned n of genetic thinking which today is dispar-d as "bean bag genetics." "Beanbag genetics" he epithet that the evolutionary biologist, ıst Mayr, employed to criticize his predeces-s' interpretation of the Mendelian principle t genes (and traits) sort themselves indepen-ıtly between generations. Early Mendelians umed that this meant that particular genes (or ait characters") were necessary and sufficient ıses for their trademark traits: "specific causes," medicine's terms. Mayr pointed out, however, t unlike colored beans drawn from a bag, ıes rarely have only one phenotypic effect, and never entirely disconnected from each other ayr 1963, p. 263). Since then, the phenomena which he referred—pleiotropy, heterogeneity, d linkage—have become foundational for ıch of modern genetics, undergirding both the ne-hunting of the Human Genome Project d the functional analysis of genes to which so ıch of basic biomedical research has turned. Despite Mayr's best efforts, however, beanbag netics has shown stubborn persistence in med-ne. "Genetic diseases" are still usually inter-eted as self-contained causal associations be-een a particular allele of a specific gene and a ıgle (though not necessarily simple) clinical ndrome, complicated at most by the magic of ysterious environmental factors (Hull 1978). As nomic research extends Mayr's arguments into ıman biology, of course, this simple "beanbag" odel for medical genetics will have to break own. Almost all the DNA-based descriptions of ew "disease genes" have underscored the fact ıat multiple alleles at a given locus can produce e same clinical phenotype, and in most cases ıultiple loci are implicated as well. The effect of is heterogeneity is to mute the predictive power f any particular genetic approach to risk assess-ıent for these conditions, and the expressions of aution that dominate most current genetic test-ıg policy statements are a reflection of this uncertainty (Benjamin et al. 1994; Holtzman 1989). It also should not be surprising that mutations at the genomic level should ramify through the body's systems in more than one direction, and end up causing widely different types of health problems. As medicine re-learns human physiology from the genome up, genetic multipotency is likely to become the norm rather than the exception: every genotypic change probably has multiple phenotypic effects, just as any particular effect is likely to have multiple genotypic causes.[2] As a result, genetic risk assessment tests for most multifactoral health problems will have modest predictive power. In fact, they will not usually be able to predict the aspects of illness that will be most important for patients: the time of onset, the severity, the duration, or the treatability of their disease experience (Juengst 1995).

What this suggests is that as an evolutionary stage in medicine's thinking about disease, the "genetic paradigm" carries its own inborn limits. If genomic science can bring medicine all the way through the simplistic "bean-bag" thinking of Mendelian medical genetics and out the other side, the allure of promoting genes as the specific causes of complex diseases should simply evaporate.

Moreover, the re-classification of diseases as "genetic" has another important set of consequences: it adds to the social meaning of these diseases, and social burdens that the afflicted have to bear. When a disease becomes reinterpreted as a genetic disease, it acquires all the peculiar cultural baggage that has traditionally been associated with genetic explanations of health problems. Three elements of this baggage seem particularly important:

1. Determinism. Since relatively few genetic mutations create easily discernible patterns of disease inheritance within a family, the clearest examples of genetic disorders (like Huntington Disease) have often been both predictable and intractable: they have appeared in highly pene-

trant Mendelian patterns in the unfortunate families that inherit them, and unfold inexorably in their individual victims. This history still affects the way many people think about genetic risk information, by leading them to assume that genetic diagnostics of any kind have more predictive power than other kinds of health risk assessments, and that all genetic health problems inevitably unfold in the lock-step fashion of our traditional models. This assumption is corroborated by popular (and academic) accounts giving genetic tests occult powers to expose individual's "future diaries" (Annas 1994). Unfortunately, overly deterministic understandings of genes can inhibit, rather than facilitate, the recipient's ability to anticipate and prepare for future illness, by encouraging unnecessary fatalism and exposing the recipient to discrimination by those who can make exclusionary use of such predictions.

2. Reductionism. Because of the causal power genetic risk factors are often (mistakenly) given, they also tend to play an disproportionate role in the social identification of those who carry them, reducing their identities to their carrier status. Genetic information can identify health risks we inherit from (and often share with) our families, and explain those risks at what seems to be a very basic biological level. Together, these facts make it easy to interpret genetic health risks as a reflection on the recipient's basic identity as a person, and to label people accordingly (Fox-Keller 1991; Brock 1992), as we do when we refer, for example, to "Down's babies," "sicklers," or "phenylketonurics." To the extent that these genotypic labels cast a (socially disvalued) health problem as a person's defining feature, this reductionistic understanding of genetic test results simply exacerbates any stigmatization that the target disease may carry (Marteau and Drake 1995; Billings et al. 1992; Saxton 1988).

3. Familial Implications. Of course, overly deterministic and reductionistic interpretations of genetic health risks are cultural perceptions which the facts of genetics do not demand. However, there is one feature of genetic risk infor tion that is relevant to almost all genetic test When genetic information reveals an indi ual's risk for disease, it immediately suggests possibility that family members are also at risk course, to the extent that this suggestion alerts atives to remediable health risks, it is one of virtues of taking the genetic approach. Howe it can also challenge families in a numbe ways. First of all, clinically useful genetic in mation about individuals often requires know the background against which the individu genome presents itself: the pattern of inherita of the traits and markers in question within larger family. This means that in order for a netic test to be useful to an individual fa member, other members of the family have to willing to provide that background, and, in process, discover their own status within the p tern. Moreover, like most medical interventio genetic testing is usually motivated by a crisis someone diagnosed with breast cancer or gene disease—which creates a sense of urgency to " the family in for testing. " For those other fam members, the decision to participate in a testi program raises a basic moral question: what a the demands of my loyalty-based obligation help my kin learn their genetic risks? In partic lar, must I sacrifice my own "right not to know" order to help my relative enjoy the "right know," and join him or her in braving the ps chosocial risks of having that personal inform tion known about me? When family membe decide to protect their own interests and decli to participate, the same question is passed "dow stream" to their children and grandchildren: those downstream kin should decide to be teste the status of the declining member could be r vealed as a simple matter of deduction. What i terests must they sacrifice, then, in order to gi the decliner the filial respect that they deserv

Finally, if a decliner's kin do become inte ested in learning their own genetic risks, but ca not do so without involving the reluctant relativ what lengths may the family go to persuade the unwilling to do their familial duty? Split decisions about genetic testing have already been observed by genetic counselors to lead to familial discord in some cases, while unanimous decisions in other cases have raised suspicions of undue familial pressure to participate.

Of course, genetic information is as much about our differences as it is about our shared traits, and illuminating those differences is another way in which genetics can challenge the familial virtue of mutual loyalty. As we are able to sort out which lineages within families, and which individuals within a lineage, carry a family's risk-conferring mutations, tension will be created between the divergent interests of the two groups. Whatever their commitment to family solidarity, the family will have to face the fact that it will be in its "normal" members' interests to reveal their non-carrier status in some circumstances and in the interests of the carriers to conceal theirs. Even if no clinical evidence of the family's condition exists in some family members, if they are not proven to be non-carriers, they can suffer from what sociologists call a "courtesy stigma," simply by virtue of their relationship to an individual who has such a condition (Malkin et al. 1990). Family members free of the mutations in question, for example, will find it in their interests to use that information to counter their family history of a disease in applying for insurance. In doing so, however, they will inevitably raise questions about their kin who do not volunteer their test results in turn. Should families be expected to stick together "in sickness and in health" as we ask of married couples, or do the "limited sympathies" of human nature give us leave to concentrate on the welfare of our own threads within the familial patterns of inheritance?

Since human families will always weave together a combination of different genetic threads, new abilities to identify those differences will continue to expose families to this kind of external pressure, as long as we live in a society that uses such differences to allocate its opportunities. These three features of genetic explanations—their deterministic reading, their reductionistic application, and their familial implications—serve to raise the stakes and animate the discussions of genetic imperialism, because together they give genetic diseases a social meaning that other health problems do not share. Moreover, they are the same social meanings that have fueled some of the worst political abuses of biomedical science over the course of the last century: the U.S. eugenic sterilization and immigration policies (Reilly 1991) and the European racial hygiene programs. Now, as then, to the extent that genes are understood to implicate patients' futures, their identities, and their closest relationships, they become centrally important to the patients' lives. In fact, as I will show below, most of the ethical, legal and social issues currently being discussed as the "downstream" risks of the Human Genome Project—i.e., the issues of genetic privacy, discrimination, and education—are direct creations of this old-fashioned "new way of thinking" about our health problems.

If the conceptual evolution that the Human Genome Project promises for medicine merely takes us to the next iteration of the research program that has guided medicine for the last century, then one of the outcomes may be the increased incidence of patients facing genetic diagnoses and their attendant social burdens. But in the process of doing that, it could have other consequences as well: as I show below, it could lead us to relabel more previously healthy people as sick, and it could lead us to interpret more human traits as pathological. The extent to which those consequences occur depends, I will argue, on the extent to which the public and the genetics community continue to rely on two other nineteenth-century pathological concepts: the notions of disease agency and constitutional predisposition.

GENETIC CONTAGIONISM

One of the major conceptual effects of the doctrine of specific causation in nineteenth-century medicine was the ontological reification of diseases in terms of their causal pathogenic agents. Both in Pasteur's germ theory and in Virchow's cellular pathology diseases were understood to be reducible to real things in the world: the pathogens or lesions which could provide necessary and sufficient targets for intervention. Under this view diseases are separable from the patients that suffer them; they are understood best as predators attacking the patient, either as invading germs or as devouring wounds (Rather 1959; Richmond 1954). Diseases like schistosomiasis and herpes fit clearly into this scheme: they are diseases identified with the invading entities that cause their clinical signs and symptoms. Explaining a set of clinical problems as a "cancer"—an abnormal body part, consuming other normal body parts—is also to use this model, as is a diagnosis of "spina bifida"—a localizable lesion in the body. On this model, the proper target for therapeutics is not the epiphenomenal clinical symptoms of the disease, but whatever the disease "agent" does to cause those symptoms: the infection, the metastasis, or the break. The great successes of the public health movement in combating infectious disease in the early twentieth-century, and the reorientation of psychiatry to look for the "organic" bases of mental illness during the same period owe much to this interpretation of disease, as does the common correlative view that health is largely a matter of being "clean" and "whole."

One of the important corollaries of this ontologically robust view of disease is that it becomes possible for diseases to be "carried" by organisms who, while unaffected themselves, serve to transmit disease to potential hosts. As historians note:

> The simplistic interpretation of the germ theory, one which many physicians embraced at first, was that a pathogenic bacteria in a human b equaled a disease. Before long it became c that some individuals could harbor large nu bers of dangerous bacteria and suffer no effe The most famous of these was Mary Mal whose gallbladder teemed with typhoid bac while she enjoyed perfect health. . . . The car state is now recognized as extremely commo many diseases (Hudson 1987, p. 164).

Moreover, the lesson of Typhoid Mary was t the "carrier state"—is also a crucial target for tervention in any attempt to forestall the spreac a disease of this sort. From the point of view preventive medicine, carriers do not enjoy p fect health at all: they are infected with dise which could either eventually blossom to ha them or spread to those around them. This ma possible the concept of screening otherw healthy people to detect their hidden diseas both for the purposes of providing them w "pre-emptive therapy" and providing others w protection from the danger they represent (Brandt 1987).

It is easy to interpret genetic diseases using t model, and to think of genes as germs or "tra missible lesions." Indeed, the "bean-bag" Me delian genetics of the 1920s and -30s made t wholesale application of this model irresistible those who were interested in extending the su cess of public health methods to solve the soci problems of rising health care costs, "feeb mindedness," crime and immigration (Paul 198 Reilly 1991). Even after immigration restrictio and surgical sterilization were rejected as legi mate means of preventing genetic infection, e genicists looked forward to the day when son biochemical means is discovered for detecti the existence within the organism of the recessi genes responsible for the emergence of defecti characters. It would then be a simple matter apply tests to all individuals and discover thos who possess the recessive factors for defecti traits. Preventing undesirables from reproduci continuing this generation after generation ls to the elimination of a considerable num- of such defectives from the population, with result that the perpetuation of the race is left hose individuals that seem to possess normal ts (Fasten 1935, p. 353).

Jnfortunately, it is not so easy to escape the aceptual legacy of this way of thinking about netic health problems. The view that genetic eases are reducible to the genetic alleles which y express is a widespread element of genetic dicine's paradigm. In fact, medical genetics ems to have finally succeeded in combining germ theory and cellular pathology in its view genetic disease. Like localized lesions, we see netic diseases as defects at the molecular level, d whose pathogenic effects are, more often n not, the progressive, degenerative, break- wn of the body. This view suggests "surgical" erventions to repair the defects through re- mbinant DNA gene therapies. Thus, "when neticists discuss one of the diseases, they are w talking about an anatomic derangement in e same concrete sense that the urologists talk out a kidney stone, or cardiologists talk about a enotic mitral valve" (Stanbury et al. 1983, p. 3). rthermore, they claim that "conceptualiza- on of disease at the level of the gene strengthens e drive to 'cure' the disease at the same level. here is something aesthetically compelling out cutting to the heart of the problem, by eating the disease at the molecular level, where originates" (Roblin 1979, p. 111).

On the other hand, like infectious diseases, e think that genetic defects can lie dormant in eir "carriers," and be transmitted to their off- ring, long before they are clinically manifest. his view suggests preventive measures to fore- all the clinical manifestation of the disease in ose already infected, and, once again, public ealth programs to contain the spread of disease enes within the population. Again, appealing to he fact that "the major successes of medicine— or example, antibiotics, immunization, vaccination, prevention of Rh disease, endocrine replacement therapy—have been where the intervention or treatment has been directed early on at the underlying disease mechanisms" (Baird 1990, p. 208), geneticists continue to endorse population screening programs designed to detect carriers of recessive genetic disease in order to "reduce the incidence" of the disease (Caskey 1993; Palomaki 1994).[3]

Like the disease agency theories that preceded it, in other words, the separation of disease and patient effected by this robustly ontological view of genetic disease allows the creation of a new class of people with genetic health problems: the "carriers" of genetic disease. Just as the emergence of localized plaques and tangles in the brain tissue can justify a diagnosis of "organic" Alzheimer's disease even before symptoms occur, and just as the presence of HIV virus makes one a reportable "carrier" of HIV disease, so the identification of the "Huntington" gene is understood to secure a diagnosis of Huntington disease, and "carrying" one allele of a recessive disease gene makes one a legitimate client for genetic services.

Unfortunately, if genes do not serve well as "specific causes," they are even less well suited to play the roles of either germs or wounds. Again, as the number and variety of different specific mutations that can all cause the same disease increases, so does the challenge of detecting and correcting them all in a patient. Worse yet, the causal complexity works in both ways: even the paradigmatic examples of clean Mendelian "single gene" disorders, like "recessive" cystic fibrosis and "dominant" Huntington's disease are turning out to be multifactoral enough that carrying one of their (multiple) pathognomic genotypes no longer guarantees that one will experience a problematic clinical syndrome (Benjamin et al. 1994; Strohman 1993). Since most prophylactic interventions are conceptually committed to a deterministic etiology of specific causation, applying this model on the basis of genetic information risks making and acting on both false negative and false positive prognoses. This means that preventive interventions also risk intervening unnecessarily in cases that the environmental forces of expression and penetrance would have naturally mitigated (Strohman 1993). Even the view of genetic defects as molecular lesions is quickly becoming outdated. Many of the "genetic factors" now being associated with disease risks are not the structural breaks, deletions, rearrangements or malformations of DNA that have preoccupied medical geneticists until now. With genome research, the "defects" identified are more often structurally sound variations of the gene, part of a range of differentially benign mutant forms that make up the "polymorphisms" of the gene. One interesting example of the strain this fact puts on our conceptual scheme is the growing practice of using the term "pre-mutations" to describe the benign products of a nucleotide repetition problem, reserving "mutations" for the disease-causing versions: it echoes neatly the manner in which oncologists discuss "pre-cancerous lesions" in attempting to use their own ontological disease language to talk about human variation (Roussea et al. 1991).

Moreover, applying the disease agency interpretation of disease to genetic disease gives the new classes of patients some additional burdensome social roles. Two kinds of problems are important.

First, just as the germ theory was used to stigmatize "carriers" of infectious disease like Typhoid Mary, gene carriers also suffer stigmatization as tainted sources of disease (Kenen and Schmidt 1978; Markel 1992; Marteau and Drake 1995). This stigmatization can manifest itself in subtle social labeling (as in the characterization of particular families of patients as "cancer families" (Malkin et al. 1990), or in frank discrimination (as in the claim that carrying particular genes amounts to a "pre-existing medical condition" for the purposes of insurance underwriting (Billings et al. 1992). Here, it is not diagnosis of a disease that triggers the reductionistic geneti[c la]beling: it is merely the identification of an i[ndi]vidual or family as a "carrier" of the disease ge[ne.] Ironically, this perception that gene carriers [are] already themselves "diseased" can be exa[cer]bated even in attempts to combat the discrimi[na]tion that perception can produce: for examp[le,] the only way that the Americans with Disabili[ties] Act can be interpreted to protect gene carr[iers] from employment discrimination is if, in fa[ct,] being a gene carrier is considered to be a physi[cal] disability (Rothstein 1992).

Moreover, disease "carriers" acquire strong [so]cial obligations not to spread their diseases, ev[en] where those duties are not enforced by the pub[lic] health authorities. In genetic contexts, where [the] disease is "vertically transmitted" from parents [to] offspring, these perceived social obligations c[an] conflict with the reproductive plans and libert[ies] of prospective parents (Faden 1994; Charo a[nd] Rothenberg 1994). To the extent that genetic s[er]vice programs are evaluated for funding in pub[lic] health terms—i. e., in terms of their success in [re]ducing the incidence of particular genes—g[e]netic service providers will have a stake in seei[ng] that their clients make the "correct" reproducti[ve] decisions: decisions not to bear children at ri[sk] for genetic disease (Clarke 1990). While respo[n]sible couples can and do take genetic conside[ra]tions into account in making their reproducti[ve] decisions, our historical experience with the e[x]cesses of the eugenics movement shows the da[n]ger of pressuring them to do so: reproductive d[e]cisions are wrapped tightly enough with a wi[de] enough diversity of fundamental beliefs and va[l]ues in our culture that, within wide limits, almo[st] any use of public health authorities to attempt [to] control them will be perceived as unjustifiab[ly] coercive.[4]

GENETIC HUMORALISM

The late nineteenth-century alternative to fin[d]ing a specific causal explanation for a clinical il[lness] s was to appeal to the doctrine of "constituːal pathology." Unlike specific causation, the ıstitution concept provided a view which alːed diseases to be related to their sufferers rinsically as well as accidentally. The elents composing the body—tissues, fluids and ces—were taken to be maintained in characistic proportions by the (formal) constraints of particular, definitive nature of that individl. Well into the nineteenth-century the constiion was interpreted as the relative balance of four humors, placing the concept in a tradin that can be traced almost continuously back Galen and Hippocrates (Ciocco 1932; Haller 31). The resulting way an individual was comsed was called his or her "physical make up" or onstitution" (Ciocco 1932). An individual's nstitution was reflected in emotional states d behavior (as the person's mental "temperaent"), and in his or her physical appearance rough the characteristic "habitus" of the body d "facies" of the face) (Stephenson 1888). More portantly, however, one's constitution also afcted one's health: Depending on the relative lance struck between the elements in one's nstitution, it could display "diatheses" or speal susceptibilities to certain diseases (Rosenrg 1976). These constitutional diseases were lled "dyscrasias," because they represented an trinsic imbalance within one's make-up. The rst edition of *Black's Medical Dictionary* inudes this definition, summarizing the doctrine:

> *Constitution*, or diathesis, means the general condition of the body, especially with reference to its liability to certain diseases. A sound constitution is one in which the structure and functions of the various parts and organs are so evenly maintained that there is no apparent liability to any disease. The term "constitutional" is sometimes vaguely applied to diseases which present knowledge does not permit of our attributing to any definite organ or system. A constitution such as the gouty constitution may be inherited, or it may develop as the result of improper food, habits and environment; or, on the other hand, a hereditary predisposition towards some disease may be gradually eliminated by a careful and regular life. (Cotmy 1906)

This definition captures a number of the important features of the concept of a constitution. First, it is a concept that was traditionally used in explanations of clinical phenomena at the level of the whole organism. It describes the "general condition of the body" as a whole, and the specific pathological predispositions that condition produces. Lower-level or more specific clinical complaints or symptoms would be explained as a consequence of the individual's intrinsic susceptibilities: i.e., in terms of the relations between the individual's form and functioning. As the "even maintenance" of a "sound constitution" suggests, the concept rests on a "physiological" model of disease-as-disequilibrium (Rather 1959).

As pathological explanation increasingly moved to the levels of tissues and cells, constitutional thought lost its theoretical foundations in the humoral doctrines. As a result, its explanations became vague, drawing more heavily from contemporary chemical notions like the "dispositions" of compounds (Mann 1964). Moreover, since many of the old "constitutional" diseases could be reinterpreted ("ontologically") as histological lesions or infectious diseases, the explanatory scope of constitutional theory was limited to illnesses for which no more concrete account could be given: it became a "pathology of the gaps." This meant that in internal medicine, constitutional terms were often used as synonyms for "idiopathic," to indicate that the cause of the problem was actually unknown. At the same time, this focused constitutional thought more squarely on the (mysterious) domain of hereditary diseases, and provided a form of explanation for the patterns of transmission that were observed. If diseases that "run in families" were to be explained as inherited traits, they had to be explained constitutionally as the result of tendencies of the hereditary "stock" or "blood" to function or dysfunction in particular ways (Adams 1814). This model provided a useful pre-Mendelian source of explanation for the observed variety in the expression of hereditary disease. A constitutional imbalance only made one susceptible to the attack of a disease, rather than directly causing it. Moreover, the imbalance itself could be rectified (or exacerbated) by environmental factors. With the rediscovery of Mendel's work at the turn of the century, constitutionalists quickly adapted Mendelian genetic explanations to constitutional pathology. By 1929, the situation could be summarized this way:

> With the World War, the doctrine of the constitution took a sudden leap forward, and was further helped out by the development of Mendelian reasoning (genetics) and endocrinology. Consideration of the soldier as a whole, and of vast outdoor clinics of men en masse tended to revive the general pathology of Hippocrates just as the pathological lesion and the bacillus forwarded special (local) pathology and specific therapy. The constitution came to be seen as the summation of inherited traits which are basic to disease. The constitution became assimilated to the genotype of Johanssen; the physical habitus and facies to the sometimes illusory phenotypes (Garrison 1929, p. 678).

Finally, as the definition above suggests, because of the explanatory flexibility of the constitutional doctrine, and the varied hereditary patterns, constitutional pathology retained from its humoral roots a commitment to the notion of the inheritance of acquired characteristics. Like the balance of humors, constitutions, and their pathological tendencies, could be influenced by the activities of the individuals that displayed them and the environments in which they were displayed. Since this seemed to fit the facts of many "constitutional" diseases, linked ther the localized pathologies of the day, and also fered a possibility for their treatment, medic clung to this view long after the other life scien had given it up (Churchill 1976).

In fact, while it is rarely acknowledged as su constitutional thinking continues to flourish genetic medicine. As Robert Murray writes, geneticists, "There is only one context in wh genetic health can be unambiguously discus (if one discusses it at all) and that is from standpoint of the individual with a genetic c stitution that clearly produces a detectable turbance of the body's equilibrium with its en ronment or accelerates the process of aging of t body or of particular organs or tissues of the boc (Murray 1974). There are two important conc tual reasons for this, both of which have be capitalized upon by the Human Genome Pr ect and its proponents.

First, while the inheritance of acquired ch acteristics is no longer part of medical gene thought (at least not until the discovery of the panding nucleotide repeat mutations! (Rouss et al. 1991), the constitutionalist's hope that i herited characteristics might be mitigated by b havioral interventions is still at the core of its a proach. Genomicists write that "ultimately, t results of the HGP ... will profoundly alter o approach to medical care, from treating disea that is already advanced to a preventative mo focused on identification of individual risk. Th should permit early initiation of changes lifestyle and medical surveillance, preventing i dividuals from becoming ill in the first plac (Guyer and Collins 1993, p. 1151).

The disease agency model that is so helpful justifying reproductive case control measur (like population carrier or prenatal screenir programs) is too deterministic to be very hel ful in explaining how genetic knowledge ca prevent disease in people who have already i herited the relevant "patho-genes." In order t promise preventive interventions that go beyon roductive interventions (with their uncom-able eugenic associations), genetic medicine eds the flexibility of constitutional concepts e "predisposition," "susceptibility," and "ge-tic loads" and "thresholds." Thus, they write t

> We have known for a long time that many common diseases such as atherosclerosis, hypertension, schizophrenia and so on are familial, but the genetic aspects have been ill defined. From the examples given, it is clear that we are learning that most common diseases are genetically heterogeneous, but susceptibility is due to major genes in many cases. Genotypes relatively unusual in the population may come to make up a large proportion of those with common diseases. An essential point is that individuals at risk can be identified for intervention, and there may be a long period to intervene.... Rather than ignore the internal genetic component to disease cause, we should evaluate the genetic input and then attempt to tailor preventive or therapeutic programs to take it into account. We will then be able to focus our prevention of disease where it will have most effect—to those who are predisposed, and before they start down the pathogenic pathway.... Our opportunities for preventing expression of predisposition, although limited now, are rapidly increasing. Technological developments are likely in the future to identify at risk individuals at relatively low cost, for example, looking for 80–100 different disease-predisposing genes in one sample from an individual at once.... We need to see our own genetic individuality as a potential origin of disease. We are all different—we are all genetically unique—which means our risk for disease is different one from another. Progress depends on realizing this and applying the knowledge to prevention (Baird 1990, pp. 207–08).

As this passage suggests, the second reason constitutional" thinking has been so tenacious n medical genetics is its utility in explaining health problems as genetic diseases without the need to show the specific necessary and sufficient genes involved. Any unusual phenotypic variation, in this case, warrants a claim of genotypic "imbalance" or "diathesis" which can be appropriated as the "internal genetic component" of the disease cause. For the complicated conditions that we continue to have to relegate to the "polygenic" or "multifactoral" miscellaneous bin of the genetic disease category, this ability is crucial, since it allows us to posit predispositions or susceptibilities where we cannot yet tell convincing specific causal stories for the mutations they find. Conceptually, this offers a catch-all category that, like most over-inclusive explanatory hypotheses, is open to, and often criticized for, overuse and abuse (Edlin 1987; Wachbroit 1994).

Moreover, one way in which this overuse manifests itself is in the creation of entirely new forms of human pathology. Since any deviation from a biological norm should have a constitutional pathological explanation (as a constitutional imbalance, a diathesis, in one direction or another), any deviation can be turned into a new genetic disease. Thus, for those who think about disease in constitutional terms, "as more and more is learned about the genetic underpinnings of various human traits, abilities and physical characteristics, some conditions, which we now regard as 'normal' variations, may come to be viewed as maladies" (Gert et al. 1996, p. 157). In other words, just as deep thought was pathologized as a symptom of the "melancholic" constitution, and heavy drinking has been pathologized as an expression of the "alcoholic" disposition, so can the identification of genetic influences on stature, aggressiveness, or risk-taking be used to pathologize shortness, "criminality," and risk aversion as newly discovered forms of "genetic disease" (Duster 1989). Troy Duster and Dorothy Nelkin's work shows the pervasive ways in which this tendency to "medicalize" (or, in this case, "geneticize" (Edlin 1987) socially problematic differences between people in order to justify efforts at social control has already crept into the culture (Duster 1989; Nelkin and Tancredi 1989). In this way, to the extent that our enthusiasm for medicine's new "preventive mode" encourages more people's "genetic individuality" to be understood as "sources of disease," the genetic paradigm will have succeeded in increasing our society's perception of its overall genetic morbidity.

The "constitutional" catch-all interpretation of genetic deviations also has its share of special social connotations. Like "carriers" of disease agents, those that are known to be constitutionally prone to pathology face a special kind of stigmatization that accidental victims of disease avoid. However, while those labeled as "carriers" can be stigmatized as irresponsible and unclean vectors of disease, the "predisposed" are more likely to be labeled as weaklings in the face of disease. For the Victorians, for example, while the asymptomatic syphilitic was to be chastised as negligent and profligate, the consumptive, the alcoholic, and the "latent schizophrenic" had to be protected from their own inability to resist disease. Today, this same "vulnerability stigma" can be seen to be animating the way we think about those at genetic risk of disease, from the grounding of airmen with sickle cell trait in the 1970s (Duster 1989, pp. 24–28) to the recent concern over the "psychological vulnerability" of children at genetic risk for colon cancer (American Society of Human Genetics and American College of Medical Genetics 1995).

Moreover, as many have pointed out, the constitutional way of thinking about genetic disease shifts the burden of responsibility to response to the disease. If particular individuals are understood to be unusually vulnerable outliers of the normal population, people whose genetic health problems are primarily rooted in "their own genetic individuality," it becomes natural to assign them the sole responsibility for discerning and avoiding the illnesses to which they are prone. In settings like the industrial workplace, where the relevant "external causes" of illness are controllable environmental mutagens and tox this way of thinking may relieve instituti from what would otherwise be their obligati to insure the general safety of their employ (Draper 1992; Duster 1989).

In summary, then, the "slow but steady c ceptual evolution" forecast by Watson and Co Deegan needs to be watched carefully. If it folds against the array of nineteenth-cent concepts we currently use to understand gene health problems, it risks exacerbating the ove morbidity associated with genetic health pr lems in three ways: (1) We risk adding to the b den of existing disease (by geneticizing them a thereby giving them the fatalism and "court stigma" that accompanies genetic diseases); we risk making more people sick with those d eases (by identifying carriers and thereby givi them the "infection stigma" and carrier oblig tions that accompany that ontological conce tion of disease); and (3) we risk creating more d eases (by medicalizing differences as diathes and thereby giving people the "vulnerabil stigma" that accompanies constitutional thin ing about disease).

CONCLUSION

How can we avoid these consequences? Throu its investment in research on the ethical, leg and social implications of genome research, t U. S. Human Genome Project has been a pi neer in experimenting with one way to deal wi the implications of Watson and Cook-Deegan evolution. The goal of that effort is to try to r duce the social burden of the (perceived) i creases in genetic morbidity that genome r search will produce, by establishing policies th can help keep personal problems—like repr ductive choices—appropriately personal, an social problems—like workplace safety—s curely on the shoulders of society. The possibi ties and limitations of that effort have been di cussed extensively elsewhere (American Socie

Human Genetics and American College of dical Genetics 1995; Billings et al. 1992; Brock 2; Duster 1989; Holtzman 1989; Juengst 1993; kin and Tancredi 1989; Nolan and Swenson 8). But efforts at making the social world safe genomics may not be the only approach that ossible. To take a phrase from the advocates of e therapy, would it not be more aesthetically npelling to "cut to the heart of the problem" l address it at its conceptual roots, "where it ginates?" Could we, in other words, actually e genetics and the Human Genome Project to nent a revolution in the ways we think about ease, beyond simply substituting "genes" for th "germs" and "humors?"

In the glare of medicine's nineteenth-century radigms, it is hard to see what that revolution ght produce. In broad outline, however, given at we are learning about the dynamics of the man genome, it would be likely to encourage e shift to a multidimensional understanding disease causation, with three consequences. rst, we should begin to see a new conceptual paration between diseases and their causes. he etiological reductionism that allows one to iagnose" the active presence of a genetic disse upon finding its pathognomic molecular dect is crumbling under the weight of counteramples, as genomic research reveals the many ays that specific clinical syndromes and molecar mutations can be mis-matched. As mutaon-based nosologies begin to fray beyond clinial utility, a return to clinically described entities ems likely. This, in turn, should mean a return taking the patient's complaints as the source of eaning for medicine, as "mere symptoms" reain their status as organizational tools for medal science, and the dangers of focusing too eavily on either populational or molecular conerns become clearer. Finally, both trends would romote the acceptance of multiple approaches health problems, via multiple causal "hanles," as opposed to the determinism with which enetic explanations are now invested. The fact that the National Institute of Environmental Health Sciences has recently announced a collaboration with the Human Genome Project to promote the study of gene-environment interactions in health and disease is a sign of this progress: far from eclipsing environmental approaches to disease, the Human Genome Project may in the end force biomedical research in that direction, by exposing the limits of the genetic paradigm that currently dominates the community. Developing these hints is a project for the philosophy of medicine that goes well beyond the aims of this paper. However, consider one example of the sort of conceptual clarification I have in mind.

One small step in the direction of this revolution would be to take more care with the terms we use in genetic medicine to describe its domain and its tools. One way in which the old models are perpetuated is through the generic use of deterministic adjectives, such as presymptomatic or diagnostic, to describe the entire range of risk assessments that genetics makes possible or reductionistic labels like "disease genes" and "gene carriers."

As a starting point for such a discussion, and the conclusion to this one, consider the following suggestions for a new genetic lexicon: the only genes that should be considered "diagnostic" of genetic disease should be those that can be used in confirming the diagnosis of an active genetic disease process, such as the use of mutation analysis to diagnose fragile X syndrome in developmentally delayed children (Roussea et al. 1991). By contrast, "prognostic" genes are capable of being used to forecast the emergence of a clinical health problem with a high degree of certainty, such as mutation analysis for Huntington disease (Benjamin et al. 1994). Such testing is only "presymptomatic" if one concedes that to carry the mutations is to have Huntington disease in its earliest stages.

Similarly, "predictive" mutations should be those that can be said to identify a true genetic predisposition to a clinical health problem: that is, a tendency or inclination to go wrong in a particular way, if not inhibited by other genetic or environmental checks. In these cases, a positive test result would allow us to predict that, unless the predisposition is controlled, the clinical problem will result. Newborn testing for phenylketonuria (PKU) fits this model of genetic testing. By contrast, genes that only confer a genetic susceptibility to disease—that is, a vulnerability to a particular environmental insult—might be called "prophylactic" genes or "contingency" genes (Nolan and Swenson 1988). For example, Alpha-1-antitripsin deficiency creates such a susceptibility: in the absence of tobacco smoke it does no harm; but in those who do smoke it represents a serious liability (Stokinger and Scheel 1973). By calling it prophylactic, we would simply be emphasizing that there are interventions to be made; that the problem is not internal or inevitable.

"Probabilistic" genetic testing would be a less determined category of genetic risk assessment. Here, one thinks of a test like the test for P53 mutations in Li-Fraumeni family members (Malkin et al. 1990); a test which can serve to alert the clients that they are at a statistically higher risk than the population for a particular kind of health problem, but cannot make stronger claims about the specific course the future will take. By contrast, "Genetic Profiling" would be the category of tests that simply identify a loose empirical association between a particular mutation and an increased incidence of a given health problem. An illustration here would be the putative-association between deletions in the gene for angiotensin converting enzyme and the risk of myocardial infarction (Cambien 1992).[5]

Medicine has always been devoted to interpreting signs in order to help patients plan their futures. To that extent, clinicians share an occupational hazard with weather forecasters and fortune-tellers: people set great store by the predictions they make, even when they are notoriously inaccurate. Much of that inaccuracy reflects the limits of technique: lab test resu barometer readings and palm line lengths are always precise and reliable indicators of thing come. But even sure signs can yield false pre tions when their meanings are misinterpre And since false predictions carry the appeara of certainty, they can be dangerous for both p fessionals and their clients.

How professionals should interpret predict signs for their clients depends upon the nature their services. Meteorologists predict the circu stances their clients will face as they go ab their lives, but not how their clients will expe ence that environment. By contrast, fortu tellers are expected to predict the course of th clients' future life experiences. Admittedly, meteorological approach to genetic diagnost strains against our modern inclination to inv genes with occult powers to determine the fate individuals. However, if genetic explanations disease can be reinterpreted as barometer rea ings rather than palm lines, their forecasts c strengthen their carriers, by giving them the o portunity to prepare for the environmental pre sures that they will face. If the purpose of medic prediction is to enhance rather than constra personal autonomy, the weather-person's pe spective may be worth remembering in trying sort through what it means to "have the genes" f the health problem that concerns us.

Scientific critics of the Human Genome Pro ect's attempts to anticipate and address the eth cal, legal and social implications of new advanc in human genetics have sometimes queried wh it should be the responsibility of the genome re search community to become the "lightening ro of human genetics" on moral and political pu poses, given the fact that the social problems genetic privacy, stigmatization and discrimin tion seem so far out of their control. In fact, how ever, the scientific community is crucial to this e fort, because it is their evolving understanding o genetic disease that animates most of our issue hey can teach the rest of us to think about dis-e in a way that avoids the old-fashioned errors genetic imperialism, genetic contagionism, d genetic humoralism, they will have suc-eded in giving us both new wineskins and new ne with which to toast the new millennium.

NOTES

1. There is no shortage of evidence that genome sci-tists see themselves as poised at the beginning of the d of history" for medical science. For example. Wal- Gilbert writes that:

> The genome project is not just an isolated effort on the part of molecular biologists. It is a natural development of the current themes of biology as a whole... The information carried on the DNA, that genetic information passed down from our parents, is the most fundamental property of the body. To work out our DNA sequence is to achieve a historic step forward in knowledge. Even after we have made that step we will still need to refer back to the sequence, to try to unravel its secrets more and more completely. But there is no more basic or more fundamental information that could be available (Gilbert 1992, p. 83).

e also Guyer and Collins (1993) and Hood (1988), r similarly eschatological claims for genome re-arch.

2. For example, the recent claims of association be-veen the APOE4 allele and Alzheimer's disease have uite complicated implications for clinical practice be-use of the already established uses of APOE4 testing r coronary artery disease risk and head injury progno-s (Mayeux et al. 1995).

3. Thus, it is not too surprising to find direct echoes f the old eugenics rhetoric in the current literature: r example, the recent editorial suggesting that, while ene therapy has little hope of reaching "the theo-etical ideal of 'purifying' the human gene pool," "a roader approach, based on systematic screening of the hole population for carriers and the elimination f new carriers among their offspring, would in principle be effective" toward that preventive goal (Davis 1992, p. 361).

4. Ruth Faden makes this point nicely in the context of prenatal HIV screening:

> Eliminating an incident of disease or disability by "preventing" the person who would have the disease or disability from being born is not an instance of prevention—not in the sense in which it is ordinarily meant and not as the term ought to be used.... It suggests that the lives of some persons with a disability or illness are not worth living, that such persons are to be understood only as social or economic drains and never as sources of either independent value or enrichment for the lives of others (Faden 1994, p. 92).

5. The point of such a lexicon is not to create watertight categories to which particular genes and genetic tests would be permanently assigned. The categories are clearly overlapping, and one test could fall into several depending on the clinical situation. For example, a HD mutation test could be "diagnostic" if it were used to rule out a diagnosis of HD in a neurologically impaired patient. Rather, the point is to develop some conventions for describing tests in ways that give the public a more nuanced understanding of their epistemic power and practical significance.

REFERENCES

Adams, J.: 1814, *A Treatise on the Supposed Hereditary Properties of Diseases*, J. Callow Publishers, London.

American Society of Human Genetics, American College of Medical Genetics.: 1995, "Points to consider: Ethical, legal, and psychosocial implications of genetic testing in children and adolescents. " *American Journal* of *Human Genetics* 57, 1233–1241.

Annas, G.: 1994, "Rules for 'gene banks': Protecting privacy in the genetics age," in T. Murphy and M. Lappé (eds.), *Justice and the Human Genome Project*, University of California Press, Berkeley, pp. 75–91.

Baird, P.A.: 1990, "Genetics and Health Care: A Paradigm Shift," *Perspectives in Biology and Medicine* 33, 203–213

Benjamin, C. M., Adam, S., Wiggins, S., Theilmann, J. L., Copley, T. T., Bloch, M., et al.: 1994, "Proceed with care: Direct predictive testing for Huntington Disease," *American Journal of Human Genetics* 55, 606–617.

Billings, P., Kohn, M., De Cuevas, M., Beckwith, J., Alper, J. S., and Natowicz, M. R.: 1992, "Discrimination as a consequence of genetic screening," *American Journal* of *Human Genetics* 50, 476–482.

Brandt, A.: 1987, *No Magic Bullet: A Social History of Venereal Disease in the United States Since* 1880, Oxford University Press, New York.

Brandt, J.: 1989. "Presymptomatic diagnosis of delayed onset diseases with linked DNA markers: The experience of HD," *Journal of the American Medical Association* 61, 3108–3114.

Brock, D.: 1992. "The Human Genome Project and human identity," *Houston Law Review* 29, 19–21.

Cambien, F.: 1992. "Deletion polymorphism in the gene for angiotesnsin converting enzyme: a potent risk factor for myocardial infarction," *Nature* 359, 5641–5644.

Caskey, C. T.: 1993. "Presymptomatic diagnosis: A first step toward genetic health care," *Science* 262, 48–49.

Charo, A., Rothenberg, K.: 1994, "'The Good Mother': The limits of reproductive accountability and genetic choice," in K. Rothenberg and E. Thomson (eds.), *Women and Prenatal Testing Facing the Challenges of Genetic Technology*, Ohio State University Press, Columbus, Ohio, pp. 105–131.

Churchill, F.: 1976, "Rudolf Virchow and the pathologist's criteria for the inheritance of acquired characteristics," *Journal of the History of Medicine* 31, 117–148.

Ciocco, A.: 1932, "The historical background of the modern study of constitution," *Bulletin of the History of Medicine* 4, 23–28.

Clarke, A.: 1990, "Genetics, ethics, and audit," *Lancet* 335, 1145–1147.

Collingwood, R. G.: 1974, "Three senses of the word 'cause,'" in T. Beauchamp (ed.), *Philosophical Problems of Causation*, Dickenson Publishing Co., Encino, California, 118–126.

Cotmy, J., (ed.): 1906, *Black's Medical Diction* 1st edition, A. and C. Black, Ltd., London.

Cook-Deegan, R.: 1994, *The Gene Wars: Scie Politics and the Human Genome*, W. W. Norton. N York.

Davis, B.: 1992, "Germ-line gene therapy: Ev tionary and moral considerations," *Human Gene T apy* 3, 361–365.

Draper, E.: 1992, *Risky Business: Genetic Test and Exclusionary Practices in the Hazardous W place*, Cambridge University Press, New York.

Duster, T.: 1989, *Backdoor to Eugenics*, Routle Publishing Co., New York.

Edlin, J. G.: 1987, "Inappropriate use of genetic minology in medical research: A public health iss *Perspectives in Biology and Medicine* 31, 47–56.

Faden, R.: 1994, "Reproductive genetic testing, p vention and the ethics of mothering," in E. Thoms and K. Rothenberg (eds.), *Women and Prenatal T ing: Facing the Challenges of Genetic Technolo* Ohio State University Press, Columbus, Ohio, 88–98.

Fasten, N.: 1935, *Principles* of *Genetics and Eug ics*, Ginn and Co., New York.

Fox-Keller, E.: 1991, "Genetics, reductionism a normative uses of biological information," *Southe California Law Review* 65, 285–291.

Friedman, T.: 1990, "The Human Genome Pr ect—Some implications of extensive 'reverse genet medicine," *American Journal of Human Genetics* 4 407–414.

Garrison, F.: 1929, *An Introduction to the History Medicine*, W. B. Saunders, Philadelphia.

Gert, B., Berger, E., Cahill, G., et al.: 1996, *Mor ity and the New Genetics*, Jones and Bartlett Publishi Co., Boston.

Gilbert, W.: 1992, "A vision of the Grail," in I Kevles and L. Hoed (eds.), *The Code of Codes: Sc entific and Social Issues in the Human Genome Pr ect*, Harvard University Press, Cambridge, Mass., p 83–98.

Guyer, M., and Collins, F. C.: 1993, "The Huma Genome Project and the future of medicine," *Amer can Journal of Diseases* of *Children* 147, 1145–1152.

laller, J.: 1981, *American Medicine in Transition:* –1910, University of Illinois Press, Chicago.

lesslow, G.: 1984, "What is a genetic disease?" in L. denfelt and B. Lindahl (eds.), *Health, Disease and usal Explanation in Medicine,* D. Reidel Publishers, ton, pp. 183–193.

loltzman, N.: 1989, *Proceed with Caution: Predict- Generic Risks in the Recombinant DNA Era,* Johns pkins University Press, Baltimore.

Hood, L: 1988, "Biotechnology and medicine of the ıre," *Journal of the American Medical Association* , 1837–1844.

Hubbard, R., Wald, L: 1993, *Exploding the Gene th,* Colophon Books, Boston.

Hudson, R.: 1987, *Disease and Its Control: The Shap- of Modern Thought,* Praeger Press, New York.

Hull, R.: 1978, "On getting 'genetic' out of 'genetic ease,'" in J. Davis (ed.), *Contemporary Issues in Bio- dical Ethics,* Humana Press, Clifton, New Jersey, pp. -87.

Juengst, E.: 1993, "Causation and the conceptual eme of medical knowledge," in C. Delkeskamp- yes and M. A. G. Cutter (eds.), *Science, Technology d the Art of Medicine,* Kluwer, Dordrecht, pp. 127–152.

Juengst, E.: 1995, "The ethics of prediction: Genetic k and the physician-patient relationship," *Genome ience and Technology* 1, 21–36.

Kenen, R. H., Schmidt, R. M.: 1978, "Stigmatization carrier status: Social implications of heterozygote reening," *American Journal of Public Health* 49, 5–120.

Malkin, D., Li, F. P., Strong L. C., et al.: 1990, Germ-line p53 mutations in a familial syndrome of east cancer, sarcomas and other neoplasms," *Science* 0, 1233–1238.

Mann, G.: 1964, "The concept of predisposition," *urnal of Environmental Health* 8, 840–845.

Markel, H.: 1992, "The stigma of disease: The impli- ations of genetic screening," *American Journal of Med- ine* 93, 209–215.

Marteau, T. M., Drake, H.: 1995, "Attributions for isability: The influence of genetic screening," *Social cience and Medicine* 40, 1127–1132

Mayeux, R., Ottoman, R., Maestre, G., et al. 1995, "Synergistic effects of traumatic head injury and apolipoprotein E4 in patients with Alzheimer's Disease," *Neurology* 45, pp. 555–557.

Mayr, E.: 1963, *Animal Species and Evolution,* Harvard University Press, Cambridge.

Murray, R.: 1974, "Genetic disease and human health: A clinical perspective," *Hastings Center Report,* 4–7.

Nelkin, D., Tancredi, L.: 1989, *Dangerous Diagnostics: The Social Power of Biological Information,* Basic Books, New York.

Nolan, K., Swenson, S.: 1988, "New tools, new dilemmas: Genetic frontiers," *Hastings Center Report,* 40–46.

Palomaki, G. E.: 1994, "Population-based prenatal screening for the fragile X syndrome," *Journal of Medical Screening* 1, 65–72.

Paul, D.: 1984, "Eugenics and the left," *Journal of the History of Ideas* 45, 567–590

Rather, L. J.: 1959, "Towards a philosophical study of the idea of disease," in C. Brooks and P. Cranefield (eds.), *The Historical Development of Physiological Thought,* Hafner Publishing Co., New York, pp. 351–375.

Reilly, P.: 1991, *The Surgical Solution: A History of Involuntary Sterilization in the U.S.* Johns Hopkins University Press, Baltimore.

Richmond, P. A.: 1954, "American attitudes towards the germ theory of disease, 1860–1880," *Journal of the History of Medicine* 9, 428–454.

Roblin, R.: 1979, "Human genetic therapy: Outlook and apprehensions," in G. Chacko (ed.), *Health Handbook,* Amsterdam, North Holland Publishing Co, 104–114.

Rosenberg, C.: 1976, *No Other Gods: On Science and American Social Thought,* Johns Hopkins University Press, Baltimore.

Roussea, F., et al., 1991, "Direct diagnosis by DNA analysis of the Fragile X syndrome of mental retardation," *New England Journal of Medicine* 325, 1673–1681.

Rothstein, M.: 1992, "Genetic discrimination in employment and the Americans with Disabilities Act," *Houston Law Review* 29, 23–85.

Saxton, M.: 1988, "Prenatal screening and discriminatory attitudes about disability," in E. Baruch, A. D'Adamo, J. Seager (eds.), *Embryos, Ethics and Women's Rights*, Haworth Press, New York, 217–24.

Stanbury, J., et al.: 1983, "Inborn errors of metabolism in the 1980's," in J. Stanbury et al., (eds.)., *The Metabolic Basis of Inherited Diseases*, 5th edition, McGraw Hill, Inc., New York.

Stephenson, F.: 1888, "Temperament and diathesis in disease," *Medical Record* 34, 362.

Stokinger, H. D., Scheel, L. D.: 1973, "Hypersusceptibility and genetic problems in occupational medicine: A consensus report," *Journal of Occupational Medicine* 15, 564–573.

Strohman, R. C.: 1993, "Ancient genomes, wise ies, unhealthy people: Limits of a genetic paradigr biology and medicine," *Perspectives in Biology Medicine* 37, 112–145.

Tauber, A. I., and Sarkar, S.: 1992, "The Hur Genome Project: Has blind reductionism gone far?" *Perspectives in Biology and Medicine* 35, 220–

Wachbroit, R.: 1994, "Distinguishing genetic ease and genetic susceptibility," *American Journa Medical Genetics* 53, 236–240.

Watson, J., Cook-Deegan, R.: 1990, "The Hun Genome Project and international health," *Journa the American Medical Association* 263, 3322–3324.

CHAPTER 25

From "Enhancing Cognition in the Intellectually Intact"

PETER J. WHITEHOUSE, ERIC T. JUENGST, MAXWELL MEHLMAN, AND THOMAS H. MURRAY

PHILOSOPHICAL ISSUES

ONE CAN NEVER BE TOO rich or too thin, ne saying goes, suggesting that at least some human characteristics have o optimum level; one can just keep getting better and better. Is cognition mong this class of characteristics? If it is not, then the debate over the so-ially and medically acceptable use of cognitive enhancers at least has ome clear boundaries: there is no reason to endorse or accept practices hat would make people too smart for their own good. The challenge would e (merely!) to try to determine the optimum level of human cognition, and o decide how far on either side of it we are willing to allow people to vary.

On the other hand, if improved cognition is a limitless benefit, the ethical and social policy questions become considerably more acute. How should medicine define the limits of its obligations to provide enhancement services to the public? How should society define the limits of what it is willing (or obligated) to pay to secure equal opportunity for its citizens? Of course, high doses of cognitive enhancers might have harmful physiological side effects that outweigh their benefits at some point. But in and by themselves, could faster thinking, more reliable memory, better coordination, quicker uptake, extended foresight, and a clever tongue ever be a bad thing?[1] Before we can be clear about the specific issues that cognitive enhancers would raise, we need to know more about what kind of human good cognitive enhancement represents.

One approach to discerning the boundaries of cognitive enhancement would be to examine what happens when humans lose their cognitive abilities, to see if that end of the spectrum holds any clues to what a "hyper cognitive" pathology would look like. With Alzheimer disease, for example, patients' cognitive failures (failures of memory, concentration, foresight, coordination, and language skills) are usually the "presenting complaints" of the disease. In severe cases, these cognitive failures manifest themselves in personality changes so striking that the patients' own families and caregivers wonder whether, in some impotent way, the patients are really still the "same person" they once knew.

By the same token, it is just as likely that, as individuals' cognitive abilities increase, their personalities will also change. Increased memory, new insights and better reasoning could all lead to new values, new perspectives on one's relationships, and new sources of pleasure and irritation. That does not mean that the enhanced literally will lose their identities and become different people, any more than someone with Alzheimer disease does. But in the figurative sense intended by caregivers of people with this disease, it may be that after some point the cog tively enhanced will no longer be recogniza by those who knew them before their enhan ment.

Personality changes are not bad in themsel of course, and there is no reason to believe t cognitive enhancement would routinely lead changes in the direction of rudeness, antisoc behavior, or moral evil. For the individual wh being enhanced, the changes are likely to be perienced simply as growth, with perhaps pains and satisfactions that accompany norm maturation. Indeed, for philosophers like De Parfit, who sees human identity itself as enou of a flux in normal circumstances to take litera the statement that "I'm not the man I was at 2 the personality-changing effects of cognitive e hancement would seem thoroughly unproble atic.[2]

On the other hand, some criticize Parfit's in vidualistic vision of human identity as sho sighted. Perhaps human identity is better und stood as defined by the web of relationships which individuals are embedded from conce tion. In this view, we are not monads of expe ence, unfolding atomistically through time. V are simply the intersection of multiple changi relationships and roles, and we cannot chan ourselves without disturbing that larger w of identities. From this perspective, personali changes are by necessity a community event a should be undertaken as such.[3] Any changes ourselves that would destroy or inhibit relatio ships important to others would need to be car fully justified to be acceptable. Requests for co nitive enhancements that promise to "make new woman of you" should be treated with th same skepticism that one would give a father's r quest to have Alzheimer disease induced so as relieve him of his familial obligations.

Of course, even in the relational model of pe sonal identity, it is an empirical matter whethe a given enhancement candidate's defining re lationships might not be flexible enough to ac mmodate the personality changes involved, l perhaps even benefit from them. That ans that, in either model, the larger challenge nains: If there is no optimum level of cognitive hancement for any individual, how should soty and the medical profession delimit their obations to provide the benefit?

A recent proposal relevant to this question is bin and Daniels' endorsement of what they l the "normal function" standard for deterning the limits of "medically necessary" (and erefore socially underwritten) mental health rvices.[4] They argue that it is not necessary, and deed it is probably fruitless, to try to draw a conptual line between legitimate "treatment" and nmedical "enhancements" by trying to limit e former to curing diseases and the latter to imoving positive health. The concept of disease is otoriously elastic, and they argue that an approiate line can be drawn simply by striving to locate fairly medical services within a population. Following Daniels' earlier work, they con rue health care as one of society's means for prerving equality of opportunity for its citizens, d they define health care needs as those serces that allow individuals to enjoy the portion society's "normal opportunity range" to which eir full array of skills and talents would give em access, by restoring or improving their abiles to the range of functional capacities typical r members of their reference class (based on, r example, age and gender) within the human ecies.

Daniels refines this definition of health care eeds by saying that the notion of "species typical nctioning" it relies on is not "merely a statistial notion" but implies "a theoretical account of e design of the organism" that describes the natural functional organization of a typical nember of the species."[5] Since "the share of the ormal opportunity range open to an individual s determined in a fundamental way by his talents nd skills," then "impairment of normal funcioning through disease and disability restricts an individual's opportunity relative to that portion of the normal range his skills and talents would have made available to him were he healthy" (p. 34).

Thus,

> Treating illness and enhancing human capabilities may both be desirable social goals, but they should not be confused with one another. The normal function model holds that health care insurance coverage should be restricted to disadvantages caused by disease and disability unless society explicitly decides to use it to mitigate other forms of disadvantage as well.[6]

The "normal function" approach is a sophisticated attempt to define the limits of social and professional obligations to provide health services. It comes close to accurately reconstructing the rationale behind many actual judgments by health care coverage plans (those using normal function rationale) and professional societies.[7] Unfortunately, this approach founders when applied to the problem of a limitlessly beneficial cognitive enhancement. In this case, two of its weakest assumptions betray it: that we have a "theoretical account of the design of the organism" that is robust enough to specify "species typical function" in the area of cognition, and that an individual's "skills and talents" are fixed as a baseline constraint on the available opportunity range by the "natural lottery" of human genetics.

On the first score, what do our theoretical accounts of human cognition suggest about "species typical" cognitive function? Statistically, of course, it is possible to draw out a spectrum of human cognitive capacities with an average middle range, a "norm" in the empirical sense that Daniels rejects as inadequate for his purposes. But theoretically? Contemporary human biology, set as it is within the context of modern biology generally, admits of very few open-ended functional goals in our organismic design. In fact, out of the traditional biological trinity of survival, reproduction, and sensation, only the last still seems important when thinking about human cognitive capacities. Indefinite individual survival, it turns out, may not be part of the species design after all, if our bodies are ultimately programmed to wind down with the aging process. Spreading our genes through reproduction, although an important goal in shaping human evolution, seems to be all but overwhelmed by the cultural artifacts our brains have created along the way, only the pursuit of sensation, originally no doubt a mere means to securing the other two, seem to remain as an innate and active guiding principle of the human design.

That is not to say, of course, that humans would rather be satiated pigs than frustrated philosophers. To the contrary, our (self) defining feature and point of pride is that the form of sensation we prize most is that which constitutes the life of the mind: cognitive experience. That's why we allow the spread of our "memes" to take precedence over the spread of our genes, and why so many of us would choose to give up continued survival if it no longer involved cognitive experience. Just as some plants can never live too long, and some animals can never have too many offspring, humans can never have too much cognitive experience. This is another way of restating the point that cognitive enhancement seems to have no obvious "down-side" for human beings, from the point of view of organisms' "theoretical design."

If that's the theory, there is no "optimum" norm for cognition in human beings, and thus no way to deny even a natural genius's claim on our cognitive enhancement services. The only alternatives would be to fall back on the statistical average cognitive capacity of the population to indicate the ceiling of legitimate requests for enhancement, or to set the ceiling by the best available example of excellent cognitive functioning and to bring people up to that level on request. These alternatives, however, raise the second problem with this account: a problem of fairness.

Daniels assumes that people's "talents and skills" (read, cognitive capacities) are inborn, largely immutable, and most often uneq
Since he is (correctly) committed to the idea t
"the general principle of fair equality of oppo
nity does [should] not imply leveling individ
differences," his vision of fair access to hea
care would yield a system in which every indiv
ual could have the services needed to realize
or her "full array" of personal talents and ski
regardless of the resulting disparities. But if eve
one's talents and skills can themselves be i
proved, it becomes difficult to resist an "equal
ing" policy that would discriminate against t
naturally fortunate. If a statistical norm is used
a goal for services, then all those born above t
norm will be denied access, even if they fall do
to the norm from their innate potential beca
of accident or disease. Even if the ceiling were
at the level of the species' cognitive champic
the less fortunate would have a disproportiona
claim on enhancement resources. To those, li
Daniels, who value the ability of each individu
to realize the "full array" of opportunities he
she can reasonably achieve, that disproportiona
claim would also be an unfair claim, and thus
bad way to define the limits of acceptable cog
tive enhancement practices.

If the "normal function" approach will n
help to define the limits of professional and so
etal obligation to provide cognitive enhanc
ments, the practice cannot be governed strictly
a medical matter. Instead, we will need to loo
beyond the health care sphere for clues and co
siderations relevant to the regulation of cogniti
enhancers. . . .

NOTES

1. For example, the lesson that the stoic and cerebr
"Mr. Spock" repeatedly teaches his Star Trek audienc
is that the price of enhanced cognition would be a co
comitant decrease in the emotions that make
human. But there is no reason to believe that there is
necessary correlation there. It is just as likely that emo
tional responsiveness would increase with cognitiv

From "Enhancing Cognition in the Intellectually Intact"

ancement, as one's powers of discernment, depth nemory, and ability to universalize grew.

2. Derek Parfit, *Reasons and Persons* (Oxford: Oxd University Press, 1984).

3. Charles Taylor, *The Ethics of Authenticity* (Camdge, Mass.: Harvard University Press, 1991).

4. James Sabin and Norman Daniels, "Determining edical Necessity' in Mental Health Practice," *Hasts Center Report* 24, no. 6 (1994): 5–13.

5. Norman Daniels, *Just Health Care* (New York: Cambridge University Press, 1986), p. 28.

6. Sabin and Daniels, "Determining 'Medical Necessity' in Mental Health Practice," p. 10.

7. Ad Hoc Committee on Growth Hormone Usage, "Growth Hormone in the Treatment of Children with Short Statures," *Pediatrics* 72 (1984): 891–94.

CHAPTER 26

Treatment, Enhancement, and the Ethics of Neurotherapeutics

PAUL ROOT WOLPE

1. INTRODUCTION

THE STUDY OF THE BRAIN has alway promised more than just the cure of disease. Franz Joseph Gall's phreno ogy, which identified 27 faculties in the brain (such as valor, cunning pride, ability to learn, ambition, and metaphysical perspicuity), was ir tended to detect the morally infirm and differentiate "higher" from "lower races. Cesare Lombroso, the 19th-century "Father of Modern Criminol ogy," argued that criminals were evolutionary throwbacks with "atavistic brains and morphological features characteristic of lower races. Craniom etry, the science of correlating brain size with intelligence, was used pri marily to create intelligence hierarchies within and between races. Nobe

Treatment, Enhancement, and the Ethics of Neurotherapeutics

ze–winning psychiatrist Antonio Egas Moniz anced lobotomy in the late 1930s and 1940s as neans of controlling aggressive or violent be-ior. These efforts, and most that came after m, were suffused with moral assumptions and ons of desirable and undesirable human char-eristics, but were believed by their proponents epresent the dispassionate pursuit of objective ence.

Neuroscience today is also built on a series of ndamental assumptions about human nature d worth. It is not possible, and perhaps not de-able, to purge neuroscience of moral presup-sitions, dealing as it does with fundamental as-cts of identity, personality, free will, and other lue-wrought concepts. As in the 19th and early th centuries, our scientific inquiry is guided by lturally determined standards of what traits we ink are valuable to explore and what behaviors think are desirable to control or eradicate. r example, imaging studies that look for mor-ological or functional differences in the or-trofrontal cortex or the amygdala of "psycho-ths" (usually defined as violent criminals with tisocial personality disorder) raise many of the me ethical and philosophical questions (if in uch more sophisticated scientific packaging) the science of earlier in the century (Abbott 001; Anderson, Bechara, Damasio, Tranel, & amasio 1999). The attempt to localize crimi-ality and explain it as the function of a specific athologized section of the brain is itself an genda of a particular cultural and historical mo-nent, and one with significant moral implica-ons.

Perhaps the most significant moral discussion n modern neuroscience has been directed at the se of pharmaceuticals to alter the fundamental ognitive and affective functions of the brain. he human desire to induce mental states hrough ingestion is, of course, as old as the dis-overy of fermentation (if not older, with the dis-overy of natural hallucinogens or stimulants), nd so is moral debate about it. Nineteenth-cen-ury America was particularly enamored of developing nutritional philosophies of health with a moral tinge, from the botanical medicine of Samuel Thompson to the non-stimulating diets developed by Will Kellogg (corn flakes were invented as a bland breakfast to avoid stirring up the passions in the morning) or Sylvester Graham (whose now-famous cracker was designed towards the same ends as corn flakes). For centuries, lay, folk, and professional movements in both Western and Eastern medicine have prescribed foods, herbs, and potions to induce proper physical and mental functioning. We still try to "eat right" to improve mood and general mental functioning, and use stimulants (caffeine), sedatives (alcohol), and mood enhancers (chocolate), and have built nutraceuticals (St. John's Wort, Kava, *Ginkgo biloba*) into a multibillion dollar market. Yet, the debates about the proper use of these substances show no signs of abating.

The ability of the new range of pharmaceuticals to alter or target mood states, levels of cognition, or cognitive skills such as memory is one of the most promising and challenging developments of the 21st century. Drugs developed for some of our most intractable diseases now promise us the power not only to treat pathology, but to improve or augment otherwise average or typical functioning; not only to arrest the cognitive deterioration of Alzheimer's, for example, but to improve cognitive functioning in the healthy. Drugs developed for narcolepsy entice us with amphetamine-free wakefulness (Bastuji & Jouvet 1988); drugs developed for depression promise to elevate our spirits in general (Kramer 1993); and drugs developed for erectile dysfunction are sold freely on the web with only a nod to medical necessity (Armstrong, Schwartz, & Asch 1999). If history is any precedent, we will enthusiastically embrace these technologies, even as we agonize over whether or not we should do so.

Debate has already begun as to the implications of these technologies for defining the difference between treatment and enhancement. There are two fundamental questions that confront us. The first, more philosophical question of enhancement is about categorization: what do terms such as "average" or "normal" functioning, or even "disease" and "enhancement" mean when we can improve functioning across the entire range of human capability? Is the typical, occasional erectile dysfunction that most men experience a "disease" (or at least a condition worthy of medical attention) now that we have a treatment for it? If Prozac can lift everyone's mood, what then becomes "normal" or "typical" affect, and will grouchiness or sadness or inner struggle then be pathologized? And if we can all be happy and well-adjusted through Prozac, should insurance pay for everyone to reach that state of bliss? The second, related question addresses a broader social concern: should we encourage or discourage people to ingest pharmaceuticals to enhance behaviors, skills, and traits? What are the social (and economic, religious, psychological, . . .) implications of using drugs or other neurotechnologies to micromanage mood, improve memory, to maintain attentiveness or improve sexuality?

2. DEFINING ENHANCEMENT

The answers to these two questions are, in large measure, dependent on how we define enhancement itself. But the more closely we examine the concept, the slipperier it appears. As enhancement is a concept that defines the boundary condition between what we consider disease intervention and what we do not, by definition the term will conform to what the culture, or medical professionals, see as the proper objects of medical intervention. In other words, what medicine chooses to treat is defined as disease, while altering what it does not treat is enhancement.

The difficulty of creating a meaningful enhancement standard to use to allocate medical care or create guidelines for clinical treatment can be illustrated by looking at one proposal. The bioethicist Norm Daniels asks what kind of m ical care should be covered for all citizens i just society, and in doing so has developed p ably the most detailed discussion of the enhan ment issue (Daniels 1985; Daniels 2000; Sabi Daniels 1994). Daniels is interested in deter ing what should be considered obligatory nonobligatory provision of care in a just soci He begins by arguing against trying to demarc a treatment/enhancement distinction to so that dilemma. First, he suggests, even if we co clearly define the two, we cannot draw a cl moral line that justifies considering one the gitimate object of medical attention and not other. Secondly, there is something ultimat arbitrary about how we draw many of our d ease/non-disease distinctions. Finally, there treatments or conditions (such as abortion shyness) that are clearly outside disease defi tions, yet that we may want to provide in our sta dard medical offerings.

Daniels illustrates his point by offering the f lowing example: imagine two boys, both whom are of short stature and are projected grow into short stature adults of about 5 ft. 3 (which is at the low end of the normal growth d tribution for males). One is short because he h growth hormone (GH) deficiency from a bra tumor, while the other is short because, thoug he has normal GH secretions, he has very sho parents. Both "suffer" from the same conditio and in both the causes are fundamentally bi logical. Yet only one is "sick"; any interventio we design on behalf of the second is like to be labeled "enhancement." Daniels pushes even further: what if we find the gene(s) th cause short stature in the boy without the tumo and discover he is short because his cells d not respond readily to GH, or because his G levels level off faster, or because he has fewer r ceptors? Is he then "sick?" And what if the othe boy has a gene that predisposes him to the tumor Now both causes can be considered genetic, ye one boy is granted full economic and social ac s to medical resources, while the other may t be.

Daniels' concern is about obligatory vs. non-igatory medical services, and its implications social justice; what services must be provided all citizens in a society that sees provision of sic care an inalienable right? What standards "medical care" do we use when we desire to tribute medical care fairly and equitably in so-ty? Why is the society ready to help the boy th the tumor reach greater stature, and not the er, and is the reasoning justified?

Daniels suggests that instead of using defini-ns of disease as our standard, which may lead to treat one boy and not the other, we should stead determine for each trait, state, or behav- what he calls "species-typical functioning." e concept implies not just a statistical accu-ulation of some average level of functioning in particular realm of human activity, but rather examination of the design of the organism to termine the "natural functional organization" its members. The "normal function model" rves as the standard of functioning that a society as an obligation to try to achieve for all its mem-ers. While a society has no obligation to provide rvices that raise any citizen's function above the pical level for the species as a whole, it does ave an obligation to provide services that, to the egree possible, raise the level of functioning of ny citizen with deficits to the species-typical vel. In such a case, if short stature can be shown cause difficulties in the lives of males of such ature (as it can, in such things as employment iscrimination and mate selection), society has n obligation to try to ameliorate that departure om normal function (i.e., male-typical height) o matter what the cause. Daniels goes on to sug-est that normal functioning is important as a aseline not because it is "natural" (a thorny con-ept philosophically) and so inviolable, but be-ause it is a convenient baseline to determine what society should owe to its members. In addi-ion, the approach resists the trend towards medicalizing problems, and sets stronger boundaries around what medicine should attend to. Pursuing some ideal of total physical, mental, and social well-being is beyond medicine's proper domain (Parens 1998).

There are a number of problems with Daniels' argument. His model has been criticized as to the difficulty in determining species-typical functioning for a host of traits (e.g., what is "species-typical" happiness, or shyness, or cognition, or even erectile function?). Remember that we need to determine this not by some statistical average, but rather by a "theoretical account of the design of the organism." How happy were we, in fact, designed to be? Other critics have pointed out the model's assumption of the innateness and immutability of talents and traits; the presumption that maximization of potential is only owed the low-functioning; and the culturally and ideologically bound determination in many traits of what should be considered "typical" or "normal" (e.g., Juengst 1998; Lachs 2000; Silvers 1998). Daniels' effort well illustrates the fundamental problem of drawing the lines between the kinds of physiological interventions that we conceptualize as curative or normalizing, and those we consider extraordinary or enhancing.

Other models have been proposed as well (see Juengst [1998], for a review).Yet, ultimately, any exclusive enhancement definition must fail, in part because concepts such as disease, normalcy, and health are significantly culturally and historically bound, and thus the result of negotiated values. The provision of services under the rubric of medicine is, ultimately, somewhat arbitrary, the product of social negotiation and historical precedent. Decisions about what to fund through insurance reimbursement, what to restrict by regulating access (through physicians, for example), and how society as a whole should regard the use of "enhancing" pharmaceuticals and other technologies will be the product of a long series of conversations in the professional literature and in public fora as these technologies develop.

The enhancement/treatment conundrum can therefore be summarized as addressing three levels of inquiry:

1. Medicine and reimbursement: what should be the proper role of enhancement technologies in medicine and those who fund it? Can a distinction be made between therapy and enhancement that is meaningful and operationalizable? Can we defend the proposition that medicine should concern itself with, or that third party payers should only fund, "treatment" and not "enhancement?"
2. Public policy: in what spheres of public policy should a distinction between disease and enhancement be maintained? Should there be rules against using certain enhancement technologies in sports, for example, or among children? And conversely, should public policy encourage use of enhancement technologies among those for whom it might aid in safeguarding the public good?
3. Normative behavior: is there a normative recommendation for how we should think about enhancement in general? Should society promote or resist biotechnological enhancement? And whatever the normative decision, why does there seem to be such initial resistance to its uses?

3. NEUROTECHNOLOGIES AND THE ENHANCEMENT QUESTION

The questions posed above are particularly trenchant when applied to emerging neurotechnologies. On one hand, human beings have always developed strategies and technologies to enhance their cognitive and affective functioning. We send our children to school, memorize poetry, develop training programs, meditate, enrich our word power, read novels, go to therapy, try to get a good night's sleep before exams, eat "brain food" such as fish, shut the door and turn off music to study—all actions that, to one degre another, are intended to create environme inner states, or improved functioning that encourage or support a desired level of neurol ical performance. We bang our heads, rub temples, snap our fingers, and try to stop think directly about a topic to recall it to memory. In dition, we drink alcohol and caffeine, take R alin and Prozac, inhale nicotine, smoke ma juana, and use other pharmacological means induce our brains to act in ways that we desire to increase memory, stabilize mood, encoura creativity, or promote attentiveness.

The enhancement question, however, ari primarily in technologies that attempt to direc moderate the neurochemical, structural, or ele trical components of the brain. The manipu tion of brain function through learning, me tating, behavioral reinforcement, biofeedbac temple rubbing, or any other mechanism that ther draws on the body's own resources, or m nipulates the external environment to indu change, do not raise the same ethical challenge What characterizes the particular ethical cu rency of the enhancement debate today is th ability to bypass these types of activities and change the brain directly.

Let us leaven our discussion with an examp of a drug with the ability to enhance norm functioning: modafinil. Modafinil (2-[dipheny methyl]-sulfinylacetamide) is a eugeroic (lite ally, "good arousal") drug that creates a wakefu alert state in those who take it. Early reports su gest that, unlike amphetamines, modafinil doe not create a "buzz," does not cycle high and low does not increase heart rate and blood pressure and is non-addictive (Bastuji & Jouvet 1988 US Modafinil in Narcolepsy Multicenter Stud Group 2000). Amphetamines create a dose dependent impairment of the sleep cycle, s that one needs more and more amphetamines t stay awake, and is ultimately more fatigued Modafinil not only does not disturb sleep, it onl ms to cause wakefulness under conditions ere vigilance is sought by the person who has en it (Legarde, Batejat, van Beers, Sarafian, & della 1995). Modafinil is generally prescribed sleep disorders, such as narcolepsy and hyper-nnia, and may be effective in the sleepiness t can accompany diseases such as Parkinson's. Modafinil, marketed under the brand name ovigil, may eventually challenge Viagra in its peal to off-label and black market usage. Also e Viagra, new sources have begun to tout the nefits of modafinil. A CBS News report trum-ted, "A Dream Come True? New Drug Tricks ain to be Awake" (CBS News 2002). The *New rk Times* ran an article emphasizing the drug's tential in "a chronically sleep-deprived na-n" (Goode 1998), and the *New Yorker* maga-ne ran a glowing piece asking whether "science n make regular sleep unnecessary" (Groop-an 2001). Cephalon, the manufacturer, has ne little to discourage the hype; in fact, the DA recently cautioned Cephalon to be more reful in its claims about Provigil in its direct-to-nsumer advertising (*Los Angeles Times* 2002).

Additionally, the potential of modafinil to be ed for non-therapeutic purposes has been pro-oted in reports citing the armed services' inter-t in the drug for use in pilots. One study that me out of the United States Army Aeromedical esearch Laboratory examined helicopter pilots ho were exposed to two 40-h periods of contin-ous wakefulness separated by only one night f recovery sleep. When receiving modafinil, e pilots scored higher on tests of performance nd physiological arousal than they did while n placebo, and also had improved self-ratings of igor, energy, alertness, talkativeness, and confi-ence (Caldwell, Caldwell, Smythe, & Hall 000).

It is not therefore surprising that the United tates Army, as well as a number of European rmed forces, are already using modafinil; up ntil now, the standard issue wakefulness drug vas Dexedrine, which causes all the side effects of amphetamines. The Department of Defense Advanced Research Projects Agency (DARPA), which is funding research into modafinil, justified the research by claiming:

> As combat systems become more and more sophisticated and reliable, the major limiting factor for operational dominance in a conflict is the warfighter. Eliminating the need for sleep while maintaining the high level of both cognitive and physical performance of the individual will create a fundamental change in warfighting and force employment, (quoted in Groopman 2001, p. 55).

The armed services are not employing the drug without at least some ethical reflection on the appropriate uses of pharmaceuticals as enhancement agents; as a United States Air Force report puts it: "The development of modafinil brings to light a crucial social question. What would be the impediment for its use, if a compound such as modafinil is more like caffeine than amphetamine in terms of safety, and yet, as effective as the amphetamines?" (Lyons & French 1991).

The "crucial social question" of Lyons and French already confronts us. The use of Viagra, for example, is common among men who would not qualify for a diagnosis of erectile dysfunction (Armstrong et al. 1999). Ritalin sales in certain school districts exceeds any reasonable estimate of children with ADHD that meets DSM-IV criteria (Diller 1996; Miller, Lalonde, McGrail, & Armstrong 2001a, 2001b). Kramer (1993) suggested that Prozac makes some patients "better than well," and prescriptions soared. Clearly, some of the top selling drugs in the world today are being used by patients who fit no traditional definition of pathology, yet still see in their own functioning a deficit that these drugs address.

Modafinil will likely follow the patterns of Viagra and Prozac, with areas of overprescribing, significant off-label usage, websites with cursory medical examination, and significant non-prescription sales. Still (or perhaps therefore?) policies need to be made, and so the enhancement question must be addressed. Should modafinil be prescribed solely as a medical drug, properly used only for those suffering from sleep pathology? If so third party payers, including government programs, should cover it. Or, should it be classified as an over-the-counter drug, available to anyone who wants it? Or, should we create a class of drugs available only to those who can show legitimate social need, those whose fatigue might put others at risk, such as airline pilots, or truck drivers? If so, we might see modafinil use as akin to reconstructive surgery, where payment is determined on perceived necessity. For those with severe injury or disfiguring birth defects, reconstructive surgery is medically justifiable and covered. For those electing to have surgery for cosmetic purposes, physicians are still free to offer it (or not), but no one is under a moral obligation to fund it. Finally, as a general social policy question, should we restrict modafinil's use in certain defined social settings, such as sports competitions (where those who use it will have an advantage), or in pediatric use (where students should be learning nonpharmaceutical attention skills), or in people in particularly high-stress jobs, such as airport traffic controllers (who might be tempted to abuse it)?

4. THE PROBLEMS OF NEUROLOGICAL ENHANCEMENT

The difficulty in deciding the questions of the correct use of neurological enhancers is, in part, a recognition that since we do not really understand the implications of enhancing neurological function, our strategies may backfire. The idea that attention is good, so increased attention is better, or that cognition is good, so increased cognition is better, may turn out to have unexpected consequences. Let us take as an example the effort to develop drugs targeted to improving memory in human beings (e.g., Furey, Pietr
Alexander, Schapiro, & Horwitz 2000). The
provement of memory sounds attractive in
abstract, and certainly is desirable for those
fering from Alzheimer's or other conditions t
affect memory functions. But there are many
knowns in the use of such drugs in the cognitiv
intact. The assumption is that memory drugs
simply increase the amount of memory we h
available, leaving all other cognitive and affect
processes unaffected. But in fact, memory is a
lective, delicate process. There are experien
and data that our brains filter out. Our cognit
processes retain specific kinds of data, un
specific circumstances, while other input is
glected. Who needs to remember the hours wa
ing in the Department of Motor Vehicles stari
at the ceiling tiles, or to recall the transient a
nesia following a personal trauma? Yet, we do n
know whether memory enhancement dru
might impair our selectivity process. Might th
improve our retention of all memories, even t
traumatic or trivial memories that the brain ten
to repress? Might we end up awash in memori
that are troubling to us, unable to forget a painf
past? And how might a memory drug affect ass
ciated mental processes—mood (which is close
connected to memory), or attentiveness (da
dreaming is often fueled by a sudden recolle
tion)? Perhaps evolution has stabilized at a pa
ticular level of memory capacity because mo
sacrifices a certain cognitive flexibility; a plast
brain may have advantages over one cramme
with memory.

The concern is not only speculative. In 199
scientists reported in *Nature* that they had gene
ically engineered mice with increased ability
perform learning tasks (Tang et al. 1999). The sc
entists inserted a gene in mouse zygotes that i
creased the production of the protein subun
NR2B, part of the NMDA receptor. The mic
also displayed physiological changes in the hi
pocampus (associated with learning) when co
pared to non-transgenic mice. However, subs

:nt research seemed to indicate that the mice h enhanced NR2B seemed to have a greater isitivity to pain (Wei et al. 2001). Though it y be that the mice do not feel the pain more itely, just learn about pain more readily and is seem to react to it more strongly (Tang, imizu, & Tsien 2001), it is troubling that even : most preliminary research on memory en- ncement has already raised the question of un- pected collateral effects. Perhaps there is a link do not understand between memory and in, either at the structural or behavioral level. hat other unexpected linkages might be dis- vered in attempts to change cognitive func- ns through induced physiological modifica- n?

While most of the "cognitive enhancement" scussed in the literature focuses on memory or tentiveness, the range of cognitive abilities, of urse, exceeds just these two traits. Learning, nguage, skilled motor behaviors, and "execu- e functions" (such as decision making, goal tting, planning, and judgment) are all part of :neral cognition, and a drug that managed to ihance a greater range of function (especially :ecutive function) may be more desirable than ie that narrowly enhanced memory alone Vhitehouse, Juengst, Mehlman, & Murray 997). But if memory drugs alone have collateral ffects, how much more so might a drug that ifluences a greater range of cognitive function- ig? It is not only the collateral effects of neuro- gical enhancement that are troublesome, but lso the nature of the change itself. For example, ie progressive loss of cognitive function that haracterizes Alzheimer's is usually described s the "loss of personality" of the person with the isease. "Dad isn't Dad anymore" because his ognitive faculties as experienced by his loved nes are considered fundamental to who he is; oss of those functions are seen as loss of his :ssence. A general cognitive enhancement may iave the same effect. Significantly improving our verall cognitive functioning may also alter aspects of our identity that are seen as fundamental to who we are. As Whitehouse et al. (1997, p.16) write:

> Increased memory, new insights, and better reasoning could all lead to new values, new perspectives on one's relationships, and new sources of pleasure and irritation. That does not mean that the enhanced literally will lose their identities and become different people, any more than someone with Alzheimer's does. But in the figurative sense intended by caregivers of people with the disease, it may be that after some point the cognitively enhanced will no longer be recognizable by those who knew them before their enhancement.

Research on patients with frontotemporal dementia, who demonstrate often dramatic changes in well-established patterns or religion, dress, style, and political philosophy, seems to indicate that some aspects of the self are functions of the frontal lobes (Miller et al. 2001a, 2001b). Lauren Slater, author of the memoir *Prozac Diary*, writes that though Prozac relieved her of her symptoms, she no longer felt any desire to read the angst-ridden psychology and philosophy books that lined her bookshelf (Slater 1998). Slater wonders what the loss of these books, that had once been sources of wisdom for her, meant for her sense of self: "who was I? Where was I? Everything seemed less relevant—my sacred menus, my gustatory habits, the narrative that had had so much meaning for me. Diminished." Even when she rediscovers her spiritual side later in the memoir, she now wonders if her calmer, more contemplative spirituality comes not from God, but from Prozac.

Neurological biotechnologies differ from others in that they ask us to explicitly consider the kind of "self" we want to have; or, to put it less dualistically, perhaps, the kind of self we want to be. For some, our astounding ability to manipulate our own biology is an integral part of who we are as human animals. For others, it is an affront to our humanity. This is an argument for which there are no right or wrong answers, emerging as it does from two philosophically different visions of human life. Yet therein lies the tension of the enhancement debate, and there is little doubt that the battlefield on which the debate will be waged next will be our ancient desire to control the workings of our own minds.

REFERENCES

Abbott, A. 2001. Into the mind of a killer. *Nature* 410: 296–298.

Anderson, S. W., Bechara, A., Damasio, H., Tranel, D., and Damasio, A. R. 1999. Impairment of social and moral behavior related to early damage in human prefrental cortex. *Nature Neuroscience* 2 (11): 1032–1037.

Armstrong, K., Schwartz, J. S., & Asch, D. A. 1999. Direct sale of sildenafil (Viagra) to consumers over the internet. *New England Journal of Medicine* 341 (18): 1389–1392.

Bastuji, H., & Jouvet, M. (1988). Successful treatment of idiopathic hypersomnia and narcolepsy with modafinil. *Progress in Neuropsychopharmacology & Biological Psychiatry* 12 (5): 695–700.

Caldwell, J. A., Caldwell, J. L., Smythe, N. K., & Hall, K. K. 2000. A double-blind, placebo-controlled investigation of the efficacy of modafinil for sustaining the alertness and performance of aviators: a helicopter simulator study. *Psychopharmacologia* 150 (3): 272–282.

CBS News. 2002. A dream come true? New drug tricks brain to be awake; military is interested. January 14 (www.cbsnews.com/now/story/0,1597,324299-912,00.shtml).

Daniels, N. 2000. Normal functioning and the treatment-enhancement distinction. *Cambridge Quarterly* 9 (3): 309–322.

Daniels, N. 1985. *Just Health Care*. New York: Cambridge University Press.

Diller, L. H. 1996. The run on Ritalin: attention deficit disorder and stimpulant treatment in the 1990s. *Hastings Center Report* 26 (2): 12–14.

Furey, M. L., Pietrini, P., Alexander, G. E., Schapiro, M. B., & Horwitz, B. 2000. Cholinergic hancement improves performance on working m ory by modulating the functional activity in dist brain regions: a positron emission tomography gional cerebral blood flow study in healthy hum *Brain Research Bulletin* 51 (3): 213–218.

Goode, E. 1998. New hope for losers in the battl stay awake. *New York Times*, November 3, F1.

Groopman, J. 2001. Eyes wide open. *New Yor* December 3, 52–57.

Juengst, E. 1998. What does enhancement mean E. Parens (ed.), *Enhancing Human Traits*, pp. 29– Washington, D.C.: Georgetown University Press.

Kramer, P. O. 1993. *Listening to Prozac*. New Yo Penguin.

Lachs, J. 2000. Grand dreams of perfect peop *Cambridge Quarterly* 9 (3): 323–329.

Legarde, D., Batejat, D., van Beers, P., Sarafian, & Pradella, S. 1995. Interest of modafinil, a new p chostimulant during a sixty hour sleep deprivation periment. *Fundamental & Clinical Pharmacolog* (3): 271–279.

Los Angeles Times. 2002. EDA reprimands 4 dr makers for misleading promotions. January 16. (w .latimes.com/business/la-000004018janl6.story?col= headlines-business).

Lyons, T. J., & French, J. 1991. Modafinil, t unique properties of a new stimulant. *USAF School Aerospace, Brooks, TX, Science News Note* 62: 432–43

Miller, A. R., Lalonde, C. E., McGrail, K. M., Armstrong, R. W. 2001a. Prescription of methylphe idate to children and youth, 1990–1996. *CMAJ, Can dian Medical Association Journal* 165 (11): 1489–149

Miller, M. D., Seeley, W. W., Mychack, P., Rose M. D., Mena, I., & Boone, K. 2001b. Neuroanatomy the self. *Neurology* 57: 817–821.

Parens, E. 1998. Is better always good? The enhanc ment project. *Hastings Center Report* 28 (1): S1–S1

Sabin, J. E., & Daniels, N. 1994. Determining "me ical necessity" in mental health practice. *Hasting Center Report* 24 (6): 5–13.

Silvers, A. 1998. A fatal attraction to normalizing treating disabilities as deviations from "species-typical ctioning. In E. Parens (ed.), *Enhancing Human its*, pp. 95–123. Washington, D.C.: Georgetown iversity Press.

Slater, L. (1998). *Prozac Diary*. New York: Random use.

Tang, Y. P., Shimizu, E., Dube, G. R., Rampon, C., rchner, G. A., Zhuo, M., Liu, G., & Tsien, J. Z. 9. Genetic enhancement of learning and memory mice. *Nature* 401 (6748): 63–69.

Tang, Y., Shimizu, E., & Tsien, J. Z. 2001. Do nart" mice feel more pain, or are they just better rners? *Nature Neuroscience* 4 (5): 453–454.

US Modafinil in Narcolepsy Multicenter Study Group. 2000. Randomized trial of modafinil as a treatment for the excessive daytime somnolence of narcolepsy. *Neurology* 54 (5): 1166–1175.

Wei, F., Wang, G. D., Kerchner, G. A., Kim, S. J., Xu, H. M., Chen, Z. F., & Zhuo, M. 2001. Genetic enhancement of inflammatory pain by forebrain NR2B overexpression. *Nature Neuroscience* 4 (2): 164–169.

Whitehouse, P. J., Juengst, E., Mehlman, M., & Murray, T. H. 1997. Enhancing cognition in the intellectually intact. *Hastings Center Report*, May–June, 14–22.

CHAPTER 27

What's Morally Wrong with Eugenics?

ARTHUR L. CAPLAN

THE TOPIC OF EUGENICS cannot be di cussed for long without encountering the Holocaust. This is as it should b When contemporary geneticists, genetics counselors and clinical genet cists wonder, as they sometimes do, why it is that genetics receives speci attention from those concerned with ethics, the answer is simple—histor

The events which led to the sterilization, torture and murder of millio of Jews, Gypsies, Slavs, and children of mixed racial heritage in the yea just before and during the era of the Third Reich in Germany were roote firmly in the science of genetics (Müller-Hill 1988). Rooted not in fringe lunatic science, but in the mainstream of reputable genetics in what wa indisputably the most advanced scientific and technological society of it

, the pursuit of genetic purity led directly to chau, Treblinka, Ravensbruck and Auschwitz. As early as 1931 influential geneticists such as tz Lenz, were referring to National Socialism "applied biology" in their textbooks (Caplan)2). As difficult as it is for many contemporary entists to accept (ibid.; Kater 1992), main-eam science provided a good deal of enthusias-scientific support for the virulent racism that eled the killing machine of the Third Reich. When the Nazis came to power they were ob-ssed with securing the racial purity of the Ger-an people. The medical and biomedical com-unities in Germany not only endorsed this ncern with "negative eugenics," they had fos-red it. Race hygiene swept through German bi-ogy, public health, medicine and anthropology the 1920s and 1930s, long before the Nazis me to power (Weiss 1987; Müller-Hill 1988; octor 1988; Kater 1992). Many in the medical ofession urged the Nazi leadership to under-ke social policies that might lead to enhancing increasing the genetic fitness of the German eople (Kater 1992).

Eugenics consumed the German medical, bi-ogical and social scientific communities in the ecade before World War II. Many physicians d scientists were frantic about threats they saw to e genetic health of the nation posed by the pres-nce of inferior populations such as Jews, Gypsies, lavs, and to a lesser extent because the threat was ore distant, African peoples (Adams 1990). The eps they took to protect against the public ealth disaster of a "polluted" racial stock were so wful, so immoral and so heinous that they have, ghtly, shaped all subsequent discussion of the hics of both human genetics and eugenics.

NEGATIVE VS. POSITIVE EUGENICS

teps to eliminate unfit or undesirable genes by rohibitions on sexual relations, restrictions on narriage, sterilization or killing, are all forms of negative population eugenics (Kevles 1995 [1985]). Nazi judges and scientists ordered children killed or sterilized who had parents of different racial backgrounds or were thought to have genetic predispositions toward mental illness, alcoholism, retardation or other disabilities. This was done to remove the threat such children posed to the genetic stock of the nation and to avoid having to pay the costs associated with institutionalization and hospitalization (Caplan 1992). Laws were enacted prohibiting marriages between those whom Nazi race hygiene theory held were likely to produce degenerate offspring.

Conversely, on a smaller scale, the Nazis tried to encourage those who satisfied Nazi racial ideals to have more children. The most extreme form of encouraging eugenic mating was the *Lebensborn* program: a National Socialist program, which gave money, medals, housing, and other rewards to persuade "ideal" mothers and fathers to have large numbers of children in order to create a super-race of Aryan children (Proctor 1988). The provision of rewards, incentives and benefits to encourage the increased representation of certain genes in the gene pool of future generations constitutes positive population eugenics (Kevles 1995 [1985]).

Nazi race hygiene theories were false. There is no evidence to support the biological views of the inherent inferiority of races or the biological superiority of specific ethnic groups which underlay the eugenics efforts of the Third Reich. There is not even any firm basis for differentiating groups into races on the basis of genetics (see various selections in part II of Harding 1993). The negative eugenics programs race hygiene spawned were not only patently unethical, since they were completely involuntary and coercive, they were also based upon assumptions about genes and race that are not true. The Nazi drive to design future generations based on what can now be understood as invalid science skewed by racism led to concentration camps, forced sterilization, infanticide and genocide.

Arthur L. Caplan

THE LEGACY OF GERMAN EUGENICS

The rapid evolution of clinical genetics in the post–World War II era has been accompanied by a strong moral commitment to the autonomy of the patient. Those who work in clinical genetics are resolute in their belief that the purpose of their work is not to tell people what reproductive choices to make but to supply them with information which will empower them to make more informed decisions (Bartels, LeRoy, and Caplan 1993; Bartels et al. 1997). Whether or not value neutrality really does characterize the practice of counseling (Bartels et al. 1997), the centrality of autonomy in the normative ethos of professionals practicing clinical genetics is a direct response to the coercive horrors of Nazi Germany and the abuses carried out in the name of eugenics and public health in the United States in the first half of the twentieth century (Reilly 1991; Kevles 1995 [1985]; Haller 1993; Caplan 1993b; Pernick 2000).

In recent years the desire to maintain a distance between the events in Germany fifty years ago and today's effort to map the human genome and apply the knowledge gained to human beings has added a new normative twist. Most of those prominently involved now in actually mapping the human genome and in attempting early forms of gene therapy are adamant in stating that they have no interest in modifying the human germline. By forswearing any interest in germline modification, those involved in the mapping and sequencing of the human genome can more easily deflect the kinds of moral concerns that would otherwise be directed toward the project as a result of the tragic history of Germany's involvement with eugenics (Anderson 1989, 1992; Garver 1991; Munson and Davis 1992; Duster 1990; Lewontin 1992; Danks 1994).

However, whether or not particular scientists or clinicians are serious or merely being prudent in publicly forswearing any interest in germline eugenics, the fact is that there is tremendous interest in American society and in other nation using genetic information for eugenic purpo (Klass 1989; Munson and Davis 1992; Herrnst and Murray 1994; Bobrow 1995; Kitcher 19 2000).

Raising the issue of the application of euge knowledge to human reproduction is sometin dismissed as histrionic moral grandstandi Why worry about this issue when it is not n possible and is unlikely to be possible for ma years to come? But the legitimacy of worryi about the impossible seems a bit easier to defe when squared against the pace of recent develo ments in genetics and genetic engineering.

Recent advances in the understanding of sp matogenesis as well as in the fields of anin cloning and assisted reproductive technolo point toward methods that would permit the sy tematic alteration of genetic information in r productive cells (Brinster and Zimmerman 199 Eugenic goals could also be advanced throu the use of embryo biopsy and the selective elin nation of embryos or the selection of sperm embryos known to be endowed with certain tra (Caplan 1995, 1998a 1998b).

Some within the disabilities community ha noted that the use of genetic information whic results in the prevention of the birth of childre with certain traits or behavioral dispositions ca be construed as a form of eugenics. Large-sca screening programs to prevent the transmissio of congenital diseases do exist. The state of Ca fornia has for many years encouraged women t be tested during their pregnancies for fetal neur tube defects. The success of the program is evalu ated not in terms of information given to mothe but rather in terms of the number of children wi handicaps who were not born. When number c births prevented is the measure of a public healt intervention it is hard to say that anything othe than negative eugenics fuels support for such pro grams (Duster 1990; Murphy and Lappé 1994)

Ethical debates about eugenics must acknow edge the horrors perpetrated in the name of eu ics in this century. But, despite the evil that been done in the name of eugenics, the de- e cannot end there. The moral permissibility eugenic goals must be addressed on its own ms. For while arguments based upon history instructive and important, those who see no alogies between our times and earlier times are likely to find warnings about the past suffi- ntly forceful to shape future behavior or pub- policy (Caplan 1992, 1994). And while the fear the imposition of eugenic programs by a total- rian regime must be taken seriously, it is not e only path eugenics might follow.

INDIVIDUAL VS. POPULATION EUGENICS

nprovement of the genetic makeup of a popu- tion can be sought through negative or positive igenics. What is less widely noted is that either rategy can be pursued at the level of individuals d their direct, lineal offspring or for large oups or populations. Efforts aimed at improv- g or enhancing the properties of large-scale pulations such as by providing incentives for rge numbers of individuals with particular traits abilities to marry and have many children or ncouraging public health testing for neural tube efects constitute versions of population eugen- s. The goal of such activities is to shift the akeup of the gene pool of future generations in articular directions.

Positive and negative eugenics can also be car- ied out by individual couples who are not in- erested in nor motivated by the overall effect heir actions may have on the societal gene pool. ctivities intended to permit individuals to en- ow their children and their subsequent offspring vith desired traits are instances of individual eu- enics. A decision to try to implant a bit of DNA ssociated with a desirable trait into an egg so as o have the trait present in one's child is an in- tance of individual eugenics. So would a decision to clone oneself for simple reasons of vanity and self-perpetuation. So too may be a decision to abort a pregnancy when a fetus is found to have cystic fibrosis or spina bifida.

Attempting to choose the genetic makeup of one's offspring with an eye toward creating a tall child is to engage in individual eugenics. A government program with the goal of creating large numbers of tall people is an example of population eugenics.

Individual and population eugenics are conceptually distinct, but procreative decisions can be motivated by both concerns at the same time. Those who want to pursue population eugenics may be able to do so either by encouraging those interested in individual genetic enhancement to pursue their individual goals, or by efforts to control or change the overall reproductive behaviors of large numbers of people. If a dictator wants to create a future population with a higher IQ, programs might be created to discourage people with low IQs from marrying (Caplan 1995). The Chinese government passed a law to this effect in 1995 (Bobrow 1995). The same goal can also be reached by discouraging people perceived as having poor genetic endowments from reproducing by changing welfare, housing and educational policies (Herrnstein and Murray 1994). Encouraging individual couples to use genetic testing or embryo biopsy and then embryo selection in order to help insure that their children have high IQs is still another road to the same destination (Caplan 1998a). If enough families pursue individual eugenic goals, a population eugenic goal may result.

In China, policies which restrict individual couples to having a single child combined with social attitudes that prevail among many Chinese favoring boys over girls have led many couples to take steps that will insure that their child is a boy. While the Chinese government has not instituted any policies that explicitly favor the creation of male rather than female children, the combination of choices made by individual couples appears to have been powerful enough to produce a shift in the overall gender composition of the Chinese population toward more males.

Population eugenics need not be coercive, but, historically, it almost always has been. A great deal of social pressure was applied in the German *Lebensborn* programs of the 1940s. More recent efforts to shift the genetic norms of populations exemplified by the attempt to encourage those with the "right" racial makeup to reproduce, as is evident in the ethnically selective pronatalist policies espoused by governments in many parts of the world, are less obviously coercive but still involve a great deal of cultural and societal pressure. The stated policies of some religious bodies, such as certain Orthodox Jewish sects or some priests of the Greek Orthodox church, that they will not bless marriages where no genetic testing for diseases has been done, constitute examples of possible coercion for population eugenic goals by non-governmental powers.

Instances of individual eugenics are harder to find. But, decisions by families to try and have boys rather than girls may represent examples of individual eugenic thinking (Caplan 1995). And there are many instances in which persons try to avoid having a child with what they perceive as a burdensome defect or disease by using genetic testing.

INDIVIDUAL EUGENICS: THE WAVE OF THE FUTURE?

It will not be long before science makes it easier to put eugenic aspirations for populations or individuals into practice. The manipulation of gamete production to identify and eliminate unwanted traits and the ability to accurately insert genetic information directly into sperm or embryo are the subjects of investigation around the world. Embryo biopsy wherein cells are removed from an embryo, cultured and their DNA content analyzed for various propensities are already being touted by a number of infertility c ics. When these techniques are identified refined, the chance to pick the biological end ments of our offspring, to give them the "b possible start in life, will have enormous app to many.

The hope of using science and medicine create children who get the best possible star their lives is very different from the forced us medical and scientific knowledge to solve so ety's perceived ills by creating biologically su rior populations or simply killing those deem inferior. There are those who would agree w the population eugenic goals espoused by founder of the so-called "Nobel Prize" spe bank, Robert Graham, the Director of the Rep itory for Germinal Choice in Escondido, Ca fornia, that we owe it to future generations to and maximize the genetic endowment of at le some of its yet-to-be-born members by carefu selecting which genes we pass along from us them (Caplan 1995). But, the real impact of ne techniques, such as the transplantation of spe stem cells, embryo biopsy and genetic testing sperm and eggs, is likely to be seen in the condu of individual parents seeking to fulfill their as rations and dreams for their children.

Genetic enhancement in the future is muc more likely to be the product of the norm th good parents make sure that their children ha the best chance possible to succeed in life, tha it is the imposition of a governmental manda that all must procreate with the goal of enhanci the presence in the gene pool of persons with particular biological phenotype. In Western so cieties with their strong normative commitmen to autonomy and privacy, individual eugenic will have a rosier future than the harsh and intr sive steps required to implement and sustai public policies aimed at population eugeni goals.

The day when we need to decide whether it wrong to choose the genetic makeup of our chi dren is not very far off. Some argue that we lac the wisdom to choose well (Lewontin 1992). Bu t hardly stops parents today from seeking to ter the lot of their children through environ-ntally mediated efforts at enhancement. In a iety that places so much emphasis on maxi-zing opportunities and achieving the most ef-ient use of resources, it is hard to believe that essures will not quickly arise on prospective rents to use genetic information and tech-ques for manipulating genes to better the lot of eir children or of future generations of chil-en.

For some, the historical abuses committed in is century in the name of eugenics are suffi-ent grounds for prohibiting or banning any ef-rts at any form of eugenics, positive or negative; dividual or group. However, negative popula-on eugenics is not individual positive eugenics. most people agree that parents have a right, if t a duty, to try and maximize the well-being d happiness of their offspring, then it is not kely that the record of historical abuses carried t in the name of negative population eugenics ill hinder efforts to incorporate genetic infor-ation into procreative decisions about our chil-ren and their immediate descendants. As it ands today, most parents, particularly those in e middle and upper classes, would probably be ore troubled by failing to use genetic informa-on to try and improve the lot of their offspring an they would by doing so.

If that is so, then what values should influence ur ideas about human normality, perfection and mpairment? Can parents really be trusted to hoose the characteristics of their children? Is he only reason that the eugenical aspirations of eople such as Robert Graham are dismissed as ooky is that those who espouse them are holding ut false hope because there is no guarantee rtificial insemination using the sperm of men se-ected for desired traits will produce these traits in heir offspring? Making false promises to people s certainly wrong, but surely there are more fun-lamental issues involved in the ethics of inten-ionally designing "better" babies than false ad-vertising.

SHOULD WE PICK THE TRAITS OF OUR CHILDREN?

Suppose it becomes easier to achieve conception reliably outside the womb, making the analysis of the genetic makeup of embryos a simple task. Would there be any reason not to allow prospective mothers and fathers to select the biological endowments of their children? This question must be answered in light of the degree to which it is now possible for parents to obtain information about the genetic makeup of their unborn children in order to minimize the chance of having a child with a lethal or disabling medical problem (Kolker and Burke 1994).

What should medicine do in the face of the strong desire most parents feel to bring their child into this world healthy? Is there any criterion or definition that would allow the sorting of human traits into desirable and undesirable categories? Even if such a classification could be done, is it part of medicine's professional responsibility to allow parents to pick and choose among the desirable and undesirable characteristics they wish their child to have?

HEALTH, DISEASE, DISABILITY AND THE AIMS OF MEDICINE

When most people think about health, they think about it as referring to the absence of illness or disease. If you are not sick, then you are healthy. But this way of thinking about health, about what is normal and abnormal, is confusing. It is possible to be free of disease and still not be seen by others as healthy. You can be out-of-shape, nervous, on-edge, lacking in self-confidence, have no stamina, feel completely awkward and unsure of yourself, and still, on the view that the absence of disease constitutes health, be considered healthy. But that seems to stretch the meaning of health to include a bit too much. Health is not simply the absence of disease and dysfunction (Caplan 1993a, 1998b).

Health means something more. Health refers to a state in which a person is flourishing, in which bodies and minds are working, not at adequate levels but at optimal levels. Health makes essential reference to a concept of optimizing, not merely reaching, some level of minimal functioning.

If it is true that health refers to optimizing the functions of our bodies and minds then it is easy to see why health is such an elusive goal. Health is an ideal, not an average or a minimal threshold. When parents say they want a healthy child, they may well mean that they only want their children not to be sick, meaning to be disease free or able to function without serious impairments or disorders. But, they may really mean they want a healthy child, meaning they want their children to enjoy the best possible physical and mental functioning. They want their yet-to-be-born children to function at optimal levels. This is precisely the sort of wish, the pursuit of perfection, that leads some men and women to want to use the services of a facility such as the Repository for Germinal Choice.

The desire for health, in the full sense of the concept, is behind parental decisions to place their children in the elite nursery schools, expensive private high schools, tennis camps or special music or art classes. These institutions are valued not because they prevent disease or dysfunction. They are valued because many parents see them as the means to developing the best possible skills and abilities in their children. They are valued as a part of health, not as a means of avoiding disease. Presume that those who do seek out eugenic services want the healthiest possible offspring. Is there anything morally wrong with pursuing perfection as the goal of reproduction?

IS THERE A PERSUASIVE ARGUMENT AGAINST INDIVIDUAL EUGENICS?

Arguments that are commonly made against the morality of trying to design perfect children fall roughly into three categories; the unavo able presence of force or compulsion, the im sition of a standard of perfection, or worries ab inequity arising from eugenic choice. The f worry is not one that seems appropriate to in vidual eugenic choice. The latter two may be especially telling against individual euge wishes either.

Coercion

Certainly it is morally objectionable for gove ments or institutions to compel or coerce the productive behavior of persons (Reilly 1991). T right to reproduce without interference fro third parties is one of the fundamental freedo recognized by international law and moral the ries from a host of ethical traditions. It is a morally wrong to allow the state to impose its sion of the future by force. However, the goal obtaining perfection or pursuing health with spect to individual eugenics is not made obje tionable by these arguments. What is moral wrong is coercion, compulsion or the use of for with respect to reproductive decisions.

The Repository for Germinal Choice and g netics counseling programs at academic medic centers and private clinics make a special point avoiding any hint of coercion or compulsion their activities. It would seem those who correct find the reproductive policies of the Nazi regim in Germany during the Second World War, th government of South Africa prior to the creatio of democracy in 1993 or the current populatio policies of China ethically abhorrent are re pulsed more by the means than the goals in volved in efforts to design future generations.

The Subjectivity of Perfection

Some who find the pursuit of perfection morall objectionable worry about more than coercion They note that it is simply not clear which trait or attributes are properly perceived as perfect o optimal. The decision about what trait or behav is good or healthy depends upon the environ- nt and circumstances that a child will face. To k traits, features or attributes in the abstract o simply reify prejudice as optimality (Rapp 8; Harding 1993).

Views about what is perfect or desirable in a man being are more often than not matters of te, culture and bias. But they are not always nply the product of subjective feelings.

There are certain traits; physical stamina, ength, speed, mathematical ability, dexterity, d acuity of vision to name only a few, which are ated to health in ways that command univer- assent in almost any cultural or social setting aginable. It would be hard to argue that a par- t who wanted a child with better memory or eater physical dexterity was simply indulging s or her biases or prejudices. As long as there is coercion or force used to compel persons to ake choices about their children that are in nformity with particular visions of what is good bad, healthy or unhealthy, there would seem be enough consensus about the relationship etween certain physical and mental attributes d health to permit parents to choose certain aits, features and capacities for their unborn ildren in the name of their health. And if no ercion of compulsion were involved, it could ven be argued that parents should be free to pick e eye or hair color of their children or other qually innocuous traits as long as their selection nposed no risk for the child and did not com- romise the child's chance of maximizing his or er opportunities.

A parent might concede that their vision of erfection is to some degree subjective but still nsist upon the right to pursue their own values. ince we accept this point of view with respect o child rearing, allowing parents to teach their hildren religious values, hobbies, and customs s they see fit, with almost no restrictions short f imperiling the life of the child, it would be lifficult to reject it as overly subjective when mat- ers turn to the selection of a genetic endowment or one's child.

A different set of objections commonly raised against the morality of trying to achieve perfection hinge on concerns about slippery slopes of various types. Some worry that allowing parents to pick the traits of their children will lead inevitably to government forcing its vision of perfection upon anyone who wants to have children. But, this argument has problems as well. For one, it flies in the face of a number of facts about the pursuit of perfection in other areas of health care.

For many years cosmetic surgeons, psychoanalysts, and sports medicine specialists have been plying their trades without any slope having developed in American society to the effect that those with big noses or poor posture must visit a specialists and have these traits altered. Some choose to avail themselves of these specialists in the pursuit of perfection. Many do not. If there is a slippery-slope from permitting individual choice of one's child's traits to limiting the choices available to parents, it is a slope that does not start with individual choice. And if there is a problem of a slope, then it must be shown why it is morally permissible to seek perfection after one is born, but why such efforts would also be wrong if engaged in prenatally.

It is certainly and sadly true that twentieth-century history brims with instances of genocide, mass murder and ethnic cleansing. These are, nevertheless, problems of politics, government and ideology. There is nothing inherent in the decision to indulge one's preferences about the traits of one's child that is morally wrong as long as those preferences do nothing to hurt or impair the child. If there are slippery slope problems that confound the morality of eugenics, they lie in the flaws of politics as well as misunderstandings about the nature of population genetics and diversity, not in the desire to have a "better" baby.

Equality

Another objection to allowing eugenic desires to influence parenting is that it will lead to fundamental social inequalities (Kitcher 1996, 2000).

Allowing parental choice about the genetic makeup of their children may lead to the creation of a genetic "overclass" which has unfair advantages over those who parents did not or could not afford to endow them with the right biological dispositions and traits. Or it may lead to too much homogenization in society where diversity and difference disappear in a rush to produce only perfect people, leaving anyone with the slightest disability or deficiency at a distinct disadvantage.

Equity and fairness are certainly important concepts in societies that are committed to the equality of opportunity for all citizens. However, a belief that everyone deserves a fair chance may mean that society must do what it can to ensure that the means to implementing eugenic choices are available to all who desire them. It may also mean that a strong obligation exists to try and compensate for any differences in biological endowment with special programs and educational opportunities. It is hard to argue, in a world that tolerates so much inequity in the circumstances under which children are brought into being, that there is something more offensive or more morally problematic about biological advantages as opposed to social and economic advantages.

It is also difficult to argue in a world that tolerates large numbers of privileged persons the right to pursue the best education for their children in situations and contexts that may well produce homogeneity in the end-results, that the pursuit of perfection or enhancement at the cost of homogeneity is allowed in schools, music lessons or summer camps when the intervention is environmental but not when it is biological. The fact that kids with privileged social backgrounds go on to similar sorts of educational and life experiences does not seem sufficient reason to prohibit the parenting practices of the upper class. It should also be pointed out that similarity is a matter of degree and that what looks homogeneous to some may appear to be very different to others. Small differences can make a big difference even in a world in which some people pursue g that will lead toward some degree of biologi homogeneity.

There does not appear to be a persuasive, principle ethical reason to condemn individ eugenic goals. At least none of those canvassec this paper provide a basis for ruling any and eugenic goals out of bounds as self-evidently i moral. While force and coercion, compulsi and threat have no place in procreative choice is not so clear that it is any less ethical to allo parent to pick the eye color of their child or try and create a fetus with a propensity for ma ematics then it is to permit them to teach th children the values of a particular religion, try inculcate a love of sports by taking them to gam and exhibitions or to require them to play t piano in order that they acquire a skill.

If there is an argument to be made against e genics, it would seem to be most persuasi against group or population eugenics. Efforts shift the composition of the gene pool wou seem to require or be more prone to slip tow the imposition of a vision by government or oth powerful institutions. In so far as coercion ar force are absent and individual choice is allowe to hold sway, then, presuming fairness in the a cess to the means of enhancing our offspring, it hard to see what exactly is wrong with trying create more perfect babies or better adults.

REFERENCES

Adams, Mark. (ed.). 1990. *The Wellborn Scienc Eugenics in Germany, France, Brazil, and Russia.* O ford: Oxford University Press.

Anderson, W. French. 1989. "Human Gene The apy: Why Draw a Line?" *Journal of Medicine and Ph losophy* 14:681–93.

Anderson, W. French. 1992. "The First Signs c Danger." *Human Gene Therapy* 3:359–60.

Bartels, D. M., B. LeRoy, A. L. Caplan, and P. Mc Carthy. 1997. "Nondirectiveness in Genetic Counsel ing: A Survey of Practitioners." *American Journal c Medical Genetics* 72:172–79.

Bartels, D. M., B. LeRoy, and A. L. Caplan. (eds.). 3. *Prescribing Our Future: Ethical Challenges in netic Counseling*. New York: Aldine de Gruyter.

Bobrow, M. 1995. "Redrafted Chinese Law Remains genic." *Journal of Medical Genetics* 32:409.

Brinster, R. L., and J. W. Zimmermann. 1994. "Spertogenesis Following Male Germ-Cell Transplantan." *Proceedings of the National Academy of Sciences* (24): 298–302.

Caplan, Arthur L. (ed.). 1992. *When Medicine Went ad: Bioethics and the Holocaust*. Totowa, N.J.: Huna Press.

Caplan, Arthur L. 1993a. "The Concepts of Health, sease and Illness." In: Bynum, W. F., and R. Porter ls.). *Encyclopedia of the History of Medicine*, 233–48. ndon: Routledge.

Caplan, Arthur L. 1993b. "Neutrality Is Not Moral-: The Ethics of Genetic Counseling." In: Bartels, M., B. LeRoy, and A. L. Caplan. (eds.). *Prescribing ur Future: Ethical Challenges in Genetic Counselg*, 149–65. New York: Aldine de Gruyter.

Caplan, Arthur L. 1994. "The Relevance of the olocaust to Current Biomedical Issues." In: Michalyk, J. J. (ed.). 1994. *Medicine, Ethics and the Third eich*, 3–12. Kansas City: Sheed & Ward.

Caplan, Arthur L. 1995. *Moral Matters: Ethical Ises in Medicine and the Life Sciences*. New York: John Viley & Sons.

Caplan, Arthur L. 1998a. *Am I My Brother's Keeper? he Ethical Frontiers of Biomedicine*. Bloomington: Iniana University Press.

Caplan, Arthur L. 1998b. *Due Consideration: Conroversy in the Age of Medical Miracles*. New York: John Viley & Sons.

Danks, D. M. 1994. "Germ-Line Gene Therapy: No lace in Treatment of Genetic Disease." *Human Gene herapy* 5 (2):151–52.

Duster, Troy. 1990. *Backdoor to Eugenics*. New York: Routledge.

Garver, K. L. 1991. "Eugenics: Past, Present, and the uture." *American Journal of Human Genetics* 49 5):1109–18.

Haller, Mark H. 1963. *Eugenics: Hereditarian Attiudes in American Thought*. New Brunswick, N.J.: Rutgers University Press.

Harding, Sandra. (ed.). 1993. *The Racial Economy of Science*. Bloomington: Indiana University Press.

Herrnstein, Richard J., and Charles Murray. 1994. *The Bell Curve: Intelligence and Class Structure in American Life*. New York: Free Press.

Kater, M. 1992. "Unresolved Questions of German Medicine and Medical History in the Past and Present." *Central European History* 25:407–23.

Kevles, Daniel J. 1995 [1985]. *In the Name of Eugenics*. Cambridge, Mass.: Harvard University Press.

Kitcher, Philip. 1996. *The Lives to Come*. New York: Simon & Schuster.

Kitcher, Philip. 2000. "Utopian Eugenics and Social Inequality." In: Philip R. Sloan (ed.). *Controlling Our Destinies: Historical, Philosophical, Ethical, and Theological Perspectives on the Human Genome Project*, 229–62. Notre Dame, Ind.: University of Notre Dame Press.

Klass, Perri. 1989. "The Perfect Baby?" *New York Times Magazine* (January 29): 22–25.

Kolker, Aliza, and B. M. Burke. 1994. *Prenatal Testing: A Sociological Perspective*. Westport, Conn.: Bergin and Garvey.

Lewontin, R. C. 1992. *Biology as Ideology: The Doctrine of DNA*. New York: Harper-Collins.

Müller-Hill, Benno. 1988. *Murderous Science: Elimination By Scientific Selection of Jews, Gypsies, and Others, Germany, 1933–1945*. Trans. George Fraser. Oxford: Oxford University Press.

Munson, R., and L. H. Davis. 1992. "Germ-Line Gene Therapy and the Medical Imperative." *Kennedy Institute of Ethics Journal* 2 (2):137–58.

Murphy, Timothy F., and Marc A. Lappé (eds.). 1994. *Justice and the Human Genome Project*. Berkeley: University of California Press.

Pernick, Martin S. 2000. "Defining the Defective: Eugenics, Esthetics and Mass Culture in Early Twentieth-Century America." In: Philip R. Sloan (ed.). *Controlling Our Destinies: Historical, Philosophical, Ethical, and Theological Perspectives on the Human Genome Project*, 229–62. Notre Dame, Ind.: University of Notre Dame Press.

Proctor, Robert N. 1988. *Racial Hygiene: Medicine under the Nazis*. Cambridge, Mass.: Harvard University Press.

Rapp, Rayna. 1988. "Moral Pioneers: Women, Men and Fetus on a Frontier of Reproductive Technology." *Women and Health* 13:101–16.

Reilly, Philip. 1991. *The Surgical Solution: A History of Involuntary Sterilization in the United States*. Baltimore: Johns Hopkins University Press.

Weiss, Sheila F. 1987. *Race Hygiene and Natio[nal] Efficiency: The Eugenics of Wilhelm Schallma[yer]*. Berkeley: University of California Press.

ACKNOWLEDGMENTS

E WISH TO ACKNOWLEDGE and thank ll of the contributors of this collection as well as ie publishers who granted us permission to re-ublish their articles. In particular, we wish to iank Jaime Ingraham and the staff and fellows of ie Hastings Center for their help in gathering permissions. We thank David Magnus for his helpful suggestions regarding the contents of this collection. We also thank Georgetown University Press for its support and guidance during the publication process.

CONTRIBUTORS

OBERT ARONOWITZ, M.D., is an associate professor in the Department of History and Sociology of Science and the Department of Family Practice and Community Medicine at the University of Pennsylvania. Dr. Aronowitz is also director of the Health and Societies Program and director of the Robert Wood Johnson Health and Society Scholars Program, both of which are also at the University of Pennsylvania.

CHRISTOPHER BOORSE, PH.D., is an associate professor of philosophy at the University of Delaware.

GEORGES CANGUILHEM (1904–1995) was one of France's foremost historians of science. Trained as a medical doctor as well as a philosopher, he blended these practices to demonstrate to philosophers that there could be no epistemology without concrete study of the actual development of the sciences, and to historians that there could be no worthwhile history of science without a philosophical understanding of the conceptual basis of all knowledge. He died at the age of 91.

ARTHUR L. CAPLAN, PH.D., is Emmanuel and Robert Hart Professor of Bioethics, chair of the Department of Medical Ethics, and director of the Center for Bioethics at the University of Pennsylvania.

SAMUEL A. CARTWRIGHT, M.D. (1793–1863) was chairman of the committee appointed by the Medical Association of Louisiana shortly before the Civil War to report on the diseases and physical peculiarities of the Negro race.

WINSTON CHIONG is a graduate student in the Department of Philosophy at New York University and is a medical student (currently on leave) at the University of California, San Francisco, School of Medicine.

K. DANNER CLOUSER, PH.D., was University Professor of Humanities (Philosophy) at Pennsylvania State University College of Medicine, where he taught medical ethics and philosophy of medicine from 1968 until his retirement in 1996. Dr. Clouser died on August 14, 2000.

PETER CONRAD, PH.D., is the Harry Coplan Professor of Social Sciences and professor of sociology at Brandeis University.

CHARLES CULVER, M.D., PH.D., is associate director and professor of medical education, Barry University Physician's Assistant Program, Barry University, Miami Shores, Florida.

ALICE D. DREGER, PH.D., is an associate professor of science and technology studies at the Lyman Briggs School at Michigan State University, and serves on the associate faculty in the Center for Ethics and Humanities in the Life Sciences at Michigan State University.

GEORGE L. ENGEL, M.D., was a professor of medicine and psychiatry at the University of Rochester School of Medicine. During a career spanning more than fifty years, Dr. Engel integrated his broad interests in biology, medicine, and psychoanalysis into a more inclusive concept of disease, the biopsychosocial model. He died on November 26, 1999, at the age of 85.

GALEN OF PERGAMUM (ca. 130–ca. 200) was a Greek physician who studied in Asia Minor and Alexandria and lived most of his life in Rome. Writing more than 500 treatises on medicine and philosophy, Galen's authority—and especially his work *On the Natural Faculties*—influenced medical research and practice and was left unquestioned until the sixteenth century.

BERNARD GERT, PH.D., is the Stone Professor of Intellectual and Moral Philosophy at Dartmouth College and is an adjunct professor of psychiatry at Dartmouth Medical School.

SANDER GILMAN, M.D., is the Distinguished P fessor of Liberal Arts and Sciences and of Me cine at the University of Illinois at Chicago.

ERIC T. JUENGST, PH.D., is an associate professo Department of Bioethics at the Case Western serve University.

R. E. KENDELL, F.R.C. PSYCH., psychiatrist, edu tor administrator, and chair of psychiatry, U versity of Edinburgh, died December 19, 20

DAVID MAGNUS, PH.D., is codirector of the Cen for Biomedical Ethics at Stanford University.

MAIMONIDES (Moses ben Maimon, 1135–120 was a Jewish physician, philosopher, and sa who worked in exile as physician to an Egypti sultan after the Muslim conquest of his bir place, Cordoba, Spain. A prolific thinker a writer, Maimonides wrote the first codified a count of all Jewish law in the Mishneh Torah well as many philosophical treatises, includi *The Guide of the Perplexed.*

JAMES J. MCCARTNEY, OSA, PH.D., is an associa professor in the Department of Philosophy at Vi lanova University, an associate fellow at the Ce ter for Bioethics at the University of Pennsylv nia, and an adjunct professor at the Villano University School of Law.

FRANCES B. MCCREA, PH.D., is a professor of soc ology at Grand Valley State University in Alle dale, Michigan.

ELLEN M. MCGEE, PH.D., is an associate for bio ethics at the Long Island Center for Ethics, C. W Post Campus of Long Island University.

MAXWELL J. MEHLMAN, J.D., is Arthur E. Petersilg Professor of Law and director of the Law-Medi cine Center at the Case Western Reserve Unive sity School of Law and professor of biomedica ethics at the Case Western Reserve Universit ıool of Medicine.

ROBERTO MORDACCI teaches moral philosophy ilosofia morale) at the Università Vita—Salute n Raffaele, in Cesano Maderno, a suburb of ilan, Italy.

THOMAS MURRAY, PH.D., is president of the Hastgs Center in Garrison, New York.

EDMUND PELLEGRINO, M.D., is the John Carroll ofessor of Medicine and Medical Ethics at eorgetown University.

ROY PORTER, PH.D., was professor of the social hisry of medicine at the Wellcome Institute, Unirsity College, London. He was the author or author of many books, including *Facts of Life* 995) and *The Greatest Benefit to Mankind: A edical History of Humanity* (1997). He died in arch 2002 at the age of 55.

JOHN T. E. RICHARDSON, D.PHIL., is on the psycholgy staff of the Department of Human Sciences Brunell University, Uxbridge, U.K. His publiıtions include *Imagery* (1990) and *Clinical and europsychological Aspects of Closed Head Inıry*, 2d ed. (2000), both by Psychology Press.

G. S. ROUSSEAU is the Regius Professor of Engsh at Kings College Aberdeen, and in 1998–2001 as a Leverhulme Trust Fellow working on literture and medicine.

DOMINIC A. SISTI, MBE, is a researcher at the Cenr for Bioethics at the University of Pennsylvaia, associate ethicist at Holy Redeemer Health ystem, and adjunct instructor at Villanova Uniersity.

RICHARD SOBEL engaged in a great deal of collaborative research with Roberto Mordacci before joining the Kibbutz Revivim, DN Halutza, 85515, Israel. His most recent publication is "The Problem of Seeing and Saying in Medicine and Poetry," *Perspectives in Biology and Medicine*, which he coauthored with Gerda Elata.

THOMAS SZASZ is a professor of psychiatry emeritus, State University of New York, Upstate Medical University, in Syracuse. He is the author of numerous articles and books, including several editions of *The Myth of Mental Illness* (originally published by Paul B. Hoeber, 1961) and *Liberation by Oppression: A Comparative Study of Slavery and Psychiatry* (Transaction Publishers, 2002).

NORMA C. WARE, PH.D., is an associate professor in the Departments of Psychiatry and Social Medicine at Harvard Medical School.

PETER WHITEHOUSE, M.D., is professor of bioethics, professor of neurology, professor of neuroscience, and professor of psychiatry in the Department of Bioethics at the Case Western Reserve University.

GEORGE C. WILLIAMS, PH.D., is a professor emeritus in the Department of Ecology and Evolution at SUNY at Stony Brook.

PAUL ROOT WOLPE, PH.D., is a senior fellow of the Center of Bioethics at the University of Pennsylvania, where he holds appointments in the Departments of Psychiatry, Medical Ethics, and Sociology. He is the director of the Program in Psychiatry and Ethics at Pennsylvania. Dr. Wolpe also serves as the first chief of bioethics for the National Aeronautics and Space Administration.

PERMISSIONS AND CREDITS

"Diseases of the Soul" and "Curing Diseases of the Soul" (chapter 2) is from *The Essential Maimonides: Translations of the Rambam* by Avraham Yaakov Finkel. ©1993, 1994 by Yeshivath Beth Moshe, Scranton, Penn. Reprinted by permission of the publisher, Jason Aronson, Inc.

"Prometheus's Vulture: The Renaissance Fashioning of Gout" (chapter 3) is an excerpt from *Gout: The Patrician Malady* by Roy Porter and George S. Rousseau (New Haven, Conn.: Yale University Press, 1998). Reprinted by permission.

"The Normal and the Pathological—Introduction to the Problem" (chapter 5) was published in *A Vital Rationalist: Selected Writings from Georges Canguilhem*, edited by François Delaporte, translated by Arthur Goldhammer (New York: Zone Books, 1994). ©1994 Urzone, Inc. Reprinted by permission.

"The Myth of Mental Illness" (chapter 6) originally appeared in *American Psychologist* 15 (1960): 113–18.

"The Need for a New Medical Model: A Challenge for Biomedicine" (chapter 7) originally appeared in *Science*, 196: 129–36. © 1977 American Association for the Advancement of Science. Reprinted with permission from the American Association for the Advancement of Science.

"When Do Symptoms Become a Disease?" (chapter 8), was originally published in *Annals of Internal Medicine* 134 (2001): 803–8. Reprinted with permission.

"On the Distinction between Disease and Illness" (chapter 9) first appeared in *Philosophy and Public Affairs* 5 (1975): 49–68. © The Johns Hopkins University Press. Reprinted with permission of The Johns Hopkins University Press.

"Malady: A New Treatment of Disease" (chapter 10) was originally printed in the *Hastings Cen-*

Permissions and Credits

ter Report, June 1981: 29–37. © The Hastings Center. Reproduced by permission of the authors.

"Health: A Comprehensive Concept" (chapter 11) was originally published in the *Hastings Center Report*, vol. 28, no. 1: 34–37. © The Hastings Center. Reproduced by permission of the authors.

"The Distinction between Mental and Physical Illness" (chapter 12) was originally published in the *British Journal of Psychiatry* (2001) 178: 490–93. Reproduced by permission of the Royal College of Psychiatrists.

"The 'Unnaturalness' of Aging—Give Me Reason to Live!" (chapter 13) is reprinted with permission. © Arthur L. Caplan.

"Diagnosing and Defining Disease" (chapter 14) was originally published as "MSJAMA: Diagnosing and Defining Disease" in *Journal of the American Medical Association* 285 (1): 89–90. © 2001 by the American Medical Association.

"'Ambiguous Sex'—or Ambivalent Medicine?" (chapter 15) was originally published in the *Hastings Center Report* (1998) 28 (3): 24–35. Reproduced by permission of the author. © The Hastings Center.

"The Discovery of Hyperkinesis: Notes on the Medicalization of Deviant Behavior" (chapter 16) is reprinted with permission from *Social Problems* 23 (1): 12–21, October 1975. © 1975 by the Society for the Study of Social Problems.

"Suffering and the Social Construction of Illness: The Delegitimation of Illness Experience in Chronic Fatigue Syndrome" (chapter 17) is reproduced by permission of the American Anthropological Association from *Medical Anthropology Quarterly* 6 (4): 347–61 (1992). Not for sale or further reproduction.

"The Premenstrual Syndrome: A Brief History" (chapter 18) is reprinted from *Social Science and Medicine*, 41 (6): 761–67. © 1995, with permission from Elsevier Science.

"The Politics of Menopause: The 'Discovery' of a Deficiency Disease" (chapter 19) is reprinted by permission from *Social Problems*, 31 (1): 111–23, October 1983. © 1983 by the Society for the Study of Social Problems.

"Aging, Culture, and the Framing of Alzh mer Disease" (chapter 20) originally appeared *Concepts of Alzheimer Disease: Biological, Cli cal, and Cultural Perspectives*, Peter J. Whi house, M.D., Ph.D., Konrad Maurer, M.I Ph.D., and Jesse F. Ballenger, M.A., eds. I 158–80. © 2000 The Johns Hopkins Univers Press. Reprinted with permission of The Joh Hopkins University Press.

"The Medicalization of Aesthetic Surge (chapter 21) was originally published as chapte of *Creating Beauty to Cure the Soul: Race and P chology in the Shaping of Aesthetic Surgery*, p 19–23. ©1998, Duke University Press. All rig reserved. Used by permission of the publish

"The Quest for Medical Normalcy—Wh Needs It?" (chapter 22) originally appeared *American Journal of Human Biology* 12 (1): 10–1 © 2000 Wiley-Liss. This material is used by pe mission of Wiley-Liss, Inc., a subsidiary of Joh Wiley & Sons, Inc.

"Concepts of Disease after the Huma Genome Project" (chapter 24) originally a peared in *Ethical Issues in Health Care on th Frontiers of the Twenty-first Century*, Stephe Wear, James J. Bono, Gerald Logue, and Adr anne McEvoy, eds. (Dordrecht: Kluwer Acad mic Publishers, 2000). Reprinted with kind pe mission of Kluwer Academic Publishers.

An excerpt from "Enhancing Cognition in th Intellectually Intact" (chapter 25) by Peter Whitehouse, Eric Juengst, Maxwell Mehlman and Thomas H. Murray was originally publishe in the *Hastings Center Report* 27 (3): 14–22, 1997 It is reproduced by permission of the authors © The Hastings Center.

"Treatment, Enhancement, and the Ethics o Neurotherapeutics" (chapter 26) originally ap peared in *Brain and Cognition* 50: 387–95. © 2002, reprinted with permission from Elsevier

"What's Morally Wrong with Eugenics?" (chapter 27) originally appeared in *Controlling Our Destinies*, ed. by Philip R. Sloan. © 2000 by University of Notre Dame Press.

INDEX

Index

Index

Index

Index

Index

Index

Index

Index

Index

Index

Index

Index

Index

Index